The MOTHER MACHINE

By the same author

The Hidden Malpractice:
How American Medicine Mistreats Women

The

MOTHER MACHINE

Reproductive Technologies
from Artificial Insemination
to Artificial Wombs

GENA COREA

HARPER & ROW, PUBLISHERS, New York
Cambridge, Philadelphia, San Francisco,
London, Mexico City, São Paulo, Singapore, Sydney

Grateful acknowledgment is made for permission to reprint:

Excerpt from *The Politics of Reproduction* by Mary O'Brien. Reprinted by permission of Routledge & Kegan Paul Ltd.

Excerpts from *Our Miracle Called Louise: A Parents' Story* by Lesley & John Brown, copyright © 1979 Chandlewise Limited (Paddington Press, 1979). Reprinted by permission.

FIRST EDITION

Designer: Sheila Lynch

Library of Congress Cataloging in Publication Data
Corea, Gena.
    The mother machine.
    Bibliography: p.
    Includes index.
    1. Human reproduction—Political aspects. 2. Artificial insemination, Human—Social aspects. 3. Women's rights. I. Title.
QP251.C78 1985   306.8'5   84-48150
ISBN 0-06-015390-3

85 86 87 88 89 10 9 8 7 6 5 4 3 2 1

*For Sandra Elkin and Andrea Dworkin,
in friendship, in admiration
and in gratitude for their work
towards the liberation of women*

Contents

Acknowledgments

Poet Robin Morgan suggested I write this book. I am grateful to her for leading me to my work, a beneficient role she has quietly played in more than one woman's life.

Over the years I worked on this book, I had many of the most wonderful conversations of my life with my agent and friend, Sandra Elkin. She has helped me with *The Mother Machine* in such varied and substantial ways that I cannot begin to describe my debt to her.

It has been a joy to work with my editor, Janet Goldstein, whose support and impressive skills have been absolutely crucial to me in completing this book. I could not ask for anything more in an editor or a friend.

Tom Marlin, whose wit brightens my darker days, gave up much free time to enable me to use a word processor. I am grateful for his constant support and encouragement. (Not to mention all the bicycle tires he's changed for me over the years.)

Pauline Bart came up with the perfect book title the same minute in which I asked her to think about it.

I am lucky to have worked with Denisce DiIanni, my search assistant, who tracked down articles for me in specialized libraries and provided other invaluable forms of assistance. She has rescued me more than once.

I feel a special gratitude to my friends Lia Coulouris Pavlidis and Abigail Connell, who, over a four-year period, read drafts of various chapters. Without their intelligent and insightful responses, as well as their encouragement, I could hardly have finished this book.

My work with Renate Duelli-Klein, Robyn Rowland, Jalna Hanmer and Jan Raymond, sister members of the co-ordinating committee of the Feminist International Network on the New Reproductive Technologies (FINNRET), has been a source of joy and strength to me. I feel privileged to know such women.

Thanks to Mary Beth McCann, who struggles and strives for her own liberation and that of all women and in the process, inspires those around her.

I thank the lesbian mothers who wrote long, thoughtful answers to my questionnaire on their use of artificial insemination by donor.

For many different kinds of help, I am deeply indebted to Kathleen Hector; Kathrin Lassilla; Rebecca Albury; Merlin Stone; Barbara Walker; Sheila Ballantyne; Jeanne Rudd; Jim Maconochie, Jr.; Sylvie Shaw; Marilyn Waring, MP; the Bloodroot Collective; Ann Gill; Hester Eisenstein; Jenna Marie Maconochie; Frances Goldin; Cynthia Merman; Chris Schillig; Anke Ehrhardt; Claudia Dreifus; Barbara Seaman; Teresa Barbuto; Jean Thompson; Charles Haseloff; Alice Wolfson; Elizabeth Corea; Jim Mason; Marie Corea; Ed Corea; Anne Simon; Rosalind Herlands; Mary Sanford; Francine Hornstein; Fred Setterberg; Karen Gustafson; Meg Kenagy; Wanda Tsafos; Mary Gustafson; Maureen Flannery; Katherine Corea; Vera Farr; Sandra Cooney;

Katherine Yih; Norma Swenson; and women at the Rape Crisis Center of Chippendale, Australia.

I am grateful to the Fund for Investigative Journalism for its grant and to Howard Bray for his continued interest in this project.

It was a pleasure working on this book at the MacDowell Colony where wonderful cooks—Rita Allison, Donna Jenisch and Bobbie Larouche—fed me vegetarian meals through three chapters.

I interviewed scientists, attorneys, ethicists and business executives involved in the new reproductive technologies as either participants or commentators. The fact that some of them will disagree sharply with my perspective on these technologies in no way reduces my gratitude for their generosity in taking time to talk with me and to help me understand their fields and their perspectives. Among those interviewed were Dr. Jerry Sherman; Roxanne Feldshuh; Thea Muller; Paul Smith; Dr. Stephen Jay Gould; Frances Hornstein; Donna Hitchens; Dana Gallagher; Annette Baran; Barbara Kritchevsky; Gordon Doak; Dr. Harold Meryman; Dr. Robert Glass; Dr. B. C. Bhattacharya; Dr. Ronald Ericcson; Dr. Paul Dmowski; Joan Oaktree; William I. Battin Jr.; Helen Battin; Dr. Roberta Steinbacher; Dr. Nancy Williamson; Gerald Markle; Patrick Steptoe; Vern Jones; Dr. Jaroslav Hulka; Dr. William Sweeney; Dr. Wayne Decker; Dr. Luigi Mastroiani; Dr. Cecil Jacobson; Dr. Michelle Harrison; Dr. John Biggers; Dr. James Mills; Patricia Hynes; Dr. Mitch Levine; Noel Keane; Katie Brophy; Dr. Richard Levine; Harriet Blankfield; William Handel; Burton Satzburg; Dr. Michael Birnbaum; Rep. Richard Fitzpatrick; Jami Warner; Dr. Philip Parker; Andrea Dworkin; David Martin; John Stehura; Dr. Richard Seed; Dr. Sarah Seidel; Dr. John Buster; Dr. Marie Bustillo; Dr. Gary Hodgen; B. J. Anderson; Michael Eberhard; Jeremy Rifkin; Dr. Davor Solter; Michael Bradbury; Dr. Janice Raymond; Jalna Hanmer; Julie Melrose; Dr. Robert Sinsheimer; Dr. E. S. E. Hafez; Dr. J. R. G. Gosling; Barbara Eck Menning; Gwen Gotsch; Beverly Freeman; Nora Coffey; and Judy Norsigian.

I will forever be grateful to the feminist writers whose work has sustained me.

Finally, I thank those who passed their imperfect genes on to me, including an Irish vegetable peddler, an Italian cobbler, a laborer in a box factory and women who, within the confines of a cruel institution of motherhood, somehow managed to raise, nurture and love their children.

Introduction

We are in the midst of a dramatic biological revolution:

—Clinics for in vitro fertilization ("test-tube babies") are springing up throughout the industrialized world.

—Physicians are artificially inseminating women, flushing embryos out of them and transferring those embryos to other women. They hope to make a postmenopausal woman pregnant soon.

—In vitro fertilization (IVF) clinics in Australia, England and the United States are freezing human embryos for later transfer.

—Plans are underway to fly embryos across country so that, for example, an embryo could be flushed from a woman in Los Angeles and transferred into a woman in Massachusetts.

—Commercial firms are offering the sale of surrogate mothers (breeders) to customers, some of whom are infertile couples, others, single men.

—Sex predetermination clinics are providing services to couples who want boy babies.

Day by day it becomes clearer that sophisticated reproductive technologies are not a futuristic eventuality but rather an increasingly pervasive aspect of our lives today. Yet what do we really know about these newest medical miracles?

If we accept what we are told by physicians and scientists (as reported in the media), we believe these technologies offer treatments for infertility or the prevention of genetic disease. If we think of medicine as an institution which exists to heal us, it follows that we think of reproductive technologies as therapeutic. When we hear terms like "treatment," "therapeutic modality" and "patient" in connection with test-tube baby programs, such terms seem appropriate. The language we have available to us—in this case, the language of therapy—shapes the way we perceive reality. Yet in attempting to grasp the new reproductive technologies, that language fails us utterly.

We have words to describe the "foreground," the surface reality, but none to describe the "Background," the underlying truths.[1] We have words to describe medicine as a healing art, but none to describe it as a method of social control or political rule.

Yet some people are grappling with this linguistic (and conceptual) blind spot. Dr. Thomas Szasz, a professor of psychiatry at the State University of New York who warns that medicine, when allied with the state, can indeed control us, gives us a word for political rule by physicians: pharmacracy. It comes from the Greek root *pharmakon* for "medicine" and is analogous to "theocracy," rule by God or priests, and "democracy," rule by the people (quoted in Raymond, 1979). This book differs sharply from most writings on the subject, since I emphasize that reproductive technologies are a political issue, and I will sometimes refer to the physicians, embryologists and others involved as "pharmacrats."

The foreground deals with such questions as: How can the maturation quality of eggs be improved before they are suctioned out of women's ovaries during surgery? Who is legally liable if this or that goes wrong? Does the fee paid to the surrogate mother constitute, for federal tax purposes, compensation or rental income? (Maule, 1982, p. 657)

The Background deals with the social and political context in which the technology is developing. Here, the technologies are seen as something created in the interests of the patriarchy, reducing women to Matter. Just as the patriarchal state now finds it acceptable to market parts of a woman's body (breast, vagina, buttocks) for sexual purposes in prostitution and the larger sex industry, so it will soon find it reasonable to market other parts of a woman (womb, ovaries, egg) for reproductive purposes.

Since we live in a society where white people are valued more highly than those of color, these technologies will not affect all women equally. There will be no great demand for the eggs of a black woman. But there may well be a demand for her womb—a womb which could gestate the embryo of a white woman and man. (See Chapter 11.)

The Background deals with such questions as: At what costs to women are we channeled into biomedically manipulated reproduction? What are the implications for women as a social group when our numbers are reduced through sex predetermination technology? What is the real meaning of a woman's "consent" to in vitro fertilization in a society in which men as a social group control not just the choices open to women but also women's *motivation* to choose? (See Chapter 9.)

Advocates often argue that these technologies do, in fact, bring women new options and choices. But feminists, looking to the Background, have pointed out that any discussion of "rights" and "choices" assumes a society in which there are no serious differences of power and authority between individuals. Where power differences do prevail, coercion (subtle or otherwise) is also apt to prevail.

These and other forces acting on women's lives within a system of male supremacy have been powerfully documented.[2] We are familiar with the repeated exposés of male treatment of women in the medical system.[3] The harm women have been subjected to through DES, the Pill, IUDs, estrogen replacement therapy, tranquilizers, unnecessary hysterectomies and cesarean sections, etc., has been catalogued. But all this seems to be forgotten when commentators discuss the new reproductive technologies. It is as if the "old" reproductive technologies (such as the IUD) and the "new" ones arose out of two separate medical systems, one of which has a clear record of having hurt women, another of which will help women. But in fact there is one system and one low valuation of women in it.

In *The Mother Machine*, I often refer to the developers and supporters of reproductive technology as "men." In doing so, I recognize the following: The overwhelming majority of reproductive engineers are male. The overwhelming majority of persons on whose bodies these men experiment are female. The technology used emerges from a science developed by men according to their own values and sense of reality. Theorist Julie Melrose's concept of male and female reality helps clarify the situation. Noting author Andrea Dworkin's distinction between reality and truth ("Reality is whatever people at a given time believe it to be. . . . Truth is absolute in that it does exist and can be found"), Melrose writes: "Males and females are treated differently literally from birth, and the experiences of men and women are likely to be significantly different from one another. To the extent that human beings are the products of our experiences, the sense of reality that we develop out of those experiences will also be different" (Melrose, forthcoming).

Reproductive technology is a product of the male reality. The values expressed in the technology—objectification, domination— are typical of the male culture. The technology is male-generated and buttresses male power over women. It is true that some women are now engaged in reproductive technology as physicians, nurses, entrepreneurs. They are accepted in this field because they abide by the rules male values dictate. Their gender is female but the reality from which they operate is male. As the technology expands, more and more women will engage in it. This will be a triumph of tokenism, providing what one author calls "the illusion of comprehensive female inclusion."[4]

Sociologist Jalna Hanmer has pointed out that women can and do act as the agents of male power. For thousands of years in China, for example, mothers bound and painfully crippled the feet of their daughters. I know that, though in much less dramatic ways (such as in defending pornography), I have acted in the past as the agent of male power. But I did not understand what I was doing. When others had helped me to understand—through their spoken words, their books, their actions—I ended my complicity. I hope that women in reproductive technology, many of whom impressed me as intelligent, compassionate people committed to defending patients, will look at their work with new eyes.

When I write the word "men" in this book, I am writing about some individuals, but also about the institution of masculinist politics, about men as a social category and dominant class. Male readers may have a hard time with this. Perhaps they are learning about many of these technologies for the first time here, feel outraged by the way they are being developed and used, and horrified that certain women in their lives might someday be harmed through such technologies. Yet they read this book and feel that they are being blamed for them. It is "men" who are doing it and they, after all, are men. Perhaps they feel some guilt at what they learn here, and then anger at having been made to feel guilty when none of this is their fault. Finally, they may dismiss the book as "strident" (a word rendered meaningless by its frequent political use to punish feminists), or as one suffused with an "antimale bias."

Men are in a difficult position here. In this book, they are faced with evidence that they, as a social group, obtain economic, sexual, and psychological gains from women at a most terrible cost to women. These are painful facts, facts that may conflict with the male reader's sense of what is right and just. The typical human response to such a situation is to come up with defensive beliefs in order to avoid painful perceptions.

Sociologist John Dollard analyzed the defensive beliefs whites in a southern town in the 1930s came up with to avoid seeing clearly the cruelty of their caste treatment of Blacks. He pointed out: "Defensive beliefs in a society, like rationalizations of the individual, make possible the avoidance of the actual situation; they tend to eliminate the problematic, offensive, inconsistent, or hostile facts of life. One clings to the defense and avoids the traumatic perception of social reality."

The male reader who wants to enter the discourse of this book with integrity needs to examine his own reactions to *The Mother Machine* to see if they are defensive beliefs he is using to shield himself from problematic facts. The judgment that this book is "antimale" and "strident" is, I think, such a defensive belief.

Other male readers may feel: "I love my daughters, my mother and my wife and I treat them lovingly and all this talk about male oppression of women has nothing to do with me." Yet one of the defensive beliefs Dollard named is that Southerners loved Blacks individually, were kind to them and took care of them. "This belief is undoubtedly used to allay the anxiety which inevitably arises over the invidious distinctions maintained against Negroes as a caste," Dollard wrote. Men who treat their wives well are not off the hook for their complicity in the way women as a class are treated.

Large numbers of male readers may not scorn, ridicule, rape or beat women or hire their bodies for reproductive or sexual services and may deplore such actions on the part of their fellow men, just as large numbers of southern white people in the 1930s did not scorn, ridicule or torture Blacks though the customs allowed them to do so. But what Dollard wrote of good-hearted whites is equally true of good-hearted men: "Their position as caste members ... is such that they cannot escape a kind of complicity in sadistic actions since such acts serve to consolidate the caste position of the liberals quite as well as that of the sadistic offenders themselves."

To avoid recognizing this, male readers could take the path of defense. Or they could respond differently to the facts exposed in this book: They might recognize the actual situation—a situation in which a masculinist political structure oppresses women—and try to change it.

People who are born into a privileged class, as men are, are not obliged to embrace its values and its privileges. They can break rank. They can become traitors to their class. They can work for social justice. I hope men will do this.

If the facts exposed in this book are painful for men, they are agonizing for women. We women, too, are apt to throw defensive beliefs up around us in order to avoid seeing facts that would require us to ask unsettling questions about our lives. It is tempting to dismiss critical views of the technology as paranoid or antiprogressive and move on to happier thoughts.

Infertile women may have a special problem with this book because they have suffered deeply. The technologies seem to promise an end to that suffering, and I come along and cast doubt on that promise. Yet, however angry these women may be with me for the unwelcome facts I report, I am with them, I am for them. Because I am for them, I must report that the vast majority of women enrolled in in vitro fertilization programs have not been helped and that many have suffered during the experimentation on their bodies. This fact has not surfaced. What has been allowed to surface is that a (white) woman in this city or that has had a baby through IVF and is extremely happy. Her photograph is published in the newspaper and she is interviewed on television. Such selective highlighting of facts has made it difficult for infertile women to evaluate the true promise of the technologies.

While these technologies have been presented as boons to women, providing, as endless headlines have proclaimed, "new hope for the infertile," it could as well be argued that they bring new despair. A few years earlier, a woman could at some point, however painfully, come to terms with her infertility, go on with her life, find a way to live it fully. Now there is no easy way off the medical treadmill. She may now spend a major part of her adult life in debilitating treatment in experimental programs. There is always a promising new program to enroll in, its low success rate played down, its "hope" played up. The years roll on.

The suffering infertility causes women is enormous and deserves to be treated seriously. I do not think that those who respond to the suffering by offering to probe, scan, puncture, suction and cut women in repeated experiments are taking that suffering more seriously than I. They are not asking how much of women's suffering has been socially structured and inflicted and is therefore not inevitable. And I doubt that every pharmacrat who takes eggs from women without their knowledge in the course of unrelated surgery, who switches embryos between women, who plans on dividing, sexing and engineering human embryos is acting out of compassion for infertile women.

I hope that, reading my criticisms of the reproductive technologies, women who have been enrolled in IVF or embryo transfer programs or who have served as surrogate mothers or egg donors do not feel that I am criticizing them as well. Most assuredly, I am not. What I am doing is naming forces that act on women's lives and lead some of us to participate in these programs. (Of course the impact of these forces varies depending on our individual circumstances. See Frye, 1983, pp. xii–xiv.)

While infertile women are now those most directly affected by reproductive technologies, this will change. According to the visions of researchers, the new technologies eventually will be used on a large proportion of the female population. (This is another of those facts kept in the shadows.) Many women—not just those with fertility problems—will raise test-tube babies to whom they bear no blood relation, the egg fertilized in the laboratory having been not their own, but that of a donor. Older women and women with genetic diseases, endometriosis, hyperthyroid or a history of miscarriage are among those envisioned as future IVF candidates. Another group, characterized by one pharmacrat as large and growing, is women whose eggs were damaged by exposure to toxins in the workplace. (See Chapter 7.) Rather than cleaning up toxic workplaces, pharmacrats suggest depriving women workers of their own children and operating on them so they can bear the babies of other women.

Ultimately, then, the issue is not fertility. The issue is the exploitation of women.

These assessments are the result of a cumulation of facts and ideas garnered over a number of years and after much research and analysis. The structure of this book mirrors this cumulative experience. In a series of chapters, I report on the technologies—their history, methods, social effects and future applications—and in a final section I place the new technologies in a larger context.*

Part I deals with artificial insemination. The first chapter introduces a concept that informs the discussion of the entire book: eugenics, the attempt to improve the human race by controlling who is allowed to reproduce. The potential use of artificial insemination in a eugenic program is discussed here. Chapter 2 deals with the

---

* Notes placed at the end of each chapter provide important additional information and clarifying examples. The Chronology provides an overview of technological developments for easy reference.

threat artificial insemination by donor sperm (AID) poses to the patriarchy. Chapter 3 describes how medicine and law have managed (however inadequately) to fit AID into the concept of the patriarchal family.

In Part II, we move to the first of several more complicated technologies: embryo transfer. Chapter 4 recounts how, under the ancient Goddess religion, the cow was worshiped. It then describes the transfer of embryos between cows on a midwestern farm. Chapter 5 explains the history of and procedures involved in embryo transfer in animals, where the technology was first applied. In Chapter 6, I describe the development of the business of embryo transfer in humans.

Part III moves on to in vitro fertilization. Chapter 7 recounts the history of IVF technology and describes the potential uses of IVF foreseen by reproductive engineers—uses far more expansive than mere treatment for infertility. Chapter 8 provides an account of the iatrogenic (doctor-induced) origins of many forms of infertility and discusses the risks of IVF to woman and child. Chapter 9 focuses on the women in IVF programs: how real the "informed consent" of these women actually is; the suffering they undergo in the largely unsuccessful IVF programs.

Part IV concerns four other technologies. Chapter 10 deals with sex determination; Chapter 11 with surrogate motherhood; Chapter 12 with the artificial womb; and Chapter 13 with cloning.

The last part is unlike any of those preceding it. In Chapter 14, I point out that through the decades, with the widespread use of the reproductive technologies, institutions will be restructured to reflect the new reality: control by men of female biological reproductive processes. We do not know exactly how this new reality will be expressed. Numerous commentators, some writing even before the appearance of these technologies, have discussed or predicted the creation of a class of professional breeders (Davis, 1937; Westoff, 1978; Scott, 1981; Francoeur, 1970, p. 106; Kieffer, 1979; Packard, 1977). Andrea Dworkin has predicted the development of reproductive brothels where women sell wombs, ovaries, eggs (1983). In this chapter, I describe how these technologies could be used in such a brothel.

In the last two chapters of the book, I draw on the important work of political scientist Mary O'Brien in presenting one theory to explain man's intense desire to control reproduction. O'Brien has pointed out that birth, like such other biological necessities as sexuality, labor (to provide food) and death, shapes human consciousness; that man's and woman's experience of this differs; that woman has a continuous reproductive experience which involves sexual intercourse, growth of the child within her body for nine months and birth; that man has a discontinuous reproductive experience— sexual intercourse followed nine months later by the birth of a child through another person's body, an event he not only does not experience, but one he need not even know about; that man's sense of separation from reproduction, his lack of a sense of connection to the next generation, has affected him deeply. I argue that, envying woman her genetic continuity and her connection to the human species, men of different times and cultures have tried to make her reproductive experience their own through a variety of means, the latest of these being the development of obstetrics and gynecology and the new reproductive technologies. Through these technologies, man is increasingly creating a continuous reproductive experience for himself and a discontinuous one for women. These two chapters provide part of the truth, a hint of an explanation for the biological revolution we find ourselves in the midst of.

In the Crystallization, I report on the early efforts of women from many countries, working together, to deal with the threat posed by this biological revolution.

Notes

1. The concepts "Background" and "foreground" were originally used by Denise Connors and developed by Mary Daly in *Gyn/Ecology* and Janice Raymond in *The Transsexual Empire*. Connors emphasized the positive dimensions of the "Background" concept, using it to signify the deepest dimensions of women's lives. These dimensions are often camouflaged by the superficial foreground images of women as portrayed in literature, the mass media, etc. However, the "Background" as managed by pharmacrats, Raymond asserts, displays a host of male-volent intentions and operations not accessible in the foreground.

2. See Mackinnon, 1979; Frye, 1983; Barry, 1979; Hull et al., 1981; Dworkin, 1974, 1981a, 1981b, 1983; Rich, 1977; Daly, 1973, 1978; Walker, 1983; Griffin, 1978; Morgan, 1970, 1982; Woolf, 1966; McNulty, 1980; de Beauvoir, 1970; Jones, 1980; Lerner, 1973; Smith, 1983; Spender 1982.

3. See BWHBC, 1984; Arms, 1975; Scully, 1980; Seaman, 1980; Harrison, 1982; FFWHC, 1981; Corea, 1985.

4. Raymond, 1979, p. 26. For discussions of the function tokenism plays in maintaining male power, see, as well as Raymond's book: Daly, 1978; and Judith Long Law, "The psychology of tokenism: an analysis," in *Sex Roles*, I (1975), 51.

Part One

ARTIFICIAL INSEMINATION

1

Eugenics:
Family (Genetic) Planning

She was a Quaker. The wife of a merchant. The infertility patient of Dr. William Pancoast. She was a woman whose name was never recorded.

Dr. Pancoast, a professor at Jefferson Medical College in Philadelphia, had already examined and tested her numerous times. Finally, he discovered that she was fertile and that the problem was her husband's: There were no sperm.

Pancoast (or maybe it was one of his students) had an idea. He called her in. He just wanted to examine her once more, he told her.

The woman lay on the table as she had been told to do. Pancoast's six medical students—all young men—stood around her body. Pancoast anesthetized the woman with chloroform. He took the receptacle into which one of his students had masturbated. With a hard rubber syringe, he inserted the student's semen into her uterus. He then plugged her cervix with gauze.

When she awoke, he did not tell her what he had done. He never told her. Nine months later, she bore a son.

It was 1884. This was the first reported human artificial insemination with donor semen.

It was a rape.[1]

1981: Joey dropped the ampul of frozen sperm into a thermos of hot water and let it thaw. Then, standing in the barn, he loaded the sperm into his gun. He placed a rod over the gun. He tightened it. Pulling a transparent plastic glove over his left hand up to his elbow, he walked into the corral.

12

Two men—the farmer and a farmhand—had already driven the 14-month-old heifer into a pen. She was Number 60N. The number was tagged through her ear. She was frightened. Her eyes were wide, terrified.

The men snapped wooden slats into place around her neck to secure her head. She tried to pull her head out.

Joey walked from the barn into the corral and then into the pen. Without a word, hardly breaking his pace, he drove his left arm into the heifer's rectum. She jumped and squirmed. She struggled again to free herself from the head catch. "Whoa!" the men shouted.

("They all fight it," the farmer had explained to me earlier.)

Joey moved his hand in the cow's rectum, found and held the cervix. With his right hand, he inserted the rod into her vagina at a 45-degree angle. He located the opening of the cervix. Twisting, he worked the rod through the cervix. He shot the gun in her.

Joey took his arm and gun out of the cow. The men released 60N's head from the lock. They opened the gate by her head so she could return to the corral.

The men talked among themselves. They did not look at the cow. The heifer began backing slowly and cautiously out the pen, returning the way she had been driven in. Her sides were shaking. Her eyes were big. She made no sound. It was as if she were tiptoeing away.

Joey looked over, saw her backing out. He kicked her. Startled, she ran forward and out the gate.

Joey "gets into" about 150 cows a year. Manager of the herd on a breeding farm in the Midwest, he inseminates the cows only when the breeder cannot get to the farm on time.

They produce calves on this farm. Then they sell them to stockers who "grow 'em out" on a high roughage diet. The stockers then sell the calves to "finishers" who fatten the animals and slaughter them.

Earlier, standing in the corral, Joey had talked to me of cattle breeding, explaining that a cow needed about two months' rest after calving before she could be inseminated again. Her uterus needed to heal from the birthing.

"You got to take into consideration they're a machine," he says as my tape recorder preserves his words.

"A machine?" I repeat.

"Well, basically. If they don't produce a live calf every year, they go down the road."

"What does 'down the road' mean?" I ask, knowing.

"Slaughter."

"I see. So the function of the cow then is to calve, to produce young?"

"That's right. That's why they're basically a machine that has to produce this marketable product or unit every year. Look at it like any type of machine. If it doesn't produce, it's going to go by the wayside."

He points to a cow.

"Now there's a *very* productive machine there. She's a tremendous cow anyway. I wouldn't be surprised if she's a [egg] donor someday. She's that good."

A cow's function is to produce calves. One of woman's main functions has been to produce children: children to carry on the names of men and inherit their property; children to become soldiers, workers and consumers; children to populate the lands of states seeking "national greatness."

Argentina has been one of those states. In March 1974, its ministry of health issued a decree restricting the sale of contraceptive pills and accusing "non-Argentine interests" of encouraging birth control and "perverting the fundamental maternal role of women." The decree was issued in the name of then President Juan Perón, who had reportedly always been attracted by the vision of a large and powerful Argentina. Commenting on the population issue, *Las Bases*, a magazine considered the official publication of the Peronist movement, wrote: "We must start from the basis that the principal work of a woman is to have children."[2]

Birth control crusader Margaret Sanger's bitter remark, made in a 1933 speech, that women were "breeding machines for men," has been valid throughout patriarchal history. In the thirteenth century, St. Thomas Aquinas declared that woman, though "defective," does have one purpose: reproduction. God made her as a helpmate to man. She was "not fitted to help man except in generation, because another man would have proved a more effective help in anything else" (Hutchins, 1952, pp. 489, 518). Centuries later, in 1851, the German philosopher Arthur Schopenhauer also argued that "women exist, on the whole, solely for the propagation of the species" (Hays, 1964, p. 209).

When European men colonized North America, they imported women into the colonies to breed. Women were sold into marriage. "Just as man bought land so that he could grow food, he bought a wife so that he could grow sons," Andrea Dworkin wrote in the feminist classic, *Our Blood.* "A man owned his wife and all that she produced. Her crop came from her womb, and this crop was harvested year after year until she died."[3] If the man died first, she had no right to the children she had birthed. A husband, Dworkin reported, bequeathed his children to another male who would have full custody rights.

Within the racial caste system, Black women had even less control over their bodies than white women. During slavery, white men measured a Black woman's worth by her ability to produce more wealth for them in the form of more slaves. Especially productive women were called breeders. Martha Jackson's aunt was a breeder woman. Jackson, an 87-year-old ex-slave interviewed during a Federal Works Project in Alabama in 1939, recalled that the master rarely ordered her aunt whipped " 'case she was er breeder woman en' brought in chillum ev'y twelve months jes lak a cow bringin' in a calf. . . . He orders she can't be put to no strain 'casen uv dat."[4]

What if a woman—Black or white—could produce no children? Then she was not a real woman, for producing children was the function that defined woman.

A woman who failed to produce a child could be reproached, ridiculed, and, during the Middle Ages, even burned as a witch. Husbands in polygamous marriages might replace her with a new wife and relegate her to the level of a servant. In many Islamic lands, they could cast her out.[5] She could be divorced, leaving her isolated, socially stigmatized, often poverty-stricken. Patriarchal societies made it easy for men to dispose of barren women. For example, under Jewish law, a husband has a right to sue for divorce if his wife is barren. But a woman may not sue for divorce on grounds that her husband is sterile.[6]

"In centuries past," wrote infertility counselor Barbara Eck Menning, "The woman who was childless was as useless and despised as a piece of land that would yield no crops. The same word was given to both—barren."

To avoid such fates, some women risked their lives. In the nineteenth century, J. Marion Sims, the American "Father of Modern Gynecology," performed life-threatening operations on women so they could (if they survived) bear children.

"Nothing, not even danger of death for the patient . . . was as important as the one great necessity of enabling childless women to emerge, rejoicing, from their tragic barren state," reported Sims' biographer.

Sims, who devoted a large proportion of his practice to sterility, wrote of his perilous surgery on uterine tumors:

> It might very well be a question whether such a hazardous operation
> ... should be performed simply for the removal of sterility.... But I
> could very well imagine cases where it would be justifiable. Suppose
> a dynasty was threatened with extinction, and the cause of sterility
> was ascertained to be an enucleable fibroid.... Or suppose an ancient
> family of great name, influential position, and large fortune, desirous
> of perpetuating these noble heritages in a line of direct descent ...

was thwarted by an infertile woman? (Harris, 1950, p. 184). While
the words "dynasty" and "family" sound genderless, in fact the
names, positions and fortunes of which he writes belong to men.

In the twentieth century, too, women have risked their lives to
produce the children required of them. At the International Conference of Women Physicians in 1919, a Dr. Kahn, then of China,
spoke of the suffering enforced childbearing caused women:

> The greatest crime that a Chinese woman is supposed to commit is
> not to have children, not to have sons, but she is to have them
> whether she wills it so or not.... Thus far I have not been able to
> help the women very much because I have not dared.... No matter
> how many children [a woman] has she must continue to bear them.
> I have known women who have borne more than a dozen children,
> one every year, and if they were to try not to have any more children
> they would be ostracized socially by their families. The husband
> would immediately take several other wives and then the wife would
> become a nervous wreck because nobody would recognize her.

Referring obliquely to contraception, a topic that in 1919 was
not considered fit for discussion at a medical conference, Dr. Kahn
continued:

> What are we to do with these cases? Many of them are my own
> patients. I have had to deliver them with forceps, one after another,
> and when they are physical wrecks and not able to have children, are
> we to help them prevent conception? Have we the right? (Proceedings
> of the ICWP, 1919)

Begetting and siring. Genesis. Procreation. These were the words
used, respectively, by Hebrews, Greeks and premodern Christians
to describe the transmittal of life to the next generation.

Today, we use the metaphor of the factory: reproduction.[7]

Man seeks to control the re-productive processes of cow and
woman to exercise "quality control" over the products we produce.

Joey, the farmer, understood the importance of quality cattle.

To him, the cow produces a "marketable product or unit."

So too does the pregnant woman produce a commodity, "a national asset."[8] In the current obstetrical literature, her baby is frequently considered a product. For example, in attempting to justify a phenomenal rise in cesarean sections (almost quadrupling from 5 percent in 1968 to 18.5 percent in 1982), physicians argue— without supporting evidence—that they are getting "better babies" through surgery. Ignoring the risks of that major surgery to the woman, Dr. Norman Thornton of the University of Virginia observed in 1976: "Obstetricians today are much more interested in the *product* [my emphasis] they deliver than the cesarean section rate" (quoted in O. H. Jones, 1976).

It had better be a good product. "What we have to do now is concentrate on quality control," Dr. Saul Lerner said in explaining a preconceptual counseling program he runs in his office. Before a woman becomes pregnant, Lerner tries to identify and minimize any "risks" to the as yet unconceived child. Lerner, then chairman of the American College of Obstetricians and Gynecologists' District I, stated: "If more babies are surviving, we've got to make sure they are better babies."[9]

The notion that life is a commodity over which men must exercise quality control is an ever-recurring theme in patriarchal history. This idea is most clearly expressed in "eugenics," an ideology established in 1869, which argues that the powerful (i.e., "the fit") should control the lives and reproduction of inferior people in an attempt to produce "better" human beings. It defines inferiority by race, class and physical condition.

Eugenics was to become an influential movement led by some of the most esteemed statesmen, academics, scientists, physicians and reformers in the United States. This particular movement would disintegrate in moral embarrassment in the 1930s after Adolf Hitler showed the world how a eugenic plan could be massively implemented.

The aim of eugenics is to improve the human race through selective breeding. This involves "the application to man of the methods developed by breeders for improving their stocks."[10]

Plato advocated this in *The Republic* long before the term "eugenics" had been coined. In his ideal state "the best of either sex should be united with the best as often, and the inferior with the inferior, as seldom as possible ... if the flock is to be maintained in first-rate condition." But the rulers, who would arrange the couplings, must keep this human breeding a secret, "or there will be a further danger of our herd ... breaking out into rebellion" (Edman, 1956, p. 412).

Plato was advocating both negative eugenics (decreasing the propagation of the handicapped) and positive eugenics (increasing that of desirable human types).

Leon F. Whitney, field secretary of the American Eugenics Society, advocated the same centuries later, in 1934. According to Whitney, the state was like an agriculturist. It cultivated not grains and animals—but its families. It must ensure that "the better type of individuals are preserved," and the seed of the inferior destroyed.

"There are figs and thistles, grapes and thorns, wheat and tares in human society," Whitney wrote, "and the state must practice family culture" (Whitney, 1934, p. 135).

How? With contraception or sterilization for those "at the lower end of the social scale." Both have been tools of those attempting to eliminate the "unfit."

From roughly 1900 to 1930, during the heyday of their movement, eugenicists often advocated the sterilization of the biologically defective. Many states, beginning with Indiana in 1907, passed sterilization laws. Under those laws, physicians operated upon thousands of people. They castrated some.[11]

Who were the "defectives"? The physically handicapped. Paupers. Drunkards. Immigrants. "Dope fiends." The venereal disease-ridden. The jobless. The "feeble-minded." Often, people of color.

Many eugenicists were blatantly racist. Others were subtly so. Examples abound. A few:

—Sir Francis Galton, founder of the eugenics movement, said in 1869 that Negroes, as judged by intelligence, are "two grades" below whites. "The mistakes the Negroes made in their own matters were so childish, stupid, and simpleton-like, as frequently to make me ashamed of my own species," he stated.

—In America in 1916, Stanford University professor L. M. Terman, the man most responsible for instituting IQ tests in this country, found that an IQ between 70 and 80 is "very common among Spanish, Indian and Mexican families ... and also among Negroes. Their dullness seems to be racial, or at least inherent in the family stocks from which they come ... from the eugenic point of view they constitute a grave problem because of their prolific breeding."

Dr. Thurman B. Rice warned in a 1929 book that the race was

endangered because "the colored races are pressing the white race most urgently and this pressure may be expected to increase." He argued that no people of color should be given permanent citizenship in America.[12]

Eugenics flourished. Nazi Germany passed a compulsory sterilization law in 1933. It created "hereditary health courts" made up of a district judge and two physicians to implement the "Law on the Prevention of Hereditary Diseases in Future Generations." A variety of diagnoses could result in forced sterilization including hereditary blindness or deafness, epilepsy, Huntington's disease and alcoholism. Many others classified as antisocial or Gypsies or "Rhineland bastards," i.e., children conceived after World War I by French North African occupation troops, were also sterilized. "This clearly shows the gradual shift towards measures aimed at racial elimination" (Pfäfflin, 1983).

Whitney approved of the sterilization law. Praising Germany for its willingness "to call a spade a spade," he commented: "Though not all of us, probably, will approve of the compulsory character of this law—as it applies, for instance, to the sterilizing of drunkards— we cannot but admire the foresight revealed by the plan in general, and realize that by this action Germany is going to make herself a stronger nation."

Even after the full atrocities of Nazi Germany were known— atrocities carried out not only by goose-stepping Nazi troops, but by highly respected, white-coated physicians—some American eugenicists remained calm. In the 1950 book, *Sterilization in North Carolina*, Moya Woodside reports the opinion of a reform school administrator on sterilization. He acknowledges that there are a lot of "theoretical" arguments against it, including "infringement of liberty," but believes one must be practical. "Otherwise people just keep coming along—the defective and delinquents reappear with every generation," he explained.

Woodside reported: "He realizes of course that many people have been 'put off' sterilization by what Hitler did in Germany; but again, you have to be practical" (Woodside, 1950, p. 81).

When Hitler brought eugenics into disrepute, and new developments in anthropology, genetics and mental testing undercut the scientific basis of the movement, many of the groups dissolved. Some American eugenicists then joined the population control groups that formed in the 1940s and 1950s. They changed their vocabularies slightly to accommodate the revamped vision of the apocalypse. The new ideology would name "overpopulation" rather than "the propagation of the unfit" the threat to the human race. But methods of averting the disaster were the same the eugenicists had employed: Birth control. Sterilization.

While negative eugenics discouraged breeding among the "defective," positive eugenics encouraged increased breeding among the "fit." Birth control and sterilization were tools of the former; the new reproductive technologies—including artificial insemination by donor, embryo transfer, in vitro fertilization, cloning and artificial wombs— can be tools of the latter. Here we will examine the eugenic uses of artificial insemination by donor semen (AID).

As we will see in the following chapters, most men greeted AID with alarm, for it threatened the very basis of patriarchal descent. While they eagerly used artificial insemination in animals, they were in no rush to set up banks for *human* sperm. But a minority of men saw the potential eugenic uses to which AID could be put, and enthusiastically endorsed such use.

Through AID, they saw, men could control the quality of the products cows and women produced. In cattle breeding, AID would produce cows yielding "quality carcasses of high cutability."[13] In human breeding, it would produce "intelligent," white and, perhaps eventually through still-developing sex predetermination techniques, male persons. "High quality" humans turned out to bear an astonishing resemblance to the eugenicists themselves.

Where do physicians look for particularly "intelligent" sperm vendors?

Among themselves. A 1979 survey of AID practitioners found that eighty percent of physicians use medical students or hospital residents as sperm vendors all or most of the time.* These and other sperm vendors "are a select group with presumably above-average health and intelligence," researchers noted in the *New England Journal of Medicine* (Curie-Cohen, 1979).

Medical school professors also sell their sperm. They and younger medical personnel "are traditional donors and preferred because of their understanding the biologic need of the program, accessibility and selection with regard to health and intelligence," an American Fertility Society report observed in 1980 (Hulka, 1980).

George Annas, chief of the health law section of Boston University School of Public Health, fired off a stinging criticism of

---

* Attorney George Annas rightly objects to the use of the term "donor" for men who sell their sperm. So I use the term "sperm vendor" for such men, reserving the term "donor" for true gift-givers.

the practice in 1979. Annas believes the physicians, in spreading their genes far and wide, are serving their own needs and not those of AID children. Lawyers, he believes, would likely choose law students as sperm vendors. Generals would view military academy cadets as superior human specimens.

"There can be little debate that physicians ... are making eugenic decisions—selecting what they consider 'superior' genes for AID," Annas writes. "In general they have chosen to reproduce themselves (or those in their profession)" (Annas, 1979).[14]

Recipients of this choice sperm must also meet certain qualifications. Fertility clinics often require that women requesting AID "therapy" be married and emotionally stable[15] and have "enough income to raise a child well."

AID, then, could be used eugenically by selecting both the sperm vendor—a middle- or upper-class medical student—and the woman who will be granted insemination—also a middle- or upper-class woman who can afford to pay for the expensive "treatments" and to bring up a child at a living standard that meets her physician's expectations.

While physicians rate their own sperm as Choice, others dream of even higher quality semen: Prime. What if such sperm, produced by men like Newton and Beethoven, were injected into women routinely?

In the very first report of AID—Pancoast's impregnation of the Quaker woman—the author suggested "a society for artificial insemination as a method of improving the species, a sort of early eugenics" (Gregoire and Mayer, 1965). Physicians commented favorably on the article; through such a society might the thorns be removed from the human race.

In 1935, Dr. Hermann J. Muller, a Marxist geneticist, advocated a voluntary program he called "germinal choice." Child quality could be improved, he argued, if women would allow themselves to be inseminated artificially with the sperm of "some transcendently estimable man."

The sperm of reputedly great men would be collected and stored. The men would die. Their sperm would wait out what Muller called a "probationary period." It would become clear during this time whether the man had truly been great or had only seemed so. Unspecified persons would then evaluate his alleged greatness and the worth of his progeny. If his life work and his children were judged superior, his sperm would be used; if not, discarded.

Within a century or two, Muller envisioned, much of the

population could "become of the innate quality of such men as Lenin, Newton, Leonardo, Pasteur, Beethoven, Omar Khayyám, Pushkin, Sun Yat-Sen, Marx . . ." (Muller, 1935). (During the Cold War, Muller scratched Lenin from his list.)

Muller, who won a Nobel Prize for his work on the effect of radiation on genes, observed in 1959 that thousands of women had already used AID. Many had been motivated by their husbands' infertility. Infertility, he wrote, provided "an excellent opportunity for the entering wedge of positive selection, since the couples concerned are nearly always, under such circumstances, open to the suggestion that they turn their exigency to their credit by having as well-endowed children as possible" (Muller, 1959, p. 30).

If the practice "of having children of chosen genetic material" expands, Muller noted, sperm banks would be necessary. The banks would originally be established for two groups:

—Men who want to preserve their sperm before undergoing vasectomy
—Men seeking to protect their germ cells from the growing radiation hazards of industry, commerce, war, space flight and "the as yet unassessed hazards of the chemical mutagens of modern life."[16]

Originally providing a kind of insurance, these banks would "eventually offer a wide choice of sperm," Muller wrote. They would increasingly be used for conscious selection of progeny.

The effects of "superior" sperm could be multiplied many-fold, Sir Julian Huxley, a leading English eugenicist wrote in 1963, through the use of what he called "E.I.D.—eugenic insemination by deliberately preferred donors." To realize such a program, he explained, AID, then under a legal and moral cloud, must be made fully respectable. The anonymity of sperm donors must be abolished. Physicians and Britain's National Health Service should keep a register of certified donors giving particulars of the donors' family history. "This would enable acceptors to exert a degree of conscious selection in choosing the father of the child they desire," Huxley wrote, "and so pave the way for the supersession of blind and secrecy-ridden AID by an open-eyed and proudly accepted EID where the E stands for Eugenic."

Dr. Jerome K. Sherman, who developed a method of freezing human sperm, was a good friend of the late Dr. Muller and approves of Muller's germinal choice plan. Sherman, now of the University of Arkansas, helped draw up the provisional guidelines for sperm banks published by the American Association of Tissue Banks in 1980—guidelines which specifically state that sperm banks could be used in dealing with both infertility *and* population control.

Sperm banks could be used in two ways in population control, Sherman explained in an interview. First, some men would only undergo sterilization if a sperm bank existed in which they could first deposit semen in the event that they later wanted more children. Secondly, sperm banks would permit the selection of superior semen for insemination. Getting better genetic donors with better attributes would be a form of controlling the *quality*, rather than the *number* of the population, he pointed out.

"Population control has come to mean not only the reduction of the number of births in our world's population explosion, but also the genetic improvement of the population," he wrote.

Some degree of chemical control of heredity and eugenics is on the horizon in man's biological destiny, he stated. Sperm banks, he added, provide an interim method for population control before genetic engineering (presumably of embryos) becomes feasible.

Among Sherman's suggested requirements (Sherman, 1964) for donor sperm banks are:

—Cross-matched cataloguing of characteristics of mind and body of the donors, available at suitable centers in various parts of the country

—A system of transport of frozen human semen from selected donors, available from all over the country and world in designated centers.

—The establishment of a clearing house with all pertinent information on stored semen, functioning in association with consultants in medicine, genetics, psychology and social work in such programs as germinal choice

In 1968, Dr. S. J. Behrman, another pioneer in the use of frozen sperm (he began working with artificial insemination more than thirty years ago), discussed the "application of semen banks as a mechanism of positive eugenics" before the American College of Obstetricians and Gynecologists. Dr. Behrman quoted at length from Muller's germinal choice plan. The success of the plan, he pointed out, depended on the widespread availability of frozen, preserved semen.

"For one hundred years," he told his colleagues gathered in Hot Springs, Virginia, "all efforts to preserve spermatozoa by freezing . . . have been dominated by a single motive, i.e., simply the desire to control fertility. This motivation is clearly acknowledged with respect to the semen of domestic animals and implied, if not clearly stated, in the efforts of those who have worked with the freeze preservation of human semen" (Behrman and Ackerman, 1969).

There were two very powerful advantages to controlling fertility by freezing germ cells, he explained. First, fertility control could be established independently of place and time. (In other words, with frozen sperm, a man could engender a child a continent away even after his own death.) Secondly, fertility can be controlled "with respect to desired qualities in the offspring."

Behrman linked semen preservation with sterilization just as Muller had done.[17] (Later, we will see the use of both embryo transfer and in vitro fertilization linked to female sterilization.) Physicians, Behrman noted, have shown great interest in the following family-planning proposal: Men, after providing sperm specimens to be frozen and stored, undergo vasectomies.

"This method of family planning offers a good many advantages," he observed. However, he cautioned, present techniques of sperm preservation were not certain or efficient enough to allow widespread use of such a practice. The same freezing technique was used for both bull and human sperm. It worked well with bulls; less well with men. A technique for human sperm must be refined.

During the discussion of Behrman's paper, Dr. S. Leon Isreal of Philadelphia expressed pessimism about the public's ready acceptance of the plan, which required frozen sperm banks "of highly selective character."

"It is obvious that such positive genetic planning as Muller's requires a dreamer's world of men beyond the capacity of a present-day average imagination," Isreal lamented. "Even though, as Greep declared, 'Man is a mighty being and is now tinkering with the universe,' we will not be ready in a mere century to engage in such deliberately selective reproduction."

Perhaps his pessimism was unfounded. By 1976, a California businessman had established a sperm bank he called The Hermann J. Muller Repository for Germinal Choice.

The businessman was Robert K. Graham, an optometrist who had made a fortune by developing hard plastic lenses for eyeglasses. Before setting up his sperm bank, Graham wrote a book that reads like an old-time eugenics tract. In his *The Future of Man,* he terms the middle and upper classes "the repositories of every nation's intelligence and wisdom" and refers to those on welfare as "indolent people of low intelligence" who produce "deficient offspring." He advocates payments to married graduate students to enable them to reproduce more of their own kind. (Superior couples who deliberately produce only one child are "reproductive malingerers," he writes.) For those on welfare, he recommends birth control. "Multibillion-dollar welfare programs are working against reducing the number of the defective and deficient," Graham wrote. "Many of the programs actually subsidize the increase of the problem-making population. . . . At the very least such persons should be discouraged from producing offspring who have a strong chance of turning out like their parents" (Graham, 1981, p. 69–70). To the argument that people have a right to reproduce, Graham responds: "To assert that people should be free to pass on their deficiencies is like arguing that a leper should be free to infect his own offspring."

Besides publishing his ideas, Graham began implementing some of them. He collected the sperm of Nobel Prize–winning men in his Repository. He planned to allow the insemination of only highly intelligent women with it. Three Nobelists had donated their ejaculates, he announced in 1980.

To Graham's embarrassment, the mother of the first "Nobel sperm bank baby" turned out to be a former convict who had lost custody of two children by a previous marriage after accusations of child abuse (*Newsweek*, 16 July 1982).

Thea Muller, widow of geneticist Hermann J. Muller, protested the use of her husband's name for the sperm bank. In the face of her continuing opposition, Graham dropped the name. In 1963, Graham had offered to finance the germinal choice plan Hermann Muller had envisioned and Muller had accepted and helped plan the bank. But before his death in 1967, Muller became concerned that the optometrist was getting reactionary people involved in the project, Thea Muller told me in an interview.[18] One of the reactionary men Graham hoped to involve, she said, was Dr. William Shockley, who has since become a sperm donor to the bank. Shockley is racially biased, Thea Muller said. Hermann Muller, who had always fought against racism and classism, cut his ties to the proposed bank in 1965. He wrote a letter to those biologists and friends involved in the sperm bank informing them that he was shelving the project. "I think this was wise of him to do," Thea Muller said.

Shockley, who won the Nobel Prize for making transistors, has argued that there is a "basic, across-the-board genetic disadvantage

in terms of capacity to develop intelligence and build societies on the part of the Negro races throughout the world." Unfortunately, he laments, improving the social condition of Blacks will not help; their misery lies, ineradicably, in their genes (Jones, Syl., 1980, p. 69).

Shockley's involvement is significant because he is part of a larger political movement espousing "biological determinism." This is the notion that people receive fewer of the world's goods and less of its power and status because part of their own bodies—genes or hormones or brain—condemn them to a deprived life. These inferior people turn out to be women of all races and men of color. The political movement of biological determinism, masking as objective science, is influential.

Shockley, who has almost no training in genetics, believes that the quality of the human race is declining worldwide. This is an oft-repeated assertion by advocates of genetic control. There is no evidence for it.

J. Jacob Bronowski brought this out at a 1963 symposium during which eminent scientists discussed, often approvingly, Muller's germinal choice plan. Bronowski, the late British scientist and author of *The Ascent of Man,* said he did not understand what problem his colleagues were trying to solve through that plan. Though he repeatedly asked, "What is the evidence that genetically the human population is deteriorating?" the only answer the scientists gave him was one sentence from Sir Julian Huxley: "The evidence is mainly deductive, based on the fact that we are preserving many more genetically defective people than before, and are getting a lot of radioactive fallout." Sir Julian hurriedly added that the real problem was not so much genetic deterioration, but rather a need to improve the gene pool.

Bronowski offered an alternative to Muller's plan: "We might achieve the same effect in a simpler way by eating the children of the unfit, as Jonathan Swift suggested that the Irish should eat their own children," thus eliminating the poor and ending poverty.[19]

In support of his "genetic deterioration" line, Shockley refers to a declining quantity of intelligence in Blacks. He would measure "intelligence"—a quality few of its worshipers even attempt to define—through IQ tests. These tests have never been demonstrated to measure raw intelligence. Although the French originator of the tests proclaimed that intelligence was too complex to capture with a single number, American psychologists ignored his warning and perverted his intentions (Gould, 1981, p. 151). They used the IQ tests to maintain the privileges of their own class. For example, at a time when the privileged feared that the unprivileged (including immigrants) would outbreed them and threaten their ascendancy, they administered IQ tests to immigrants arriving on Ellis Island. In 1912, the IQ tests found that 83 percent of the Jews tested, 80 percent of the Hungarians, 79 percent of the Italians and 87 percent of the Russians were "feeble-minded." For this defect, many aliens were shipped back to their homelands.[20]

Shockley, developing his theory on a shabby intellectual basis, donated his ejaculate to Graham's "smart man's" sperm bank. Through such a bank, he noted, "hopefully, one would be able to build more ideal human beings . . ."

His hopes may be dashed. Dr. Shockley was 70 years old when he donated sperm. Any children he now engenders have about 40 times greater risk of suffering genetic mutations than do the offspring of men aged 19. The incidence of new mutations in the offspring of men over 40 years old is about 1 percent, the same as that for Down's syndrome in the children of women over 40.[21]

Did Shockley's own three children, engendered when he was younger, turn out to be brilliant, "more ideal" human beings? Measured against himself, he judges, his children "represent a very significant regression." But that does not mean his sperm is faulty. The eggs were to blame: "My first wife—their mother—had not as high an academic-achievement standing as I had," he said (Syl Jones, 1980).

When I began writing *The Mother Machine*, I planned to discuss this question in the first chapter: Should women enjoy re-productive freedom? The freedom to bear children at will; to choose the father of our children; to refrain from producing children? This appeared to be a crucial question. How society answered it would tell us much about the ways in which men would use the new reproductive technologies they were developing.

But it is the wrong question. I came to see that. It is a question that assumes the full humanity of women. Given the present power structure, the real question is: Should the machine (the woman) be the one to decide whether, or how often, or with what materials, it goes into production?

Obviously not.

Machine owners can say this openly when they speak of cows. A cow is "basically a machine" that must "produce this marketable product or unit every year." Few of us feel horror at this view of our sister animals. Most of us eat their young, their "products."

But machine owners must be more cautious when they speak of women. We women insist on viewing ourselves as living beings with dignity and spiritual worth, despite our long history—in Margaret Sanger's words—as "breeding machines for men." The machine owners must pretend to share that view of us.

So they say that decisions to re-produce are not an "individual" matter. They say such decisions affect the whole society. They say "society" (which is the white-dominated patriarchy) must share in that decision.

"I do not see why people should have the right to have children," Francis Crick, co-discoverer of the cell's DNA structure, said at the 1963 symposium on "Man and His Future," a symposium in which only one woman participated. "I think that if we can get across to people the idea that their children are not entirely their own business and that it is not a private matter, it would be an enormous step forward" (Wolstenholme, 1963, pp. 274–298).

His colleague, biochemist Norman W. Pirie, agreed: "Taking up Crick's point about . . . whether one has a right to have children, I would say that in a society in which the community is responsible for people's welfare—health, hospitals, unemployment insurance, etc.—the answer is 'No.'"

At this symposium, attended by top scientists in the biological fields, the voice of British biologist and writer Alex Comfort was a decidedly lonely one: Pirie "says that people do not have the right to produce children. What I am sure of is that no other persons have the right to prevent them."

But Crick, Shockley and many others were thinking up ways to do just that: Schemes to tax children; to provide cash incentives for sterilization; to license women for the number of children they may bear and men for the sperm they may deposit in seed banks; to put sterilants in the food or water supply.

It would not be difficult, Crick maintained, for the government to put something into food so that nobody could have children. Hypothetically, the government could give another chemical to reverse the effects of the sterilant.

"Only people licensed to bear children would be given this second chemical," Crick said. "This isn't so wild that we need not discuss it."

If there were a licensing scheme, Crick suggested, the first child "might be admitted on rather easy terms. If the parents were genetically unfavorable, they might be allowed to have only one child, or possibly two under certain special circumstances."

Shockley (not present at the symposium) favored another plan: The temporary sterilization by means of time-capsule contraceptives, of all young women and of every woman after each delivery. The contraceptive would be reversed only upon government approval (Djerassi, 1979, p. 180).

Joshua Lederberg and Crick independently came up with another scheme. They thought it might become socially acceptable. (Lederberg, now president of Rockefeller University, was formerly professor of biology and genetics at Stanford University.) The plan, Crick explained, was "simply to encourage by financial means those people who are more socially desirable to have children."

The obvious way to do this was to tax children. Those with money could afford to have children and pay the tax.

"It is unreasonable to take money as an exact measure of social desirability," Crick observed, "but at least they are fairly positively correlated."

So selected women would be allowed to bear children. When they conceived through artificial insemination, should they also enjoy the complete freedom to choose the inheritance of their children?

Muller himself thought that participants in his germinal choice plan, repudiating the "haphazard," "willy-nilly" method of procreation (sexual intercourse) and accepting controlled reproduction, should be rewarded. They should be granted the "privilege" of having a "major voice" in selecting the sperm donor.

Crick thinks it reasonable "up to a point" that those involved in AID have a choice. He does not describe that point.

Nobel Prize–winning geneticist Lederberg has "serious doubts" about the social controls that seem necessary for implementing reproduction control plans. They are "dangerous." But individual choice would not be "technically effective."

"And if people [read *women*] are allowed to choose the fathers of their children, will they not choose just the more notorious projections of their own images, exaggerated by the publicity given to advertised [sperm] donors?" he asked.

Physician and Anglican priest Herbert Trowell, who does not reveal his own position on reproductive freedom, comments: "If one rejects these [Christian] ethics, as many have done, then I think one must question whether a woman has the right to choose the inheritance of her child. On a purely humanistic basis are we not designing for the future of the race? We may have to say that a

particular woman is not suitable to have any children and another
woman is only suitable if linked with certain specified spermatozoa."
   These are top scientists speaking. Men with power.

Notes

1. I am not alone in viewing such an act as rape. When the report of this feat
was published by one of Pancoast's students after the doctor's death, an Oregon
physician protested. As *Fertility and Sterility* reported: "He personally had known
Dr. Pancoast and, in his estimation, the late physician was a gentleman, who would
never have stooped to the raping of a patient under anesthesia." The student's
account, however, has been accepted as valid (Gregoire and Mayer, 1965).

Furthermore, French law regards the use of artificial insemination by donor
sperm without the woman's consent as an act of rape. (*JAMA*, 11/15/47, p. 729.
Cited by T. Hall, 1979.)

In 1934, Dr. Hermann Rohleder reported: "Mantegazza regarded the injection
of strange semen without the knowledge of the woman a worse crime than infidelity
(of course this sort of insemination is a crime on the part of both husband and
physician)" (Rohleder, 1934, p. 176).

2. Kandell. 1974. Michael Debré, former prime minister of France, also clearly
believes woman's function is to produce children for the state. As *The New York
Times* reported, Debré "does not believe that France can achieve national greatness
unless it doubles its population to 100 million in the next century." He believes
women should not be allowed contraceptives and abortions. To prod them into
producing three or more children, he advocates a program of bonuses, well-paid
pregnancy leaves and tax advantages (Kandell, 1978).

Women's bodies have also been seen as munitions factories for the production
of weapons. Consider the Bible's Psalm 127, as quoted by Margaret Sanger:

> "As arrows in the hand of mighty man,
> So are the Children of Youth,
> Happy is the man that
>   hath his quiver full of them:
> They shall not be ashamed,
> When they speak with their enemies in the gate."

"Men are advised to have sufficient children to hurl at their enemies just as
the militarists of Europe today clamor for an increased population to enlarge their
armies," birth control advocate Margaret Sanger noted, commenting on this Psalm
in the 1930s. (See Sanger's papers in the Sophia Smith Collection, Smith College.)

3. Dworkin, 1976, pp. 80–84. Author Ann Jones refers to the ruses used to
assemble young women for shipment to the colonies where they could be sold as
wives. She mentions the case of William Robinson, cited by historian Carl
Bridenbaugh. Robinson was a chancery clerk convicted in 1618 of counterfeiting
the Great Seal of England. He used the false commission "to take up rich yeomen's
daughters (or drive them to compound) to serve his Majestie for breeders in
Virginia" (Jones, 1980, pp. 21–27).

4. Lerner, 1973, pp. 47–48. The children of Black women, no longer slaves, are no longer prized as economic assets. These days, Black women, rather than being encouraged to reproduce, are the victims of sterilization and of such dangerous contraceptives as Depo-Provera. (See Corea, 1985.)

5. Feldman, 1975. For information on the lot of the childless married woman, see: Menning, 1977, pp. xi, 87, 90–91; Rich, 1977, pp. 254–257; Rohleder, 1934, p. xiii; Kitzinger, 1978, pp. 42, 55, 200, 202 and 207. Describing the woman of the Indian, Mediterranean and Jewish cultures, anthropologist Kitzinger reported that she "can only justify her existence when she marries and bears children."

6. A man's right to divorce a barren wife is a legal corollary of the commandment "Increase and multiply, fill the earth and subdue it," writes David M. Feldman, author of *Marital Relations, Birth Control, Abortion in Jewish Law* (1975, pp. 53–54). This commandment, he continues, applies only to man and not to woman, "to the one whose business is to subdue rather than to be subdued." A woman has no comparable right to sue for divorce on grounds that her husband is sterile because, not being "commanded," she has no automatic claim.

7. Leon Kass and Paul Ramsey have both made this point. See Ramsey, 1970, p. 137, and Kass, 1972.

8. "In this day, when the laity is discussing eugenics, and legislatures are enacting laws for the betterment of the race, it behooves us as medical men to consider the value of the potential mother and her unborn babe as *a national asset* [my emphasis] and ascertain wherein their status can be benefitted," wrote John Fr. Moran, M.D., in "The Endowment of Motherhood," *JAMA*, 1/9/15, p. 122.

9. Callahan, 7/1/81. Ethicist Dr. Joseph Fletcher also speaks of "quality control." The ability to choose the biological quality of one's children, through voluntary choice of frozen sperm and eggs, is a great boon, Fletcher believes. "It buttresses quality control ..." he wrote (Fletcher, 1974, p. 161).

10. L. L. Cavalli-Sforza and W. F. Bodmer, *The Genetics of Human Populations*, 1971. Quoted by Marc Lappe in "Why Shouldn't We Have a Eugenic Policy?," *Genetics and the Law*. For more complete discussions of the eugenics movement, see: Howard and Rifkin, 1977, pp. 47–82; Chase, 1980; Gordon, 1977, pp. 116–158; Gould, 1981; Corea, 1985.

11. Information on sterilization, including castration, appears in "Biennial Report of the Eugenics Board of North Carolina," July 1, 1966–June 30, 1968, Sue L. Casebolt, executive secretary. See Table 12, "Operations Performed Annually, by Sex and Type of Operation, July 1929–June 1968." Most books on eugenics cited in note 8 also contain information on sterilization.

12. The quotes from Galton, Terman and Garrett appear in AASPEC, 1977, Woodward, p. 42 and Lewontin, p. 12. The quote from Rice appears in Rice, 1929. Guy Irving Burch also revealed his racism in a 1934 letter to an official of the Southern Baptist Convention who was opposing a current birth control bill. In trying to persuade the official to change his stand, Burch wrote: "Birth control ... will give classes within each nation the birth rates which the economic and social position of each warrant.... If birth control is permitted to spread to the lower classes unfortunate conditions among those classes and the Negro population will

be accompanied by a slower growth, while the more fortunate (especially when the economic burden of the luxurious breeding of dependent and defective elements are taken from their shoulders by birth control) will be accompanied by a more rapid increase." Burch's letter is in the files of the Planned Parenthood Federation at the Sophia Smith Collection, Smith College.

For information on current academic racism, see Mehler, 1983.

13. "Beef Cattle Reproduction with A. I. and Lutalyse: The Dawn of a New Era in Cattle Breeding Management," booklet copyrighted 1979 by The Upjohn Company, p. 23.

14. Geneticist Dr. Hermann J. Muller has challenged the notion that physicians are an intellectual elite. Medical students and interns were often used as multiple sperm vendors, he noted, "without regard for the fact that U.S. Army I.Q. tests have indicated this group to have the lowest mental ratings of all professions tested" (Muller, 1959, p. 30). Because I do not share the eugenicists' obsession with "intelligence," and consider I.Q. tests worthless, I find Muller's point irrelevant.

15. Some infertility clinics require that couples considering AID undergo psychologic evaluations before acceptance into their programs. There is no evidence that these evaluations are useful (Shapiro, 1981). Forcing a woman and a man to pass such evaluations provides a form of social control over them. Pharmacrats also exercise social control over women in "screening" them for surrogate motherhood and in vitro fertilization programs.

16. Muller, 1961. Like Muller, Sir Julian Huxley worried that nuclear fallout might lead to eugenic deterioration. Quickly passing over the option of a nuclear weapons ban, he notes that we could deal with the threat by freezing sperm and, as soon as technically possible, eggs. Then we could build deep shelters for the sperm banks. "Shelters for sperm banks will give better genetic results than shelters for people," he wrote, "as well as being very much cheaper." Huxley, "Eugenics in Evolutionary Perspective," *Perspectives in Biology and Medicine,* 6, Winter 1963, p. 178.

17. Muller wrote: "sterilization by vasectomy, when complemented by storage, constitutes the most efficient means for the long-term control of conception" (Muller, 1961, p. 648). Ethicist Dr. Joseph Fletcher also linked sperm preservation with sterilization: "Sterilization, the most reliable method of contraception, need no longer entail inevitable childlessness, now that we have cryogenics (freezing of sperm); a combination of both sterilization and fertility is possible now" (Fletcher, 1974, p. 161).

18. Muller himself had never been a typical eugenicist. In 1935, he had described eugenics as it has come to be known—as a "hopelessly perverted movement. . . . It does incalculable harm by lending a false appearance of scientific basis to advocates of race and class prejudice, defenders of vested interests of church and state, Fascists, Hitlerites and reactionaries generally" (Muller, 1935).

Muller was an idealist who, while not underestimating the effects of environment on human beings, believed that upgrading human genetic quality would lead to a better world where people, *by nature,* as well as by training, had weaker tendencies toward anger, fear, jealousy and egotism, and stronger tendencies toward "kindliness, affection, and fellow feeling in general" (Muller, 1959). Muller's proposals, however, were never effective, nor could they have been. Even if it were possible to identify people of "better genetic stock" (whatever *that* means), there is no effective way to spread their supposedly good genes throughout the world population of four billion people. Besides, decency isn't in one's genes.

19. Wolstenholme, 1963, pp. 284–289. For an excellent critique of the notion that the genetic quality of the human species is deteriorating, see Lappe, 1972. Imminent "genetic deterioration" of the species is a red herring, Lappe maintains. He further concludes: "The need for genetic intervention is today justified on the basis of the same unsubstantiated analysis of 'genetic deterioration' that characterized the eugenics movement of the late nineteenth century."

20. L. Kamin, *The Science and Politics of IQ,* New York: Halsted Press, 1974. Quoted in AASPEC, 1977, Lewontin. For further, excellent reading on biological determinism, see Hubbard, Henifin and Fried, 1979. For more information on the IQ tests, see Gould, 1981.

21. Dr. Jan M. Friedman, head of the division of clinical genetics, University of Texas, Southwestern Medical School in Dallas, found in a review of the literature that the risk of new autosomal-dominant mutations is about 40 times higher in the offspring of men over age 40 as in men age 19 (Mullan, OGN, May 15, 1980; also see Chatterjee, 1983). Furthermore, the provisional guidelines for sperm banks published by the American Association of Tissue Banks in November 1980 state (p. 38): "Age should be no more than 35 years to minimize chances of aging-related potential for genetic abnormalities."

2

The Subversive Sperm:
"A False Strain of Blood"

Although artificial insemination with donor sperm (AID) has been technologically possible for at least the past one hundred years, the practice has developed at a snail's pace. The fact that AID could be used in a eugenic program to control the "quality" of human beings produced has not been enough to recommend it. It alarmed men that a husband's sperm need not be used to inseminate his wife, that another man's could be. At a symposium on artificial insemination physicians and lawyers held in Chicago back in 1945, one participant suggested that AID was as startling as the atomic bomb and needed legislation accordingly (Greenhill, 1947). Bills were proposed in the Federal Republic of Germany and in Italy in the late 1950s which would have made human AID a criminal offense (Feversham, 1960).

In a paper he wrote in 1953, Dr. Jerome K. Sherman, American pioneer in sperm freezing, wondered why, after the introduction that year of a simple, effective sperm preservation method, many frozen sperm banks were not established. (Even today, only seventeen such banks exist in the United States.) He offers as one possible explanation that "there was a hesitancy on the part of physicians to try something as new as frozen semen, something which introduced another unphysiologic factor into the insemination procedures" (Sherman, 1973).

But there has been no comparable hesitancy on the part of physicians to try something as new as the conception of babies in laboratory dishes, a far more complicated procedure. With the first tentative success, in vitro fertilization clinics popped up all around the world. While in 1974, twenty years after the birth of the first child through frozen sperm, the American Medical Association declared that use of frozen human sperm "must still be recognized

34

as experimental," within four years of the first test-tube baby's birth, physicians were proclaiming that in vitro fertilization was no longer experimental (Callahan, 1982).

Sperm banks have developed slowly, not because pharmacrats fear a "new" technology, but because they recognize that artificial insemination by donor sperm poses a threat to the patriarchal family and to male dominance.

Before discussing these threats, let us review the development of this technology. Artificial insemination was possible at all only when the role of sperm in reproduction was grasped. Anton van Leeuwenhoek first described spermatozoa in human seminal fluid but, peering through his microscope in 1677, he did not know the sperm's function.

In 1779, the Italian priest and physiologist Lazaro Spallanzani showed experimentally for the first time that in order for embryos to develop, the egg and seminal fluid must come into actual physical contact. In his laboratory, Spallanzani artificially inseminated frogs, fish and dogs.

With this new knowledge on the sperm's role in reproduction, the first attempt to artificially inseminate a woman was made in 1790. The famous Scottish anatomist and surgeon John Hunter successfully inseminated the wife of a linen draper using her husband's sperm (AIH).[1] In the nineteenth century in Britain, Germany, France and the United States, AIH was reportedly practiced to a limited extent. The first recorded case using donor sperm rather than the husband's took place in 1884 in Philadelphia. In the next forty years, there was some discussion of AID and a few cases were reported in medical journals in the United States and Germany.

It was in the 1930s that physicians in Britain first seriously discussed the possibility of artificially inseminating the wives of infertile men. Small groups of gynecologists inseminated women during the Second World War but few people knew this. The practice was only beginning. A mere fifteen artificial inseminations using the husband's sperm and fifteen using donor sperm were reportedly performed in Great Britain in 1945 (Langer, 1969); by 1960, only an estimated twenty physicians were regularly performing it.

In Holland the practice was embraced no more heartily. From 1948, when the practice began, until 1960, there were fewer than ten AIDs (Levie, 1972). In the United States, 5,000 to 7,000 AID children were born every year, according to a 1960 estimate. Almost twenty years later, that estimate had expanded little: 6,000 to 10,000 births per year (Curie-Cohen, 1979).

The ability to freeze sperm expanded the potential use of artificial insemination. In 1949, A. S. Parkes and two fellow British scientists developed a method using glycerol, a syrupy substance, to protect semen from injury during the freezing.[2]

Farmers employed this method in the breeding industry. The use of frozen human sperm, however, was ignored until 1953 and 1954 when Sherman and his co-workers reported their research. They introduced a simple method of preserving human sperm using glycerol with a slow cooling of sperm and storage with solid carbon dioxide as a refrigerant. They also demonstrated for the first time that frozen sperm, when thawed, were able to fertilize an egg and induce its normal development.[3]

Despite this demonstration, few rushed to establish sperm banks. In the decade after the Sherman reports, only two frozen sperm banks or "cryobanks" opened—one in Iowa City and the other in Tokyo. The first human being conceived with frozen semen was born in 1954. By 1965, a mere twenty-four babies born in the United States and Japan had been conceived through frozen-thawed sperm. (Yet just six years after the first test-tube baby's birth, an estimated 200 babies had been born by in vitro fertilization.) In 1970, the first commercial human sperm cryobank in the United States was established and the largest one in the world, Idant, opened the following year in New York City. By 1973, the clinical use of frozen semen had resulted in only 571 births.[4]

By contrast, use of AID developed rapidly among farm animals. In Russia about 1900, scientists began studies on AID, primarily in cattle and sheep. They immediately saw its usefulness in breeding. They could inseminate thousands of females with the sperm of a few prize animals.

But how to get the sperm? Giuseppe Amantea, professor of human physiology at the University of Rome, had an idea. In 1914, he devised an artificial vagina ("AV," they came to call it) to collect dog semen. Russian scientists soon developed AVs suitable for the stallion, bull and ram. The men would sexually stimulate the bull by exposing him to a teaser animal and allowing him false mounts. Right before ejaculation, they would guide the bull's penis into the AV.

Sometimes an animal could not "serve" the AV. In 1948, scientists developed the electroejaculator, "a useful innovation for collecting from reluctant or disabled bulls and rams" (Bearden, 1980, p. 140). An electrode is placed in the rectum of crippled or old bulls in such a way that the reproductive system is stimulated.

If neither the AV nor electric current methods work, drugs can be injected to induce ejaculation. If all fails, a final option remains: "the recovery of spermatozoa from the male reproductive tract after slaughter."[5]

In 1936 in Denmark, cattle breeders formed the first cooperative AI association for the purpose of sharing the sperm of their prize bulls. The next year, Danish veterinarians developed the method of insemination (recto-vaginal) now widely used.

During World War II, the artificial insemination of farm animals accelerated rapidly and by the late 1940s, there were many AI organizations breeding cows all over the United States. The availability of frozen semen led to the widespread use of AI in the mid-1960s. Today, thirty-seven companies sell cattle semen. In the United States in 1980, 60 percent of dairy cows and 2 to 4 percent of beef cattle were inseminated artificially. These animals have never experienced their natural sexuality.[6]

While pharmacrats were enthusiastic about the use of AID to increase their control over the breeding of farm animals, most viewed the prospect of AID in women with alarm. There are two reasons for this. It poses a threat to patriarchal descent and it provides women with a means of rebellion.

AID desecrates sperm, the holy seed from which blossoms forth the power of the patriarchy. In introducing another man's "donor" sperm into a husband's wife, AID jeopardizes patriarchal descent. How can a man pass on his name and goods to his son if that son is not really *his*?

For many centuries before the establishment of patriarchy, man did not realize that he played any part in the creation of a baby (see Chapter 15). When paternity—the connection between sexual intercourse and the birth of a child—was discovered, man had a motive for subjugating woman.* If he could control his woman, allowing no other man to impregnate her, he could pass his name, power and property down through his sons. In this way, he could achieve immortality and a sense of connection with generations to come.

Subjugated, a woman became chattel, the movable property of men. She served as the womb of her husband and held a status comparable to that of cattle. She was required to bear only "legitimate" children, that is, offspring containing the seed of the man who owned her.

A woman can never legitimate her own child because "legiti-

---

* No one knows exactly when paternity was discovered. The observation that males were necessary for reproduction, Elizabeth Fisher suggests, may have been loosely made during the early stages of animal keeping, about 11,000 years ago (Fisher, 1979, p. 192).

macy" is a concept invented by men for men. It controls women who might defy male rules for reproduction. Men punish both rule-breaking women and their out-of-wedlock children. In Colonial America, a woman who bore a bastard could be fined, publically whipped and bound into indentured servitude.[7] Her bastard child could also be bound into servitude for twenty-one years or even for a lifetime. Bastardy, unlike rape or wife-murder, was an unforgivable crime. Theodore Sedgwick called it "the only crime which good society never pardons. . . . Shame, ridicule, infamy, exile attend it" (Jones, 1980, p. 44). To Jean Jacques Rousseau, the father of the Romantic revolution, bastardy was treasonous. Explaining that a faithless wife is worse than a faithless husband, he wrote:

> She destroys the family and breaks the bounds of nature; when she gives her husband children who are not his own she is false both to him and them, her crime is not infidelity but treason. To my mind, it is the source of dissension and of crime of every kind. Can any position be more wretched than that of the unhappy father who, when he clasps his child to his breast, is haunted by the suspicion that this is the child of another, the badge of his own dishonour, a thief who is robbing his own children of their inheritance? (From *Emile* in Figes, 1970, p. 74.)

To avoid punishments (such as public whippings and enforced servitude) devised by men who thought as Rousseau thought, thousands of seventeenth and eighteenth century women killed their own children. They murdered the babies men labeled "illegitimate." They stuffed their infants into sewers, threw them into rivers, hid them in trunks, buried them in the garden, in the cellar. Many were caught. Many were hung (Jones, 1980, pp. 42–57).

This is the key question AID posed to the patriarchy, the one to which courts solemnly devoted their attention: Is an AID child a "legitimate" child? Even when delivered by a man's wife, the child does not spring from the man's own loins. If an AID child is "illegitimate," has the mother committed adultery in conceiving it? Is an AID child entitled to receive a man's property, the patrimony?

Early on, the answer to that last question was no. Early on, men saw only the threat AID posed to them.

"What husband or wife, no matter how intense their longing for an heir, will consent to an injection of strange semen?" Dr. Hermann Rohleder wrote in a 1934 book on artificial insemination. "Thank God that most people still have that much tact, decency and moral feeling."

An Italian physician, he reported, had been entreated by a

childless married woman to inseminate her with the sperm of a fertile man. "He told his patient the evil contained in her suggestion," Rohleder wrote, "and pointed out to her that the artificial introduction of the semen of a strange man would be just as much of a sin as if she had herself consorted with a strange man" (Rohleder, 1934, p. 167).

And nine years later, in 1943, a physician wrote in the *American Journal of Obstetrics and Gynecology:* "The happy wife, contented through attaining a baby by means of homologous artificial insemination [i.e., with her husband's sperm], may give voice to her joy and win approbation. But the woman, made pregnant by the use of donor semen, who even whispers out of turn, on a single occasion, becomes a medical curiosity. She is envied by the primitive and wanton-minded, pitied by those gifted with easy fertility, shunned by her relatives and perhaps unfortunately by her own child" (Folsome, 1943).

In early cases, courts in England, Canada and the United States ruled that AID children were illegitimate and that the practice of AID was equivalent to adultery. As such, AID provided grounds for divorce and possible criminal prosecution.

Adultery, then, did not require sex. It was any act that might result in illegitimate conception. A Canadian case dealing with a woman who had allegedly agreed to AID without her husband's consent made that clear. In 1921, the Supreme Court of Ontario defined adultery as "the voluntary surrender to another person of the reproductive powers or faculties of the guilty person."[8] The essential element of adultery is not so much "the moral turpitude of the act of sexual intercourse," as it is "the possibility of introducing into the family of the husband a false strain of blood," the court ruled.[9]

An attorney presenting a paper at that AI symposium in Chicago in 1945 agreed with this ruling. Some courts had held that anything short of actual sexual intercourse—no matter how indecent the acts—did not constitute adultery, attorney James F. Wright pointed out. That fact strengthened the view that it is not moral depravity that is at the core of adultery, he said, "but the invasion of the reproductive function. There can be no adultery so long as nothing takes place which can by any possibility affect that function." Securing a man's property and, thereby, his immortality is really what the adultery prohibitions are all about.[10] It is not surprising then, that Wright indignantly asks from whom the AID child should inherit land and wealth. "Would he inherit from the husband of his mother, when the husband had nothing to do with producing this offspring?" (Greenhill, 1947). AID, Wright declared, should be declared by the courts to be adulterous.

The Superior Court for Cook County obliged him. In 1954, it held that regardless of a husband's consent, AID was "contrary to public policy and good morals," and constituted adultery on the mother's part. A child so conceived was born out of wedlock and was therefore illegitimate. The court added: "As such it is the child of the mother, and the father has no right or interest in said child."

As late as 1963, a court held that an AID child was illegitimate because the sperm donor was not married to the child's mother. Regardless of her husband's consent to AID, the court declared, the woman's insemination had constituted adultery.

In Britain, as in the United States, AID alarmed men. In 1948, a commission of inquiry set up by the Archbishop of Canterbury recommended that AID should be made a criminal offense. In the late 1950s, the British government appointed the Feversham Committee to inquire into AI practices and regulations. The committee, completing its report in 1960, recommended that a woman's conception by AID without the husband's consent be made a new ground for divorce. It found that AID was undesirable because it is a threat to the institution of marriage and to the resulting children. Those AID children, it found, should continue to be labeled illegitimate. "Succession through blood descent is an important element of family life and as such is at the basis of our society. On it depend the peerage and other titles of honour, and the Monarchy itself."[11]

If commissions and courts reacted to AID with distress, the response of male religious and medical leaders bordered on the testicular.* After reviewing the literature on artificial insemination, Dr. Bernard Rubin noted that it evoked "an intense emotional response" which had not changed in almost two hundred years. He thought the writers were unconsciously associating AID with incest. I think he need only have taken the writers literally. Listen to Dr. Rubin summarize their fears:

"It has been stated that AID 'endangers the family,' 'it is socially monstrous,' it endangers 'marriage, family and society.' 'It may well lead to radical revolution in which such concepts as father, brother, family descent, and the like, lose every vestige of their meaning.' There were fears of 'an anonymous world'; 'it should never be recommended.' The British Medical Association felt it was an 'offense against society'" (Rubin, 1965).

Such a response to AID is understandable if we grasp how

---

* I choose the adjective "testicular" rather than "hysterical" (a word relating to "womb") in respect for the gender to which I here refer.

terrifying to men was the prospect of "an anonymous world," that is, one without genetic continuity for men. "Grieving the loss of genetic continuity" is one of the difficult issues surrounding AID cited by infertility counselor Barbara Menning. She quotes one 30-year-old man who suffered that loss: "I did experience tremendous narcissistic hurt thinking that there would never be a child who looked like me or carried my genes. I recall that when I first considered AID, I had hoped that my wife would deliver a girl, whereas before, I had always expressed no preference. Somehow in my mind a son would highlight my loss because he wouldn't be a small version of me" (Menning, 1981).

AID posed a second threat to patriarchy. It not only jeopardized the mechanism of patriarchal descent, it also provided women with a means of rebellion. If AID were readily available, women could have families with children, but without men. This threatens the family, the community and men, sociologist Jalna Hanmer points out, and patriarchal religious leaders recognize that.

The Rev. Don McCarthy does: "Should not physicians and other health care personnel be prevented by law from using technology to impregnate unmarried women or from providing in vitro fertilization for unmarried couples? If the state is concerned to protect life, perhaps civil law ought to be equally concerned to protect marriage. The [Roman Catholic] Church stands firmly opposed to non-marital procreation" (McCarthy, 1980).

Men can hardly prevent women from performing AID. No physician is needed, nor is any complex equipment. "The technique of artificial insemination is simple," Dr. Wildred Finegold wrote in a 1964 medical text. "In fact, one of the hazards of the procedure is the ease of its performance."

Hazard to whom? Not to women. Then, to men?

Recognizing that "hazard," one man wrote to the AID Research Project: "God, you're making us less and less useful and necessary. It is frightening."

As attorney Russell Scott observed in 1981: "If reproduction by AI became the norm, it would follow that the human male would cease to be socially necessary. . . . The human species could easily be reproduced from stored sperm, or from sperm taken from a small number of selected living donors. The social implications of the disappearance of the historic role of the human male are difficult to imagine" (Scott, 1981, pp. 213–214).

Not surprisingly, men have attempted to limit the access of unmarried women to AID. Physicians quickly claimed that AI was a "medical" procedure over which they, and only they, should exercise control. The American Medical Association declared in 1974: "Because human artificial insemination is a medical procedure, the medical profession should exert its influence and efforts to the fullest extent necessary to ensure that the procedure is performed only by individuals licensed to practice medicine or osteopathy" (AMA, 1973). In 1980, a committee of the American Fertility Society recommended model legislation which provides imprisonment and fines for nonmedical persons performing AI.[12] Georgia passed a law legitimizing the AID child but only under certain conditions, among them, that a physician had performed the insemination. If a woman refuses to hire a physician, the child she bears is a bastard; if she goes to a doctor's office and takes her medicine, her baby is legitimate, sanctioned by the patriarchal state.

Most laws concerning AID now stipulate that the insemination should be performed by a doctor.

In Quebec, physicians write prescriptions for sperm. It is a "medicine." The Quebec Order of Pharmacists classified it as such in 1980 so that it could be considered a prescription drug cost under the Medicare program (AMN, 1980).

"In practice, if not in law, it's very similar here," comments Francie Hornstein, originator of an AID program at the Los Angeles Feminist Women's Health Center. "You need a doctor to formally requisition the sperm. You can't get it on your own. You register at the sperm bank. Each time you want to get the sperm, the doctor's office has to call."

Male medicine has certain criteria for women allowed what it calls the "therapy" of artificial insemination. The main criteria is that they be married. As attorney Barbara Kritchevsky observes, the very terms used to describe AI reveal the intent to limit its use to marriage: There can be no such thing as AIH—artificial insemination by husband—for a single woman.[13]

The possibility that unmarried women could choose pregnancy by AI has been mentioned in the legal literature since the 1940s "with great concern and distaste," Kritchevsky reports. She cites two articles published in 1949 that recommend legislative bans on AI for unmarried women.

Ninety percent of physicians queried in a 1979 survey had never used AID for unmarried women; 10 percent had. Physicians performed fewer than 1 percent of all artificial inseminations for the single (Curie-Cohen, 1979).

Many physicians have simply refused to inseminate them. "We do not offer the program [AID] to single women," doctors noted in *The New England Journal of Medicine* (Strickler, 1975).

Some doctors fear the practice is illegal. (It is not.) Others disapprove of bringing a child into a fatherless home or believe that unmarried women and lesbians should not be mothers. For example, Dr. Finegold believes an unmarried woman's interest in AI is "indicative of psychological distress" (Kritchevsky, 1981).

"I would refuse AID for a spinster," a British fertility clinic director wrote in 1972, "or for a couple of mixed colour or even of mixed religious denomination" (Sandler, 1972).

In 1962, the Royal Dutch Medical Association declared: "Artificial insemination of an unmarried woman is in conflict with the social order, and inadmissible on medical ethical grounds."

Similarly, the Feversham Committee expressed unqualified disapproval of AI for women unattached to men: single women, widows and "married women living apart from their husbands."

But in 1980 a woman challenged the right of physicians to refuse her AID on the grounds that she was unmarried. For such an alleged refusal, she sued a clinic in Detroit. She dropped the suit when the clinic, a division of Wayne State University's School of Medicine, announced that marital status would not be a factor in selecting "patients" for the procedure.

The reaction to this announcement overwhelmed the clinic. For several weeks, the obstetrics and gynecology department at Wayne received more than a dozen calls a day from single women, department chair Dr. Tommy N. Evans reported. "A lot of people have the idea that they can just walk in and get inseminated," Evans told *Ob/Gyn News*, "and that's just not the case at all."[14]

True. So some women began to take AI into their own hands, stating that childbearing was as much a woman's reproductive right as was abortion. "AID has a tremendous potential for expanding the options women have in living their lives," says Hornstein. "I think a lot of people get married solely because they want to have children. And maybe now those people—mostly women—won't feel that they have to get married."

The women using AI come from all walks of life. They are physicians, teachers, nurses' aides, social workers, psychotherapists, business executives, stewardesses, clerical and factory workers, principals, editors and secretaries. Some are feminists, others not at all consciously political.

Ever since approximately 1976, increasing numbers of heterosexual career women have been using AID, Annette Baran, a clinical social worker and co-founder of the AID Research Project, reports. These women are able to take care of themselves. They want a child. They are in their thirties. They have no guarantee they will ever meet, love and marry a man who will also want a child. So they go ahead on their own and bear a baby.

"They're a whole different breed," Baran says, "They're all Virgin Marys. There's no sex involved. They're bragging about it all over the place."

They do not feel like unwed mothers, Baran notes, because they did not get pregnant through an "illicit" sexual relationship. "They share it with their Board of Directors or their friends. They talk to everybody about it. They are very proud that they're a kind of pioneer woman."

Lesbian women started using AID at about the same time. It began small. A lesbian in Vermont wanted a child. A photographer who had graduated from Vassar College and obtained a master's degree from Johns Hopkins, she recalled: "I knew that the technique [AID] existed and that married women with infertile husbands were doing it and I figured maybe I could find a way for myself." For a year she kept careful records of her menstrual cycle so she could predict her ovulation, the optimal time for insemination. "I got very good at that," she observed.

Her physician father is proud of what she has done. "He sees that the choice made sense for me and is proud that I struggled to find a way to make it happen," she wrote on a questionnaire I distributed among lesbian AID mothers. "My mother views it as 'science fiction' and is sad that I did not live out her story-book fantasy of being married, etc. But she is so pleased with her granddaughter that those feelings have not surfaced since I first told her early in the pregnancy."

That same year, 1976, a lesbian in Los Angeles bore an AID baby. Rather than use a sperm bank, she and her lover found donors on their own. Then they went to the Los Angeles Feminist Women's Health Center. Staffer Francie Hornstein showed the women how to examine themselves using a speculum, flashlight and mirror and how to insert the sperm.

"She was the first woman I ever knew who actually went ahead and got pregnant by AID on her own," Hornstein recalls.

The Vermont Women's Health Center, the Los Angeles and the Oakland Feminist Women's Health Centers all now offer donor insemination programs. They began their programs, respectively, in 1975, 1979 and 1982. The Oakland center also has its own sperm bank.

"We've had three health center babies," reports Vermont staffer Dana Gallagher.

Attorney Donna Hitchens, who has written on donor insemination for the Lesbian Rights Project in San Francisco, says that AID is now in fairly extensive use among lesbians. "I'm seeing it a lot, especially in lesbians between 30 and 36 years old," she says. "In the Bay Area, we probably have two hundred children." The first such children in any numbers were born in 1979, she estimates.

A few books and articles offer how-to advice on "alternative fertilization" or "self-insemination," terms the authors prefer to "artificial insemination." They describe how to pinpoint ovulation so the woman can inseminate herself at the optimal time for fertilization. They report how women have found sperm donors (often, through friends) and what problems these women have encountered. Some women, they note, know who their sperm donors are, feeling this knowledge is important should their children someday want to learn about or form a relationship with their fathers. (One woman who filled out my questionnaire wrote that her sperm donor is a co-worker who regularly sees the child, acting as the child's friend, not father.) In many other instances, women try to keep the sperm donor anonymous for fear of a child custody suit by him later.

Gordon Prince of the Department of Child and Family Psychiatry at King's College Hospital in London is one of the many who disapproves of a lesbian using AID. A lesbian's motive for wanting children concerns him, he stated. Possibly that motive stems from aggression? Prince wonders if a lesbian's desire for AID might arise from "a basic hostility to men or to the traditional male pattern of society."* The issue needs study, he concluded. Earlier, in a 1978 case conference on lesbian use of AID, Prince had commented: "The hostility and fear to what we are discussing is very deep" (JME, 1978).

Lesbians know that. Many worry about what effect that hostility and fear may have on their children. Mary N., who eventually bore a son, Andy, is one of them: "The one thing that made us [her partner and herself] take so long in deciding to do donor insemination was fear for Andy's suffering. Was it really fair to him to do this? Finally we decided that if you think something is right—if you believe it is a woman's right to have children regardless of whether she's a lesbian or a celibate heterosexual—then it would be better to do the insemination and fight to make it acceptable. But it still scares us. It's scary thinking that your child is going to have pain."

It is still too early yet to know the full range of difficulties and

* In a brilliant analysis of heterosexuality as an institution, Adrienne Rich writes that part of the lie promulgated by that institution is "the frequently encountered implication that women turn to women out of hatred for men" (Rich, 1980).

joys these female-headed AID families will experience. All lesbian mothers who filled out my questionnaire or talked with me were very happy they had had a baby through AID. But their responses did indicate some of the complexities of their situations: the insecurity felt by the partner of an AID mother because she, who also loves and mothers the child, may have no legal or socially sanctioned relationship to that child or any right to see the child again if the relationship with the mother ends; a fear that, as lesbians, they will be declared unfit mothers and have their children taken away from them, a fear causing them to be secretive about the AID to the outside world while telling their children the truth about their conception; the guilt any mother feels ("Am I doing it right?") exacerbated, for the single lesbian, by the messages she gets that a single parent family is incomplete and undesirable; the uniqueness of the AID family's relationship with grandparents—often supportive, sometimes uneasy.

Since many of the women started their families independent of physician-controlled donor insemination services, they, unlike married couples using AID, are not so readily available for study. Many of the lesbian mothers I talked with thought it would be useful to themselves, to other lesbians considering AID, and to AID children to have information about their experiences compiled, perhaps by one of themselves. Aware of societal hostility and of the effect that hostility might have on the way any study of themselves was constructed and its results evaluated, they would be careful about which researchers they allowed into their lives.

Notes

1. Hunter artificially inseminated the linen draper's wife before it was understood that the essential requirement for fertilization was the entry of the sperm into the egg. Martin Barry, an English embryologist, suggested this possibility in 1840. It was seen for the first time in 1854 in frogs (Timson, 1979).

2. In 1776, Spallanzani was perhaps the first to report the effects of cooling on human sperm, noting that sperm cooled by snow became motionless. In the nineteenth century, Mantegazza experimented unsuccessfully with freezing sperm. From 1938 to 1945, a number of scientists observed that some human sperm could survive freezing and storage at temperatures as low as 269 degrees below 0°. Under the Parkes method, developed in 1949, a mixture of semen and glycerol is poured into a container that looks like a drinking straw. Then it is chilled in liquid nitrogen to 383 degrees below zero. Before use, the semen is thawed.

3. About 67 percent of the sperm they froze survived after storage for at least three months.

4. In 1963, Sherman introduced a new method to freeze-store human sperm using the vapor of liquid nitrogen for freezing and its liquid for storage. He reported that the survival rate of thawed sperm with this new nitrogen-vapor method was superior to that with the original "dry-ice" method.

Not all sperm survive either freezing process, however. Moreover, the conception rate for frozen sperm is estimated to be anywhere from 15 to 33 percent lower than that of fresh sperm. The length of time sperm can be stored also remains controversial. Evidence suggests that, with time, the sperm's motility (ability to move) declines. While pregnancies after ten years' storage have been reported, such reports of pregnancies using sperm in long-term storage are sporadic and do not provide data on success rates. No long-term follow-up of children conceived with frozen sperm has ever been conducted. Sources for the section on frozen sperm include: AMA, 1974; OGN, 6/1/80; Bunge, 1954.

5. Artificial insemination is not widespread outside the cattle industry. However, CBS reported that in 1978, the following animals were created by AI: 136 million turkeys; 300,000 swine; 35,000 horses; and 3,000 goats (McMullen, 1979).

6. Interview with spokesman for the National Association of Animal Breeders, July 1, 1981.

7. A more recent punishment for out-of-wedlock mothers has been the loss of their children through adoption. In recent years, these "birthmothers" have begun to organize and to declare that many of them had not wanted to surrender their children to strangers. Denied all forms of social and economic support, they had had little choice. Carole Anderson of Concerned United Birthparents wrote of the situation in the 1960s: "In order to convince us to surrender, they told us we would be ruining our children's lives by keeping them. Children of single parents, they said, would be ridiculed at school as bastards, or grow up to be homosexual because they lacked a father image, or would live in poverty forever because no decent man would marry us." In the 1960s, Anderson reported, most high schools and colleges expelled pregnant students. Employers rarely hired single mothers. Even if mothers could get jobs, few could find day-care centers. "Denied education, denied jobs, and denied any knowledge of financial assistance, few of us had any option but to surrender our children," Anderson wrote. Some of those social conditions had changed by 1981. The attitude toward unwed mothers became less punitive. Schools encouraged pregnant students to continue their studies. Subsidized day care and job training were available to some single mothers. While in 1970, more than 90 percent of single mothers had surrendered their children, by 1981, fewer than 10 percent did so (Anderson, 1981).

8. The case was Orford v. Orford. It, along with subsequent cases discussed, are reported on in these articles: Kritchevsky, 1981; Katz, *Appendix*, 1979, pp. 5–6. British courts sometimes ruled differently on this issue. See Scott, 1981, p. 206.

9. A 1939 editorial in the *Journal of the American Medical Association* (JAMA) observed: "The fact that conception is effected not by adultery or fornication but by a method not involving sexual intercourse does not in principle seem to alter the concept of legitimacy. This concept seems to demand that the child be the actual offspring of the husband of the mother of the child." If the husband's semen was used, the child would seem to be legitimate; if not, illegitimate, JAMA argued. (It suggested that a couple adopt its AID child to safeguard its inheritency.) (JAMA, 5/6/39)

10. The comments of an unnamed woman who, in a recent year, was artificially inseminated with donor sperm, reveal her failure to understand that the unfaithful act consists—not in sexual pleasure without her husband—but in using his property (i.e., her own body) to produce children that are not his: "I asked my husband repeatedly to assure me that I was not going to commit an unfaithful act. Despite his wholehearted support, I could not really believe him." She adds that she was glad he was present on the first day of insemination. "I am so glad he could witness my terror, that he heard the physician ask me three times to relax before he could even get the speculum in, that he realized this experience was certainly not sexually enjoyable for me" (Menning, 1981).

11. Feversham, 1960. The form recommended by Britain's Medical Defense Union for authorizing the doctor to inseminate a wife with donor sperm required the couple to assure the doctor that the birth of an AID child to them "will not defeat the claims of any person to any titles, estates, interests or funds".

12. As of August 1981, the American Fertility Society had not formally approved the model legislation.

13. AIH also refers to "artificial insemination homologous," use of the husband's sperm. AID is also called "artificial insemination heterologous," use of a donor's sperm. The use of the terms "homologous" and "heterologous" in these contexts is curious. Certainly the terms do not scientifically describe the procedures.

A husband's sperm is considered homologous to his wife. My medical dictionary partly defines homologous as: "Derived from an animal of the same species but of different genotype, as a homograft." A husband is a being of the same species as his wife?

Heterologous means: "1. Made up of tissue not normal to the part.   2. Derived from an individual of a different species or one having a different genetic constitution." A man who is not a particular woman's husband is "of a different species" to that woman?

Una Stannard's work gives some insight into what is going on here. In her book, she points out that not so long ago, when a woman married, she was considered to become a part of her husband in ways so literal we can scarcely grasp it today. The woman was subsumed within her husband's person; she became an actual part of his body, his womb which produced his children (see Stannard, 1977). She was "homologous" to him, "heterologous" to all other men.

14. OGN, 12/1/80. Dr. Tommy Evans, chair of the obstetrics and gynecology department at Wayne State, is quoted in this article as saying that by settling out of court "we at least limited the scope of this thing. We avoided setting a legal precedent that could be applied to other institutions." Dr. Evans noted that although the clinic is obligated to abide by the agreement, no physician can be compelled to perform any medical procedure against his principles. Attorney Kritchevsky doubts that the suit will have much effect on fertility clinic practices.

3

The Socialized Sperm:
Institutionalizing Artificial Insemination

In 1980, a gay man who had donated sperm to a lesbian I will call Susan filed a paternity suit seeking visitation and custody rights to the child Susan subsequently bore. Three years later, a California Superior Court judge declared the sperm donor to be the legal father and gave him visitation rights. The first such case in the country, it will, when an appeals court rules on it, probably set a precedent.

Faced with the aberration AID presents—a family without a father—the courts and medicine are beginning to find ways to fit that aberration into the patriarchy in a nonthreatening way. The strategy revolves around the definition of the sperm donor's role, a role that expands or contracts depending on the circumstances.

When an independent woman like Susan is involved—a woman without a primary man in her life—then the sperm donor's role expands. From early rulings in such cases, it appears that courts are beginning to change the donor's status from that of an anonymous semen source to that of a father with rights over his issue. This would curtail a woman's freedom to bear a child outside male control.

But when a married couple is involved and another man (the husband) is present to take on the paternal role, then the sperm vendor's status shrinks to one akin to a blood donor's. He supplies a bodily fluid and, still nameless, disappears. Fatherhood does not reside in that man's sperm, the courts and medicine declare.

Men did not immediately hit on these legal and medical techniques for dealing with the threat AID posed to the social order. That threat was serious so it is hardly surprising that use of artificial insemination by donor has developed slowly.

rsham Committee, as we have seen, issued its highly
on AI in 1960. In 1973, the Peel Report, issued by a
by the British Medical Association, looked more
AID. It recommended not only that the government
vide AID within the National Health Service (it now does so),
but that AID children be deemed legitimate if the husband had
agreed to the insemination. (Despite that later recommendation, AID
children remain "illegitimate" in Britain.)[1]

In the United States also, men were slowly changing their views.
Courts were less quick to brand the AID child a bastard. In 1964,
Georgia became the first state to pass a statute legitimizing children
conceived by artificial insemination if both the husband and wife
consent in writing. While most states have yet to decide if an AID
child is "legitimate," fifteen states have passed laws concerning AID.[2]
Many statutes are based on the Uniform Parentage Act proposed in
1973. That act provides that if a wife is artificially inseminated with
donor semen, under a physician's supervision and with her husband's
consent, the law treats the husband as if he were the natural father
of the AID child. The statutes make it clear that a man giving sperm
to a physician is not the legal father of any children conceived with
that sperm.

"As fatherhood is legally held to reside in the genetic contribution, the acceptance of AID children as legitimate is a break with
a particularly ancient tradition, one at the very root of patriarchal
social orders," sociologist Jalna Hanmer commented.

Men can make that break now because they are finding ways
to fit AID into the patriarchy by insisting upon locating a man to
play the role of father.

Courts dealing with AI, attorney Barbara Kritchevsky observes,
"do come out with some pretty blatant statements like, 'The most
important thing is to find this child a father and since we don't
know who the father really was, this man who at least consented to
the child's birth is going to be the father.' "

Two court rulings are relevant. The 1968 People v. Sorensen
and the 1977 C.M. v. C.C. rulings both articulated a strong policy
of finding the child a father. While a 1945 oral opinion in an Illinois
case had broken precedence with other court rulings and held that
AID was neither adultery nor grounds for divorce, it was not until
1968 that a court ruled the AID child was legitimate.[3] Donor
insemination, it further declared, was not adultery. In the Sorensen
case, the most complete judicial treatment of AID to date, the
California Supreme Court upheld the criminal conviction of a man

for not supporting the AID child conceived with his consent during his marriage. Sorensen claimed the child was not his. He had no obligation to support it, he maintained.

The court ruled that the sperm donor was not the child's father. The donor had no more responsibility for the use of his sperm than a blood donor did for his blood. "Since there is no 'natural father,'" the Court noted, "we can only look for a lawful father." That was Sorensen.[4]

Fatherhood, then, was no longer contained only in the sperm.

A 1977 ruling also articulated a policy in favor of finding the child a father. This case could give sperm donors power over single women and the children they bear. Rendered by a court in Cumberland County, New Jersey, it was—until the 1983 ruling in Susan's case—the only court decision dealing with AI of an unmarried woman. The court stated that in New Jersey the natural father of an illegitimate child was entitled to visitation. It was in the child's best interests, it declared, to have two parents whenever possible.

The somewhat odd circumstances of the case were these: C.M., the sperm donor, had been dating C.C. and they had been discussing marriage. C.C. wanted to have a child but did not want to have intercourse before marriage. When she considered asking a friend to donate sperm, C.M. volunteered his sperm and C.C. accepted. In about the third month of her pregnancy, they stopped seeing each other. After the child's birth, C.M. sued for visitation rights.

The court ruled that the sperm donor was entitled to visitation rights and also had the duty to support the child. In later court action, the donor was given the right to be designated the child's father on the birth certificate. These court decisions concerning a single AID mother sharply differed from those rendered in cases where the donor provided sperm to a married woman. In these later cases concerning custody, support and visitation of AID children, court decisions have declined to view the donor as the legal father (Kern and Ridolfi, 1982).

The court's insistence in C.M. v. C.C. that a child's best interest can only be served by finding the child a father, Kritchevsky notes, must trouble those who believe an unmarried woman has a right to conceive by AI. The court's decision could be extended to hold that a known sperm donor must be recognized as the father of an unmarried woman's child in a case where neither party intended the man to do more than provide semen, she further observes. The danger presented by the C.M. v. C.C. case—that the courts will impose a "marriage" relationship on an unmarried woman whenever the male parent presents himself—would be especially disturbing to lesbian couples planning to raise the child, she notes.

On the basis of this case, Kritchevsky predicted in 1981 that a judge may give the sperm donor paternal rights, saying, "We want this child to have some sort of male parent to identify with." Her prediction came true two years later in Susan's case.

The sperm donor who filed a paternity suit against Susan wants to be a parent to her child, Eric. Susan believes that the man's feelings about donating his sperm changed over time. Originally he had agreed to give the sperm and bear no responsibility for, or rights to, the child, she said. He had told her he was curious to see what an offspring of his would look like, but he wanted to work and travel, not care for a child. Perfect, she said.

"My impression is that things changed for him once I began showing pregnancy," she told me. "He didn't know his reaction to seeing his sperm incarnated. Obviously he had much more attachment to it than he thought he would initially. His ego became involved in seeing this person that was part of *him*." The fact that his incarnated sperm turned out to be a boy seemed to increase his interest in the child, Susan feels.

During the pregnancy, the donor said several things that made Susan nervous. He expected his name to be on the child's birth certificate; he wanted to be appointed legal guardian; he wanted a written agreement naming him as father. Susan refused. Shortly after the child's birth, he said he wanted his last name to be the child's middle name. No, Susan said.

When the donor could not win from her the access to, and claim on, the child he now wished, he brought the paternity suit.

The court treated the suit like a divorce case. It served notice on Susan not to leave the state with her child. It ordered her and the donor—who are little more than strangers—to meet in conciliation court. In a sense, as Kritchevsky feared, the court was imposing a "marriage" relationship on an unmarried woman.

That "every child should have a father" is very much an underlying value in any custody proceeding, one of Susan's attorneys, Donna Hitchens, observes. "That bias is assumed to be good for the child regardless of what disruption it creates in the child's *real* family," she said. Whenever a written agreement between a woman and a man is lacking in an AID case, and the two parties state differing versions of the oral agreement, "there's going to be a tendency on the part of judges to believe that everybody intends their child to have a father," she notes.

Other women who have borne AID children outside medical control watch this case with alarm. "Even women who have used anonymous donors are petrified," Susan explains. "If my donor can do this, then any donor can."

When a man gains the rights of access, custody and guardianship of children, he also gains some control over the mother, as sociologist Hanmer points out. If men (in this case, sperm donors) are given rights to their "illegitimate" children, a kind of polygyny could develop. "What is to stop men having control over a number of children by different women (and in this way to gain control over the women)?" Hanmer asks.[5]

Her sperm donor has certainly gained some control over Susan's life. The judge gave him summer, holiday and overnight visitation rights, so Susan must make her holiday plans around him. She must tell him if she plans to move. She must inform him of major decisions around the child's medical care and schooling.

"She's basically forced into a family relationship with this man for the next sixteen or so years," comments Hitchens.

"If Susan had been married," she notes, "or if she had gone to a doctor for the insemination, there would have been no way, under our statutes, the judge would have held this man to be the father. The only reason he did is because she is a single woman who didn't use a physician. This is a constitutional violation of equal protection."

Susan is appealing the judge's ruling.

I have discussed one method of squeezing AID into the patriarchal family: expanding the sperm donor's role into that of a "father" when a single woman has artificially inseminated herself. When the woman is married, the technique, largely handled by the physician, changes. He performs a disappearance act with the sperm vendor.

The doctor's emphasis on anonymity and secrecy throughout the AID procedure is largely an attempt to render the sperm vendor invisible so that the husband can more closely identify himself as the father. The doctor is also initiating a conspiracy to cover up the husband's sterility—"weak" sperm, in a patriarchal value system, being shameful.

Physicians obliterate the sperm vendor in a variety of ways:

—They insist that AID is therapy for infertility in which they give a female patient a magic shot and, "cured," she bears a child. In this medical construct of reality, the sperm vendor is no longer a human being. He is a pharmaceutical resource, like a plant from which one extracts medicine.

—They match the sperm vendor closely to the husband so the child can more easily pass as the natural offspring of that husband. As a result of this close matching, Idant sperm bank administrator Roxanne Feldschuh notes, "the child will appear physically to belong to this family unit."

—They may fraudulently sign a birth certificate naming the husband as the father. Alternately, they may refer the woman to an obstetrician instructing her not to reveal that she conceived by AID. This allows the obstetrician, in good conscience, to sign his name to a falsehood.

—They often advise AID couples not to tell the AID child or their family or friends how the child was conceived. "The majority of couples—something like 99 percent—choose not to tell anyone that this child was conceived through AID," Feldschuh told me in an interview. "And for all purposes except for the biological seed, this man is the father of the child. He's there during the pregnancy. He's there for support. And he's there to love and take care of that child. This is fatherhood. So it's important that there be no physical deviation within that family group."

—They destroy all donor records to preserve confidentiality. (Seventy percent of physicians did this, according to one survey [Curie-Cohen, 1979].)

—They inseminate the woman two or three times each menstrual cycle using semen from a different donor each time so no one is sure who the genetic father is.

It was not the couples who were asking for secrecy, although some, if given a choice, may have wanted it, comments Annette Baran who, with her colleagues in the AID Research Project, conducted extensive interviews with AID families. It was the medical institution that set the tone of secrecy in which AID took place. This tone hurts the AID family, she believes.

"It is our feeling that there is something different about those families, that on some unconscious level the children do know that something is askew. But they don't know what." Such a secret has a way of causing problems, of acting destructively. "Secrets gnaw at people," Baran explained. "One is afraid they will come out."

On an emotional level, Baran reported, many husbands equate AID with infidelity and adultery. (As we have seen, male courts and physicians have had the same response to AID.) The men feel their wives are having another man's baby. In truth, they are.

Some wives have fantasies about the man whose baby they are carrying. They feel that sperm vendors are supermen—studs chosen for their superior intelligence and health. The husband's repressed feelings concerning AID show up in family relationships. He may feel hostility or jealousy toward the child. Baran cites this case: "The boy was a handsome superchild and the father found nothing but fault with him. After the divorce the mother said, 'Look, there's nothing wrong with you. The reason your father didn't like you was that you weren't his son and he was jealous of you.' "

When Baran and her colleagues did a computer search of all the studies conducted on AID families, they found nothing. No research. How then can physicians assure couples that AID, conducted in secrecy, may be a fine solution to their problems when no one had looked to see what actually happens inside AID families?

Baran does not oppose AID. She argues that it should be practiced honestly, with no pretense that it will do for men what it, in fact, does not do. It does not give a man a child of his own seed. Physicians can say that that does not really matter. Apparently, in many cases, it does.[6]

Because secrecy surrounds the practice of AID in women, much remains unknown about it. We do not know how many doctors are performing it or exactly how many children have been born of it or the procedures doctors use or how they select donors or how many times they will use the sperm of one donor. Studies are inadequate. Follow-up research on AID children is almost nonexistent.

"The lack of evidence on which to base opinions and the need for follow-up research has been emphasized by all the committees which have been set up to inquire into AID," commentators noted in *New Scientist* (Snowden and Mitchell, 1980).

Physicians conduct the practice in secret, one AID practitioner told me. They feel vulnerable because of AID's uncertain legal status; no laws govern the practice at all in most states. We do not even know if physicians are screening sperm vendors for venereal disease, he said. There are indeed a few cases on record in which gonorrhea has been transmitted through AID.

The first real attempt "to unveil the long-shrouded technique" of AI was made in 1979, as the *Journal of the American Medical Association* observed.[7] Researchers from the University of Wisconsin Hospital published their excellent survey of 379 physicians practicing artificial insemination (Curie-Cohen, 1979). In a report highly critical of AID practice, the researchers concluded that such practice involved:

—A lack of uniform standards.
—"Woefully deficient" record-keeping practices. (Only 37 percent kept records of AID children and 30 percent on AID donors. As a minimum, the researchers argued, doctors should keep records on the outcome of pregnancies and on paternity.)
—A nonchalant attitude toward multiple use of sperm vendors, a practice that could lead to the inadvertent mating of blood relatives.[8]
—Inadequate screening of donors.[9]

The Wisconsin study further found that most screening for genetic diseases was performed by physicians who were not trained for this task. They showed a poor knowledge of genetics. For example, 71 percent of the physician respondents wrote that they would reject a sperm vendor who had hemophilia in his family. But it would be impossible for him to transmit this X-linked gene unless he was himself affected.

The essence of this fourth finding is that physicians are inefficient in their selection of germinal material. Hornstein looks askance at this criticism: "People don't really screen the partners they have children with that well before they decide to marry them. I wonder how many women and men talk about their family health histories before they get married or before they have children."

But efficiency in selecting choice sperm will undoubtedly improve. And other refinements will come. The development of methods to separate spermatozoa into various categories, including male-engendering and female-engendering chromosomes, would "complement" the AI technique and "increase its use," one scientist wrote in the British journal *Nature* (Jones, 1971). Sperm banks, then, could be used in programs to predetermine the sex of babies. Already Idant announces the following service: "Semen separation for male sex selection (couples accepted on a research basis only)." The ability to predetermine a baby's sex would advance man's ability to exercise child selection.

Geneticist H. J. Muller observed in 1961 that it was then possible, through AI, to exercise selection by choosing the source of the germ cells of one's children. "At present," he wrote, "this choice is confined to the male germ cells but there are indications that with a comparatively small amount of research it might in some degree be extended to those of the female as well" (Muller, 1961). (The specter of eugenics returns, a specter that looms larger as ways are found to reduce AID's threat to men and fit it into the family.)

Ten years later, in a discussion of AI, *Nature* reported: "Alternatively, if it proves practicable to transfer ova (eggs) or embryos to foster mothers and to develop suitable methods of superovulating females, fertilizing ova in vitro (in the lab) and deep freezing ova or embryos, their use might, to some degree, supersede that of artificial insemination" (Jones, 1971).

Notes

1. Peel, 1973. As the law now stands in Britain, the AID child is illegitimate. However, no court in Britain has considered the legitimacy of such a child. Most AID babies are registered as legitimate. It is thought that the court would presume the child born within a marriage to be legitimate unless evidence to the contrary were presented.

2. As of August 1981, thirty-five states had no legislation that either defined the legal status of AID children or covered the practice of AI. Fifteen states have passed some form of legislation, mostly brief statutes declaring the AID child "legitimate." Many of the laws are based on the Uniform Parentage Act, which was approved by the Commissioners on Uniform State Laws in 1973 and approved by the American Bar Association in 1974 (OGN, 1/1/1980). States having laws concerning the status of AI or of AID children are: Alaska, Arkansas, California, Florida, Georgia, Kansas, Louisiana, New York, North Carolina, Oklahoma, Oregon, Texas, Virginia and Washington (Curie-Cohen, 1979).

Kritchevsky notes that the entire issue of illegitimacy becomes increasingly irrelevant as states such as Oregon and those that have adopted the Uniform Parentage Act strive to eliminate the disabilities arising from that status. Courts, she added, are increasingly curtailing the right of states freely to distinguish between legitimate and illegitimate children. She observed: "The Supreme Court has held that while states may render children born out of wedlock illegitimate to create an incentive for citizens to enter 'legitimate' family relationships or to discourage 'spurious claims against intestate estates' [1978], it has sharply curtailed states' power to pass discriminatory legislation where no sufficiently important state interest is at stake" (Kritchevsky, 1981).

3. The 1945 Illinois case was Hoch v. Hoch.

4. The policy concerns of the court in People v. Sorensen have been reiterated in subsequent cases, Kritchevsky notes. However, attorney Barbara Katz warns that simply because some modern courts have adopted liberal interpretations does not mean that AI and related reproductive technology have been removed from the context of present adultery and legitimacy laws. Legislatures need to clarify the issues (Katz, 1979, p. 11).

5. Hanmer makes her point in discussing a legal change recommended by a 1979 report of Britain's Law Commission. British women now have undisputed

custody of illegitimate children. The law change would extend rights over these children to men. Hanmer asks: "Is the child the desired object of this proposed legislation or is the woman?" (Hanmer, 1981).

6. Baran believes that when a man donates sperm, he has a responsibility, though not a legal one. He ought to be willing to be identified in the future for medical or emotional information the child may feel she or he needs. He could be protected so he has no other obligations to the child. But in 1980, the American Association of Tissue Banks issued provisional guidelines for sperm banks that stress the need to maintain the donor's anonymity (AATB, 1980). "Special precautions" are "absolutely necessary" in this area, it states: Code identification for sperm donors must be used; only the sperm bank director or his designate should have a list linking donors' names with their identification numbers; no records should exist in either the physician's office or the sperm bank identifying donor and recipient together by name.

Dr. Jerome Sherman, pioneer in sperm freezing, oversaw the development of these guidelines. He disagrees with Baran's contention that a sperm donor should be willing to be known to the child. This is "naïve and an incorrect way of looking at it." He added: "If anything, that would weaken the family rather than strengthen it. In other words, 'Here is my daddy who pays for my food and here is my real daddy who is responsible for my short nose. Now who is my real daddy?' "

7. JAMA, 3/23/79, p. 1219. An earlier survey of physicians doing AI, published in 1941, was severely criticized for its lack of documentation.

8. While the average number of children per sperm vendor is small, the researchers wrote, few physicians have policies limiting the number of times they will use a single vendor. This fear of incest among siblings comes up repeatedly in the literature on AID.

9. Beyond choosing donors from a "select" group—the medical and academic communities—there is little further screening, the researchers found. Often the screening consisted of nothing more than asking a vendor if any genetic disease existed in his family or in giving him a short check-list of common familial diseases. "A number of doctors expected medical students and hospital residents to screen themselves before donating semen," the researchers reported.

Screening depends on vendor honesty, they observed. But the potential vendor knows that he could lose an easy source of income if he disqualified himself by reporting a genetic disease in his family. By analogy, the researchers observe, blood vendors appear to be less honest than blood donors.

Physicians providing AID are responsible for finding and screening donors if they use fresh sperm. If they use frozen sperm, the sperm bank from which they obtain it screens the donors.

Part Two

EMBRYO TRANSFER

4

The Goddess and the Cow

I

The cow was one of the oldest forms in which the ancient Goddess was known.* In Mesopotamian Sumer, she was Ninhursag, the Wild Cow, Regent of Heaven and Earth, who shattered the very air with Her presence at the beginning of time. In northern Canaan, the goddess Anath, Mistress of the Lofty Heavens, was depicted with the horns of the cow. In Greece, the goddess Gaea who "gave birth to all else that exists," was associated with the Primeval Cow. The imagery was later connected to the goddess Hera. Even as far north as Iceland the earliest writings tell of the Primeval Cow, Audhumla, She who existed before all else. Seals from Harappan India from about 3000 B.C. reveal images of the Goddess with cow horns much like those of the Near Eastern artifacts, images perhaps linked to the reverence for the cow as sacred in India even today.

In Egypt, the goddess Nut is depicted as the very heavens, the Celestial Cow upon whose body shine the stars, which were believed to be the souls of the dead that She had taken to Her. The name of Hathor evokes much the same imagery, the body of the cow with woman's head, the body of a woman with the cow's head, or even simply the image of the horned cow as the Goddess who gave all life. In the Egyptian Book of the Dead, She is known by the name

* Merlin Stone, author of *When God Was a Woman*, and Barbara G. Walker, author of *The Woman's Encyclopedia of Myths and Secrets*, read this and other material critically for me and provided me with much more information. I am grateful for their generous help.

Meh Urit or Methyer, the Sacred Cow that stands upon the mountain of heaven waiting to receive the souls of those who have been tested and found worthy.

The sanctity of the cow as Mother of All is also to be found among the Alur people of Zaire. Thus from Africa to Iceland, the cow was not only considered to be sacred but was most often regarded as the source of all life, She who was present before all else.

Under Goddess-centered religion, animals were viewed not as objects to be used at man's pleasure, but as beings that, like us, were filled with spirit. The Great Mother is believed to have birthed all living beings and to have infused Her spirit into each of them. Every object and every being on earth, then, is Her child. A stallion is our brother, a heifer our sister, for the spirit of the Goddess shines in their souls as well as in our own.

In this Great Circle of Being, all forms of life hold equal worth. Our kinship with animals is real, our respect for their knowledge profound. Priestesses prophesy with the aid of the serpent; shamans speak with the language of birds and animals.

In God-worshiping societies, there was not a Great *Circle* of Being where life was equally valued, but a Great *Chain* of Being, a hierarchy where each object manufactured (rather than birthed) by the Father God submitted to "higher" objects and dominated "lower" ones. Animals were declared to be lower than man.

Before the discovery of paternity, in the time of the Goddess, one way women were thought to conceive children was through having eaten animals. So humans felt a kinship to animals as ancestors, as totems. They saw animals as blood relatives with whom they shared the soul of the Great Goddess. True, they hunted and ate animals, but their relationship with them was roughly equal. Weapons were primitive; hunting an equal contest. Later, as Elizabeth Fisher recounts in *Woman's Creation*, we established a vertical, master/slave relationship with animals. We took animals in. We fed them. We befriended them. We killed them. We ate them. In the course of this Betrayal, the slaughter of beings we had first befriended, we killed some sensitivity in ourselves.

> When they [humans] began manipulating the reproduction of animals, they were even more personally involved in practices which led to cruelty, guilt and subsequent numbness. The keeping of animals would seem to have set a model for the enslavement of humans, in

particular the large scale exploitation of women captives for breeding and labor. (Fisher, 1979, p. 197)*

The breeding of animals, Fisher believes, suggested to men the idea of controlling women's reproductive capacities.

II

They had just begun the embryo flushing when I entered the barn. Joe, a midwestern farmer, had hired a company to transfer fertilized eggs to host, or recipient, cattle. Two weeks earlier, he had super-ovulated #300, the cow who would serve as egg "donor." Later, he had artificially inseminated her. The cow was now bound in the squeeze chute, a metal contraption used to restrain cattle. A tag labeled #300 had been stapled in her ear. The men had placed the cow's calf, #133, before her to calm her. A hypodermic needle containing an epidural anesthesia was stuck in the cow's back.

"The cow can't move," Joe explained to a neighbor who had come to watch the transfer. "The chute's got all kinds of adjustments. She just can't move a muscle in it."

Five men, mostly farmhands, stood behind the cow silently watching Michael, the veterinarian, and his partner, Bob, both from the embryo transfer company. George stood among the men. At a recent auction, George had paid $20,000 for three quarters of the cow and her calf. He was paying three quarters of the transfer bill and would own three quarters of any embryos implanted. Joe kept ownership of one quarter of each animal.

Michael, the veterinarian, was a heavy-set man in his forties. He wore overalls, boots and a plastic shield and long glove to protect him from dung when he stuck his arm into the cow's rectum. He smiled and spoke amiably. A pleasant man. (Twice during the day, he gently soothed a cow while he was hurting her, saying, "I'm sorry, honey.")

Twisting slowly, Michael inserted a Foley catheter into the left horn of the cow's uterus. A flushing solution contained in a bottle hanging high from a rafter in the barn would flow through the catheter and into the uterus by gravity. A graduated cylinder on the barn floor would catch the solution and eggs as they flowed out of

---

* Animal keeping began shortly after plant cultivation commenced. Sheep and goats were the earliest herd animals to be domesticated. Villages that practiced mixed farming and collecting, hunting and animal herding, developed in the Near East between nine and eleven thousand years ago (Fisher, 1979, p. 191).

the cow. Bob sat on a box by one of the cow's legs and held the cylinder.

They flushed each horn seven times.

The calf gamboled. Her mother, head restrained by the squeeze chute, watched. At one point, the calf strayed off. Agitated, her mother mooed and moved frantically in the restraining chute.

Joe yelled to a farmhand, ordering him to bring the calf back within sight of its mother.

"I think that calf is retarded," Joe said, disgusted.

George grinned. "Do they pay you more for beef if the calf is smart?"

As they flushed, they joked about the microscopic supercows that might be flowing into the cylinder. Watching the flowing water, Bob quipped: "That's a million-dollar bull just went by."

They expected to get from six to twenty embryos. Joe was holding six host cows in a nearby corral to receive the transferred embryos. If there were extras, Michael and Bob would bring them back to the company farm and immediately transfer them into company cattle. If those cattle became pregnant, Joe and George would own the fetuses. But they would have to purchase from the company the host cows carrying the fetuses.

After the flushing, the men released cow #300 from the squeeze chute. Michael and Bob took the container into their camper. There, they would screen the fluid for fertilized eggs using two dissecting microscopes they had set up on a table. It would take them about two hours to get the eggs, they estimated.

During the egg search, Joe and the farmhands went off to their chores. George and I waited by the camper. With much money riding on this embryo transfer, George was impatient for results. He wanted to know how many eggs Michael and Bob had found so far.

"I wish they had a number system set up for the camper the way bakeries do," George said. "When they've got four eggs, they'd place a number '4' on the camper window. Then '5.' Then '6.' "

He walked over to the camper, calling in through the screen door: "Got any yet?"

Bob shouted out: "Not yet."

George paced. One of the men would return. "None yet," we'd report and off he'd go again.

The third time George had received a discouraging report, he asked Bob: "How much of the fluid have you been through so far?"

"All of it."

George was speechless.

"But we haven't given up yet," Bob reassured him, returning to his microscope.

"It never occurred to me that they wouldn't get *any* eggs," George said to me, stunned by the news. He had been hoping for twenty. The more fertilized eggs they found, the more money he would make.

By noon, most of the men were assembled outside the camper, talking worried talk. Michael and Bob were still at it. The men would look through the camper window again and again and ask: "Anything yet?"

Again and again: "Not yet."

Gloom in the barn.

"You can't fool around with Mother Nature," Joe said.

"You really can't," added a farmhand.

"Look," George snapped, "if we'd gotten twenty eggs, we'd be saying, 'This is great.'"

Joe lamented his wasted labor. Using hormones, he had synchronized the cycles of the donor and host cows. All that work for nothing.

Joe walked to the camper window to get another report and then turned to us, grinning.

"They've got one!"

Male spirits lifted.

Later they found one more. One bull embryo. One heifer embryo.

At 2:30 P.M., we walked onto the dung-covered barn floor to begin the actual embryo transfer. Joe had purchased six crossbreed Brown Swiss polled Herefords to serve as hosts for the embryos of cow #300. He considered them suitable hosts because they were larger than the egg donor, cycled better, produced abundant milk for feeding the calves and had roomy uteri.

Michael would select two of the six cows, choosing those that had heat (estrous) dates closest to that of the donor's so their reproductive cycles were well synchronized. He would also manually examine the ovaries of each cow to help him assess which cows would make the best hosts.

Bob strung electric cords over the rafters in the barn to power the shavers he would use in preparing the cows for surgery. Noticing him, one man said: "The electrician is here."

"You bet," said Bob. "Making babies."

George, Joe and Bob began herding the potential host cows from the other side of the barn to the operating area where the squeeze chute was. They whooped and hollered. They yelled at the cows, hit them on the side and twisted their tails to make them move. Bob compared the cow herding to football playing.

Several cows balked at the squeeze chute. They would let themselves be herded right up to the chute. Then they would stop. Cow #236 resisted the most.

Bob said to her: "What's the matter with you, woman? Step up!"

After much effort, when they had finally gotten her partly into the chute, they blocked her exit by placing two-by-fours across railings. She stood in extremely confined space, metal bars against each side of her. Men surrounded her, shouting at her to move forward. Suddenly she flipped herself completely around. It was astonishing: a lumbering animal turning around in such tight space. Stunned, they had to let her go.

"Nasty cow," one man said.

Michael drew on his long plastic glove, gently drove his arm up the rectum of each cow, and palpated the ovaries. He chose two animals as the embryo hosts: One was a docile cow named Smokey. The other was the rebellious #236. They tranquilized both animals.

They placed Smokey behind #236 and tried to get her to push her sister cow into the squeeze chute. They prodded her.

"Go, you son of a bitch!" Joe yelled at Smokey.

Bob turned to me as I scribbled in my notebook: "Don't write that down."

Joe to Smokey: "Smokey, push her in, goddamn you!"

They finally prodded #236 in amid a lot of hollering ("Twist her tail!") and running around. Bob was holding the rope for the head gate. As she ran in, he yanked it hard and fast and two metal sheets shot up from each side of the chute, locking her head in place.

Yelling, running, yanking, pushing, slapping her sides, twisting her tail, clang of metal, the cow's terror, her crying out, struggling to free her head, foam flying from her mouth: my whole body tensed with the violence of it.

Cow #236 was ready for the embryo transfer.

Bob shaved the hide of #236 over the uterine area. As the machine buzzed loudly, the cow jerked, mooed, pawed in the chute. Next, Bob scrubbed her. Again she reacted.

"Oh, I know how terribly painful this soap and water is," he said to her sarcastically.

He poured disinfectant on the shaved hide. Then he and Michael gave both cows a local anesthetic.

On the farm, each cow at birth is tagged in the ear with a number. Bob had an extra tag for each host cow. The tag for #236 contained the cow's heat date and the numbers "300-1," signifying that she contained the first transferred embryo of cow #300.

Bob had a big stapler to attach the special tag to #236's free ear. When the cow saw him with the stapler, she tried to pull her head back but of course she could not, it being locked in the head gate. When he punched that tag in her ear, she cried and pawed in the chute and shook her head back and forth wildly. In contrast to #236, Smokey was extremely quiet. Yet when Bob stapled the tag in her ear, she too protested.

A visiting neighbor sat on a fence watching the procedures. She turned to look at the cows in the corral, the ones who had not been chosen as surrogate mothers.

"The other cows are getting as far away as they can get," she said.

Joe nodded toward a distant hill. "If we opened that gate," he replied, "they'd be up that hill."

Michael scrubbed up. He drew on white surgical gloves. He slit a six-inch incision in the cow's side, cutting through muscle first, and then the peritoneum. Blood dripped out.

"Hear that gush of air?" he asked us. "That means we're in."

The embryo transfer, he said, was simply the reverse of a cesarean section performed nine months early.

Michael inserted his arm up to his elbow through the gaping red slit of the cow's side. Bob walked to the camper to get an embryo, asking Harvey: "Who do you want the heifer in and who do you want the bull in?"

"Put the heifer in #236," Joe told him.

Michael pulled the uterus out to the edge of the slit and punctured a hole in it. Bob returned with the embryo in a tube placed on a syringe. They worked together, their four hands at the cow's slit. Bob pushed the plunger, inserting the embryo into the uterus.

"There she be," Bob said, stepping back. "One cow is pregnant. Eight days pregnant."

Cow #236 resisted even as Michael stitched her up with catgut. "It's like trying to mend a pair of boots," he said.

Following that first embryo transfer, Bob commented on the baby-making ability of himself and his male partner. "Everything's fine," he said at one point. "Made her pregnant." And later: "Michael and I wanted to make babies today."

Donor cow #300, who had had her eggs flushed out that morning, stood in the pasture. She and her calf walked over to us and watched as Michael stitched up #236's perineum and her hide. Joe turned to the donor: "Yes," he told her, "these are your babies."

Blood had dripped onto the squeeze chute.

"Ready to try the next victim?" Bob asked Michael.

"Sure 'nuf."

Smokey was so quiet they decided they did not need to herd her into the squeeze chute. They tied a halter around her head and neck and then positioned Joe at her rear to help restrain her if that became necessary. It did not. While Smokey remained motionless, Michael cut into her.

"I'll go get a baby, Michael," Bob said.

He fetched the bull embryo from the camper. They inserted it. Returning to the metal cart on which they kept their equipment, Bob asked, in what appeared to be a set routine: "Is it Monday, Michael?"

"Then we must be making babies," Michael responded.

(They usually transferred embryos on Mondays, they explained to us.)

As Michael stitched up Smokey and the men chatted and joked, I moved close to Smokey's head. She had been so quiet, it had been easy to forget her living presence throughout the embryo transfer. We had all focused our eyes on the slit. There was her head, bound in a rope halter, the halter tied to a railing. Her eyes were wide open.

It had been painful to see cow #236 struggling to get out of that chute and away from these men. Painful to see her jump out of her skin in terror each time they did something to her: shave; scrub; tie tail; inject needle; tag ear; cut; puncture; insert embryo; stitch. Suddenly Smokey's silence seemed more terrible. Those big eyes open, that body still, while they did those things to her.

All around me, the men were chatting.

"Next time," George said, "I want to do the embryo transfer."

The men laughed.

"I'd do it if I weren't afraid of the cow."

Laughter.

It was only his fear of the cow that held him back, George explained, adding: "The cutting doesn't bother me. I'll practice it on my dog. Get a beagle out of a cocker spaniel."

5

The Cow Industry:
Embryo Transfer in Animals

Companies have been formed to take an embryo from the body of one animal and transfer it into the uterus of another. The companies serve the livestock industry. The names some entrepreneurs have chosen for their firms give us a peek at our future: MOM Ova Transfers, Inc.; Reproduction Enterprises, Inc.; Gibson's Custom Collection and Embryo Transfer Service; OvaTech Inc.; Genetic Engineering, Inc.; Select Embryos; The Quality Embryo Transfer Co. Ltd.; Trans-Ova; Silveira Bros. Embryonics; Treasure Valley Transplants; ReproTech, Inc.; Twin Brook Genetics, Inc.; McKellar Embryos (run by Dr. Lee McKellar); International Embryos Ltd.; and Sunshine Genetics (IETS, 1981).

In researching the history of embryo transfer technology, I was astonished at the speed with which discoveries in reproduction were followed by manipulation of those processes. Men discovered the mammalian egg in 1827 and in 1875 observed the actual fertilization process for the first time. Only fifteen years after that, Walter Heape of Cambridge transferred an embryo from the body of one female (a rabbit) to the body of another. A research team repeated Heape's triumph in 1922. Others extended his experiments. Throughout the 1930s, 1940s and 1950s, various researchers successfully transferred embryos within seven different species. Later, in the 1970s, they moved on to the horse, baboon, woman (as part of the test-tube baby procedure), cat and dog.

Essentially no embryo transfers were performed commercially before 1972. But by the decade's end, embryo transfer had become a multimillion-dollar industry largely concentrated on cattle and centered in North America. While this procedure is now performed on less than 1 percent of cattle in the United States, it may, with some refinements in technique, partially replace artificial insemination within a few years.[1]

In 1974, the International Embryo Transfer Society (IETS) formed to help practitioners in this new field exchange information and increase the use of embryo transfer throughout the livestock industry (IETS brochure). It boasts 271 members in twenty-four nations. According to an IETS survey, fifty-two members are specialized companies offering embryo transfer while another fifty-five are veterinarians who perform transfers as part of their practice. A few transferred embryos in horses, sheep, goats, swine and other species. (The "other species," IETS reports, included laboratory and companion animals, nonhuman primates, exotic species, and women.) But most transferred embryos in cows.

Cattlemen use embryo transfer to increase their wealth, to get more calves from valuable cows. It is, however, not easy to tell which cows are the valuable ones, a problem an IETS survey lists as one of the embryo transfer industry's biggest (IETS, 1982). A researcher from Colorado State University does have some suggestions for identifying a superior cow. One assesses, among other factors, the cow's maternal ability, the structural soundness of her udder, legs and feet, and the carcass traits of her offspring (Elsden, undated). Another researcher defines a valuable cow this way: "True genetic value is the ability to transmit desirable traits, such as meat or milk production, to offspring since . . . cattle are intrinsically worth only the meat or milk they produce" (Seidel, April 1975).

Pharmacrats consider the eggs and embryos of cows property as their language makes clear, for example in the phrase "inexpensive embryos."[2] To see exactly how, through embryo transfer, one increases the property value of cows, we will look at each stage of the embryo transfer process.

Synchronization

Estrus, a term derived from the name of the Celtic goddess Oestris, is "the urge to mate, to regenerate ourselves," according to one author.[3] It is both the recurrent period of sexual excitement in female mammals and the cycle of changes in the reproductive organs produced by hormonal activity of the ovary. In nature, the estrous cycle controls mating. When the female goes into heat—and *only* then—the male becomes eager to copulate with her.

In embryo transfer, the reproductive cycles of donor and recipient cows must be in accord so that when the donor cow ovulates, and her uterus prepares itself for the implantation of a fertilized egg, the uterus of the recipient cow is also prepared to receive an egg. Farmers use recipients that are naturally or artificially synchronized at estrus with the egg donor.

The first report on the alteration of an animal's estrous cycle came in 1948. Since then, researchers have experimented with various methods of synchronizing or "readjusting" the cycles of cows, including the injection of progestogens under the cow's hide at varying intervals.

Normally, mammals release (ovulate) only a limited number of eggs per cycle. Researchers in embryo transfer want many eggs "for efficient operation" (Murray, 1978, p. 292). Increased "efficiency" is possible through superovulation, a development that began with the 1927 discovery that hormones produced by the pituitary gland affect the ovaries. It occurred to men that they could inject such additional hormones into a female and force the growth and ovulation of an abnormally large number of eggs from follicles, the small sacs that enclose the eggs. They tried it out in mice the very same year they demonstrated the pituitary-gonad link: 1927.

Dr. Gregory Pincus, who later developed the contraceptive pill used in women, superovulated a rabbit in 1940. Throughout that decade and the next, men hormonally "bombed" the ovaries of species after species: 1940, cows; 1943, sheep; 1949, goats; 1950, rats; 1957, monkeys. By the 1950s, they were superovulating women. It was an experimental therapy for infertility. In England in 1968, the superovulated Sheila Ann Thorne underwent a cesarean section for sextuplets.

In superovulating animals, men have used follicle-stimulating hormones (FSH) extracted from sheep, swine, and pregnant mares and women. To force the follicles to rupture and release eggs, they administer another hormone preparation.[4]

The full effects of this hormone bombardment on the oviducts and uterus and on embryos developing there are unknown. With time, the percentage of abnormal embryos recovered from these animals does increase. "This is circumstantial evidence that the environment in the reproductive tract of the superovulated donor is harmful to embryos," wrote one researcher in embryo transfer (Seidel, 1981).

In 1959, after working with adults, researchers moved on to baby animals, whose ovaries had not matured. They superovulated young rats and can now do the same to calves. Men want to do this because by getting eggs out of animals that have not yet matured (as well as out of females too elderly to carry a pregnancy), they extend the animals' period of usefulness to them.

But the ovaries of calves are not yet functioning and must be "induced" to function through hormones. Sometimes researchers overstimulate the ovary, which can enlarge more than 100 times (Seidel, 1975 Dec.). So many follicles—fifty or sixty—burst open in her body that she hemorrhages. The ovary can get stuck to other organs inside her. There is scar tissue on the ovary and what an IETS official calls "incredible adhesions." Adhesions—fibrous bands connecting surfaces that are usually separate—can cause pain in human beings. Presumably they can hurt the calf as well.[5]

Superovulation, however, is "a rather inefficient method of harvesting oocytes [eggs]," Dr. George Seidel wrote. As an alternative, he suggests using enzymes to eat up the tissue holding the ovary together. This would "free the hundreds of thousands of oocytes in the ovary" (Seidel, BARC). These eggs, he continued, might be frozen for future use. Most would have to be matured in the lab before they could be fertilized.

Ova Recovery

After superovulating the cows, men fertilize their eggs, usually through artificial insemination, and then recover the embryos. Early collection techniques involved killing the females and cutting out their oviducts. "Slaughter of donor animals augments the consistency of [egg] recovery," researchers reported (Avery, 1962). In their study, these researchers slaughtered cows two hundred yards from the University of Minnesota dairy barn. Usually within fifteen minutes of the animals' death, they had removed its reproductive tract. In the laboratory, they flushed the contents of that tract into petri dishes and searched the dishes for ova with a microscope. About 48 hours before they slaughtered the "donor," they procured blood from her external jugular vein to use as a medium in which to transfer the ova.*

As an alternative method of egg recovery, men surgically removed the oviducts from a live female 72 hours after she ovulated.

* Pharmacrats choose the benign word "donor" to describe a female whom they often slaughter or maim in an attempt to extract her "gift."

Then they flushed the oviducts to obtain her eggs.

But killing or sterilizing a superior donor cow to get the eggs she produced in just one cycle seemed "self-defeating" so researchers devised other methods. First, they tried surgery. They recovered a high percentage of eggs but because the surgery caused trauma, it could only be repeated a few times. Frequently the females were left "problem breeders," or even sterile due to surgical damage (Elsden, 1978). So men moved on to a nonsurgical method. Using a two-way flow catheter, they flushed fluids into her uterus and collected those fluids—along with the eggs—in a receptacle. This is the method frequently used today. (They had also tried relocating the ovaries so they could get at them more easily, and keeping small tubular instruments inside the females' reproductive tracts continually so the eggs would pass into the instruments and out of the bodies. But these egg collection methods had been "found wanting" [Betteridge, 1981, p. 8].)

Embryo Evaluation

After recovery, men inspect the embryos under dissection microscopy, eliminating those considered unfit for transfer and ranking the acceptable ones according to quality. This is what Finnie A. Murray of the Ohio Agricultural Research and Development Center terms "embryo evaluation."[6]

Embryo Transfer

Finally, men transfer the embryo from the donor cow to the recipient. Sometimes they do this nonsurgically, inserting a catheter through the cervix to deposit the embryo in the uterus. But the resulting pregnancy rate is only between 30 and 60 percent. (Some technicians do better.) More often, they transfer surgically, impregnating 50 to 70 percent of the cows.

When the pregnant cows approach full term, veterinarians often perform cesarean sections on them "since the calves are usually large and the recipients are generally heifers of smaller breeds" (Seidel, 1975, April).

Those are the basic procedures, but developing technologies—the freezing, twinning and sexing of embryos—will increase the versatility and therefore the use of embryo transfer.

Freezing

By freezing and storing embryos, cattlemen can wait until a scrub cow's uterus enters the proper stage for implantation. Otherwise, when relying on natural synchronization of donor and recipients, they must keep hundreds of scrub cows ready just so they will have some in the right stage of the estrous cycle.

Researchers began trying to freeze animal embryos at the end of World War II. (Pioneer M. C. Chang recalls that publication of his early successes with cooled rabbit embryos in 1947 "was one of my happiest moments, and I still remember the excitement" [Betteridge, 1981, p. 8].) Success in actual freezing came in 1971. The first mammalian embryos frozen and thawed were those of mice.[7] Only two years later the British journal *Nature* was announcing: "The first deep-frozen bull has been born." Birthed in Cambridge, England, Frosty was the first large mammal to be born after having been frozen as an embryo. In 1974, researchers demonstrated that they could compactly transport animals, stored as frozen embryos, around the world.[8]

A researcher in the Netherlands devised what two American colleagues termed "a clever alternate method" for embryo freezing. It avoided the need to collect embryos before freezing them and thereby saved time. One simply removes whole oviducts from pregnant mice and freezes them, along with the embryos they hold. When researchers want the embryos, they thaw and flush the oviducts (Leibo and Mazur, 1978, p. 187).

Half the commercial embryo transfer outfits do some embryo freezing, as one IETS official estimates. About one third of embryos are killed or severely damaged by freezing. If these losses can be reduced to less than 20 percent, most cow embryos will be frozen between collection and transfer, according to one prediction (Seidel, 1981a, p. 353).

"It is our aim to develop techniques by which a farmer or rancher can order a frozen heifer or bull carried in a straw [the embryo would be placed in a strawlike container as frozen sperm is now] and transferred into his own recipient on the farm, just as a cow is inseminated with bull semen today," wrote one transfer expert (Elsden, 1979).

Twinning

The production of two identical animals from just one fertilized egg is another developing technology.

According to one researcher in the field, "The advantage of twinning is the more efficient production of meat" (Seidel, 1975 Dec.). Dr. Sarah Seidel, executive secretary of the International Embryo Transfer Society and that researcher's wife, agrees: "The advantage of this is that you double—reliably, easily, fast, cheaply—the number of embryos a valuable donor produces. In addition, you could apply a progeny-testing technique by freezing one of the half-embryos until you see what the other one is like. If she is good, you transfer the second one."

If she is bad? What do they do with embryos they do not want either because they are of the wrong sex or are otherwise judged inferior? The trend now, Dr. Seidel explains, "is to transfer them for beef production as a second embryo in an already-established pregnancy so you get twice the number of calves born." Ireland and Japan are looking at the embryo division technique seriously because they have limited grazing space and a large demand for beef, Seidel adds.

This is how pharmacrats "twin" sheep. First, they collect a two-cell embryo from a superovulated "donor" ewe. Next, through microsurgery, they separate the embryo's blastomeres—the cells produced by cleavage of the fertilized egg. Then, holding the embryo by suction with a pipette, they rip open the layer surrounding it (the zona pellucida) with a fine glass needle, and suck out the blastomeres (Willadsen, 1979).

Now they need two containers for the separated blastomeres. So they take two eggs collected from sheep ovaries after slaughter, evacuate their contents, and insert one blastomere into each of the two newly improvised containers (Willadsen, 1980). Then they embed these embryos in a protective cylinder and place them in the oviducts of living sheep to culture them. Finally, they transfer the pair of embryos into the surrogate sheep mother who will bear the twins.

So there are four sets of females used to produce these young: the egg donors; the slaughtered sheep from whose corpses eggs are scavenged to serve as blastomere containers; the primary recipients in whose bodies the embryos are cultured; and the secondary recipients in whose bodies the twin fetuses come to term. The animals need not be of the same species. In one experiment,

Willadsen and colleagues injected the divided embryos of cows into evacuated pig eggs "collected from slaughter-house ovaries." Later, they transferred the embryos into the oviducts of ewes. Finally, through surgery, they inserted the cultured embryos into cows (Willadsen, 1981).

In a separate experiment, men transferred the first halves of twin embryos immediately and froze the others. They subsequently thawed the second halves, transferred them and produced three lambs who were the twins of animals born a month or two earlier. Such a procedure, the scientists wrote, allows "the production of genetically identical sheep of differing ages." In the future, pharma-crats speculate, it may be possible to freeze one twin embryo, thaw it and transfer it into the other one when she becomes sexually mature. In this way, men could have a female animal giving birth to her own identical twin (Seidel, 1981a).

So far, researchers have achieved twinning in sheep, mouse, cow and pig embryos. Beginning with the division of two-cell eggs, they moved on to four-cell and eight-cell embryos. Their experiments with cows demonstrate the high efficiency of the technique used (Willadsen, 1981).

In the future, human embryos could also be twinned. One of the pioneers in the test-tube baby technique referred to microsurgery on animal embryos and pointed out that by using the same procedure on human embryos "the chances of conception and twins could be increased in infertile couples" (Wood and Westmore, 1983).

Sexing

The sexing of embryos is the third technique that adds versatility to embryo transfer. Cattle breeders would like to produce bulls or heifers at will. Sperm carries the sex-determining factors, the Y and X chromosomes. When the male Y combines with the X in the egg, a male is produced. When his X combines with the egg's X, a female is conceived. So researchers have attempted to separate X-bearing and Y-bearing sperm and then artificially inseminate a cow with one or the other preparation. So far, they have not notably succeeded.

However, with an expensive and time-consuming procedure, they can determine the sex of an embryo *after* its formation and discard it if it is of the wrong gender. Damaging the embryo slightly, they snip off a small piece and place it in a test tube where its cells multiply. Then they kill, stain and squash the cells on a microscope slide (Elsden, 1978). Under the microscope, they can identify the X- and Y-bearing sex chromosomes and determine whether the embryo is male or female. The remaining portion of the embryo, if it is of the ordered sex, is transferred to the recipient cow. Though most biopsied embryos continue growth, the pregnancy rate obtained with them is slightly lower than that with unsnipped embryos.

Generally, men want heifers, which can be used to breed new calves every year or to produce milk. Men need only a few high-quality bulls as sources of semen for artificial insemination. Other male embryos then, would be "discarded," used for research purposes, or transferred to produce bulls for fattening (Seidel, 1981a).*

Several research teams are working on an alternative sexing method that may be more efficacious than the current one (Seidel, 1980). Also, research is being conducted on biopsy at an earlier stage of development, one that is optimal for the best subsequent pregnancy rates.

"When better techniques are developed, one will probably be able to sex 90 percent of the embryos, transfer those of the desired sex, and freeze the rest for research or twinning," Dr. George Seidel writes (Seidel, BARC, p. 206). He estimates that determination of the sex of embryos, twinning and in vitro fertilization will probably have commercial application before 1986 (Seidel, 1981b, p. 324).

Men see embryo transfer as a method—not only to get more calves from valuable cows, but to save endangered species, both in natural habitats and in zoos. In 1981, for the first time, pharmacrats successfully used a domestic animal as a surrogate mother for a wild species. The Bronx Zoo transferred the embryo of a gaur, a wild ox native to India, into the uterus of a Holstein dairy cow. In August, the cow gave birth to a gaur. Habitat destruction and hunting in India had drastically cut the gaur's numbers, William Conway, director of the New York Zoological Society, explained (Webster, 1981).

According to *The New York Times,* reproductive biologists and

---

* Men's fear of being superfluous, which, Elizabeth Fisher writes, is deeply engrained in men's consciousness, may be heightened when men see their own treatment of male animals. It is the *female* animals they want—the ones who bear young and produce milk. They regard most male animals as expendable. With the domestication of cattle and the discovery of castration, Fisher writes, a certain pattern was set, which influences human psychology for millennia to come: one bull, many castrates, many cows. Seeing this pattern, how could a man not develop a "sense of superfluity" in creating offspring and how could that not contribute to his "already shaky sense of self"? (Fisher, 1979, p. 27, pp. 190–200, p. 256). We saw that fear of superfluity in Chapter 2. "God, you're making us less and less useful and necessary," a man wrote to the AID Research Project. "It is frightening."

wildlife specialists looked upon the successful embryo transfer as a "major step toward being able to more freely reproduce wild and endangered animals in captivity." With embryo transfer, they could get six to eight animals a year from just one gaur. It was, as the *Times* reported, only the second time that an interspecies embryo transfer involving a wild animal had resulted in a live birth. In 1977, a domestic sheep at Utah State University gave birth to a mouflon, a wild Sardinian sheep. That was merely the beginning. Scientists and zoo keepers envision getting Arabian oryxes from gemsbok antelopes; rare pygmy chimpanzees from common chimps; wisents, yaks and elands from cows; cheetahs and leopards from lionesses.

Duane C. Kraemer of Texas A & M University produced a baboon, the first nonhuman primate, through embryo transfer in 1975. He hopes that common animals can be made to serve as "hatcheries" for the eggs of dwindling zoo species (Randel, 1981).

So men endanger some species by killing them or destroying their habitats. They enclose other animals in zoos where, due to whatever biological or spiritual cause, the animals tend to go on procreative strike. Zoo species "are hesitant to reproduce in captivity for reasons unknown," an IETS official told me. Pharmacrats come in and forcibly extract offspring from the captured animals.

Notes

1. More than 25,000 bovine pregnancies were produced in the United States in 1981, according to one estimate (IETS, 1982, p. 33).

2. The view of embryos as property is also clear in the phrases "if embryos cost $200 each," "the stockpiling of viable embryonic material," "the export and import of embryos," and in this statement from *Nature:* "Equally the technique of embryo freezing would allow genetic characteristics that are in danger of being bred out of cattle for economic reasons to be kept in cold storage for the day when these characteristics may again become commercially important" (Bullseye, 1973). And in this from a researcher: "The principal advantage of embryo transfer is that one can increase *the number of offspring per unit time* [my emphasis] from cows" (Seidel, 1975). Jackson Laboratory in Bar Harbor, Maine, keeps some of its "mouse assets" frozen in a bank, partly because it costs less to freeze embryos than to care for living animals (Schmeck, 1981).

3. Thorsten, 1980, p. 197. Each spring, in honor of Oestris, Thorsten writes, children hunted for eggs and received presents from the rabbit, "that fertile darling of the Goddess."

4. Prostaglandin, or gonadotrophic hormone preparations or luteinizing hormone from the cow's pituitary.

5. One research group superovulated newly born calves. Then, in order to observe the ovaries' response to the hormones, the researchers killed the calves. "Apparently ovaries of neonatal [newborn] calves are not capable of responding to superovulation treatment," they concluded. But they did succeed with calves as young as one month (Seidel, Larson and Foote, 1971).

6. These evaluations, generally judged to be accurate, are not perfect. Many embryos that appear normal are, in fact, not capable of developing into calves, while some that appear degenerate are not. One poorly looking embryo developed into a calf sold at auction for $131,000 (Seidel, 1981b, p. 29).

7. Live young were obtained from a high proportion of mouse embryos that had been stored in a medium with a protective agent for up to eight days at sub-zero temperatures (Whittingham, 1971).

8. The researchers flew mouse embryos, which had been stored for up to eight months, from the United States to England (Whittingham and Whitten, 1974).

6

The Woman Industry:
Embryo Transfer in Humans

Embryo West, Inc. Ovatrans International Corporation. Portable Embryonics. Perhaps within a few years firms with names such as these will be handling—not the eggs of cattle, but of women. For embryo transfer technology has been applied to us. Physicians flushed an embryo from one woman and placed it into the womb of another in April 1983 at Harbor–UCLA Medical Center in Torrance, California. They delivered the resulting child, a boy, by cesarean section in January 1984.

The experiment was financed by Fertility and Genetics Research, Inc. (FGR), a firm founded by two brothers who had been transferring embryos between cows since 1970 in their cattle breeding business.

The brothers, Dr. Randolph W. Seed, a surgeon, and Dr. Richard G. Seed, a physicist, plan to open up a string of twenty to thirty for-profit human embryo transfer clinics across the country. FGR officials intend to connect the clinics through a national data base. This will help solve one of the industry's biggest problems: finding enough human egg donors. With the computer link-up, a clinic will not be limited to egg donors in its immediate area but will instead have access to a national pool of women.

"You understand that this is done in the cattle business all the time," Dr. John Buster, an ob/gyn who headed the human embryo transfer team, explained to me. "There's nothing new in all this. It's all very feasible. It's just a case of setting it up."

Here is how this would work. An infertile or genetically "deficient" woman in Akron, Ohio, could be matched for blood type, hair and eye color with an egg donor in, say, Baton Rouge, Louisiana. The ovulation times of the two women could be synchronized either naturally or through the administration of hormones. Sperm from the husband of the Akron woman could be flown to Baton Rouge. When the physician believed both women were ovulating (with current technology, it is still not possible to know definitely), he would inseminate the donor. The released egg would spend the next three days traveling from the ovary to the uterus through the oviduct. The sperm may fertilize the egg during this time. The egg would then float freely in the uterus for another two or three days. Five days after the insemination, the doctor would attempt to "wash out" the egg (now an early embryo) by flushing the uterus using plastic tubing and about two ounces of fluid. (The procedure is called uterine lavage.) The embryo would then be flown to Akron to be transfered into the recipient's body.

Memorial Health Technologies (MHT), a firm in Long Beach, California, plans to open the first clinic early in 1985. Shortly thereafter, it will open and manage other embryo transfer centers throughout the United States for FGR.

This move from cows to women is logical, as the first book on reproductive physiology suggests. That book was published in 1910 by F. H. A. Marshall and dedicated to Walter Heape of Cambridge, the man who performed the first embryo transfer in an animal. Marshall, the scientific heir of Heape, opened his book with the statement that "generative physiology forms the basis of gynaecological science, and must ever bear a close relation to the study of animal breeding" (Betteridge, 1981, p. 1).

The Seed brothers were not the first to attempt to recover eggs from women's bodies nonsurgically. In 1972, researchers led by Dr. Horacio B. Croxatto reported in the pages of the *American Journal of Obstetrics and Gynecology* that they had conducted egg recovery experiments on young women attending a contraceptive clinic in Chile. They wanted to determine when women ovulated and how long it took the egg to get down the oviduct, information that would be useful in developing contraceptives. (One could experiment to see how various compounds affected egg transport.)

Some of the women in the clinic were being experimented upon in two ways. Researchers implanted silastic capsules of a synthetic progesterone under the skin of the women's forearms to test out a new contraceptive. Among the effects of the drug experienced by some women were abdominal pain* and abnormal bleeding (Croxatto

---

* Eight out of 97 women suffered from abdominal pain, but "the relevance of this symptom is not known."

et al., 1969). While some of these women lay on a table, hormones coursing into their bodies from the implants under their skin, researchers, in a separate experiment, attempted to flush eggs out of them, using various improvised tubing.

At one point, researchers used two polyethylene tubes, one larger than the other, tied together with nylon. The advantage of this type of tubing, they stated, "was its availability in various sizes, but unfortunately it was not easy to introduce the pair without scratching the cervix and endometrium with the tips. This produced slight bleeding, *thus making the search for ova more difficult*." (I emphasize that last clause to draw attention to what it does *not* say, i.e.: "thus discomforting the woman and increasing her risk of infection.")

Although Croxatto had suggested that egg flushing might provide a tool for infertility treatment (Croxatto et al., 1972, p. 667), the Seed brothers were the first to implement that idea. Randolph Seed was chief of surgery at Grant, a large community hospital in Chicago when, around 1976, he and his brother began to consider applying their animal research to women. They expected opposition to their work. Two later events proved this to have been a reasonable expectation: Right-to-life organizations tried to prevent an IVF clinic in Norfolk, Virginia, from opening; a British physician raised ethical objections to embryo transfer on the ground that it posed risks to the women egg donors (OGN, 1983, Dec. 1). (See discussion of risks later in the chapter.)

"We decided we wouldn't even approach the hospital to do it there, that there would be so much objection that we wouldn't even bother," Richard told me in an interview in his office in Chicago in 1980. "We just decided we'd set up this separate little office-clinic here to do it. That way, we would not subject the hospital or anybody else to any stress or strain."

In 1978, they opened up the Reproduction and Fertility Clinic, Inc., amid boutiques, gift shops and restaurants in Chicago's fashionable Water Tower Place. (FGR is a research subsidiary of this clinic. Croxatto became one of FGR's medical consultants.) They began offering the experimental technique.

"Our reception by and large has been quite favorable but we structured it in such a way that there wasn't much negative that could be said about it," Seed said.

Partially because they gave no one at the hospital the power to object to and stall the project, they never experienced the adverse publicity they had anticipated, Richard said. "We expected we'd have pickets," he added. "We planned for pickets. It didn't happen."

At their clinic, the Seeds paid donor women fifty dollars a uterine lavage. The women would get a two-hundred-dollar bonus when a fertilized egg was recovered.

From the beginning of their experimentation, the Seeds presented embryo transfer as if it were a safe technology ready to be used in women. Describing the work to a government ethics board holding hearings on in vitro ("test-tube") fertilization in 1978, Randolph Seed spoke, for example, of "the primary breakthrough which makes this embryo transplantation now possible," naming as that "break-through" the development of nonsurgical embryo flushing and embryo transfer. Yet, at the time he made this statement, he had succeeded *only once* in flushing out an embryo and had not yet even attempted to transfer an embryo. How then had it been demonstrated that the technology had indeed been successfully developed? (Several years later, they were still trying to develop tubing that did not leak.) Again, he outlined what he called "the typical procedure for an embryo transplant" in women at a time when no one had ever carried one out.

He minimized the possibility of abnormalities in the children born of embryo transfer. "There is not yet any scientific evidence which would demonstrate this in the many experimental animals that have been used," he said. "In our own work, we have had over 300 calves born through transplants and we have had no gross abnormalities" (Seed and Seed, 1978).

Yet there has never been any study comparing animals born of embryo transfer and animals born naturally (Seidel, 1981).

Concluding his statement, Randolph Seed noted that he and his brother had concerned themselves with the ethics of their work: "On balance, we have reached the personal conclusion that a risk/benefit analysis of artificial embryonation [embryo transfer] based on existing medical data indicates that it is an acceptable procedure which needs to be offered."

His egg recovery rate was then 1.5 percent. His brother had estimated that the rate would have to be 90 to 95 percent before embryo transfer would be a practical technique. Two years later, when I first interviewed Richard Seed, they had recovered only three unfertilized eggs and one embryo. Experts in the field, they had not yet been able to perform this "acceptable procedure."

The Seed brothers worked on. Then Dr. John E. Buster, an ob/gyn and chief of the division of reproductive endocrinology at Harbor–UCLA Medical Center, heard that they wanted to transfer embryos between human beings and thought it was a great idea. In June 1980, he went to Chicago to talk it over with them. He found that they "had thought the matter through rather well."

Buster wanted to work with them.

If he and his team of physicians at UCLA were to help implement the Seeds' idea by experimenting on women, they needed money. "There was no way we could charge the women for something that was so totally experimental like this," Buster told me in an interview. (Yet when the Seeds were on their own, and had, in their program, achieved not a single pregnancy, they had indeed expected infertile women to pay them. Embryo transfer would cost each couple "as much as a new car," Richard Seed told *The New York Times* in 1980. "It should be painful to them, otherwise it isn't worth our effort to work with them for a year or two" [Fleming, 1980]. They would make some accommodation for couples unable to afford their prices, Richard told me that same year, though, in general, their clients are "middle class couples who can afford a certain amount of medical treatment.")

Buster tried unsuccessfully to get research money from the National Institutes of Health and from hospitals in his area. Then Richard Seed introduced him to Lawrence Sucsy, an investment banker in Chicago. Sucsy, who is now chairman and chief executive officer of FGR, had proposed a way of financing the human embryo transfer program that involved the formation of a partnership and the pooling of investment money. Sucsy, Buster and others put together a private offering for a partnership and spent a year and a half trying to sell it to investors, who would purchase a share in a partnership. "I literally walked on the concrete on Wall Street along with Mr. Sucsy and Randy Seed," Buster recalled. Investors were unconvinced that the business would make money. They argued that women would not agree to have sperm put in their bodies and eggs flushed out of them, that infertile women would not want the technology, that no woman was so desperate she would take a donated egg.

"Sucsy had to compete for the same [investor] dollars that are normally spread into oil and gas and gold," Buster said. "That's hard competition because investors don't care really what you're doing. They just want to be sure to get the money back." Buster thinks that the birth of the first American test-tube baby in 1981 may have helped them in finally getting investors to treat their proposal seriously. By December 1981, they had raised the necessary money.

In an effort to thwart competitors, FGR had applied for patents on its catheters (tubing) and on its embryo transfer process. This has aroused controversy.[1]

"Ordinarily when you develop a new medical procedure, it's reported in the scientific literature and if it has merit, it receives wide dissemination," B. J. Anderson, associate general counsel at the American Medical Association, told me. "You don't attempt to commercialize it and limit it to a few in order to gain an economic advantage."

Meanwhile, in Torrance, the UCLA team was documenting the animal research on embryo transfer, meeting with psychologists who developed tools for screening women egg donors, consulting lawyers and ethicists, writing consent forms, and developing catheters for the procedure. Then, with a $400,000 repayable grant from FGR, the team was ready to begin. It needed egg donors. That was a problem.

"We know that they [egg donors] are out there, that there are thousands of them," Buster told me. "But early in the program, because we were concerned about a bad image for the university, we were very quiet about all this."

Rather than seek publicity to recruit egg donors, they quietly placed a few newspaper ads. "Help an Infertile Woman Have a Baby," their ad began. Although 380 women responded, all but forty-six were immediately screened out, some because they lived too far away. The forty-six took a standardized personality test. The team's psychologists found that abnormal psychological traits were threefold to sixfold more common among these volunteers than would have been expected among the general population. The results also suggested that "only" one third of the women were interested in the program for altruistic reasons while most of the others sought novelty and excitement or wanted to improve a poor self-image. After this test, the psychologists screened out nineteen more women and interviewed the remaining twenty-seven.[2] More than half the candidates interviewed had a history of abusive and/or alcoholic parents or other childhood problems. "Given the nonsupportive, if not traumatic, histories reported by many candidates, this project may have been seen as a chance to increase self-esteem and compensate for disappointment in themselves and their parents," commented one team member (OGN, 1983, Dec. 1).

Many of the women appeared to have difficulty cooperating with authority figures, a trait incompatible with this type of project, he said (OGN, 1983, Dec. 1). (One can see why compliancy in a donor would be important to the team. Among the researchers' requirements was that the donors "be available on a fairly regular basis" [*People,* 1983, Aug. 8]. Women not awed by authority figures might place limits on their availability.)

So the newspaper ads did not bring to the program many women who could pass the screening process. "The lesson was that newspaper ads are not the way to go," Buster said.

What was?

Buster listed several. The infertile woman could find her own egg donor (perhaps her sister) and bring that donor into the program. Also, brochures on embryo transfer could be left in doctors' waiting rooms where women patients could read them. "We think that once they know this can be done, they'll come to us in large numbers," Buster said.

The researchers are writing the brochures.

Richard Seed had had another solution to the problem when I talked with him in 1980: "We try to set up a system similar to a blood bank's in which every recipient must provide one or two donors for the egg bank."

(While researchers associated with the embryo transfer industry and the public relations firm hired by that industry speak of "egg" banks, "egg" donors and "ovum" transfer, in fact they are really referring to *embryo* banks, *embryo* donors and *embryo* transfer. The fact that these researchers have chosen such terms, knowing their inaccuracy, suggests they are aware of the potential public relations problem they have.)

The conceivable: A woman is infertile. She learns that she can only be accepted into the embryo transfer program if she delivers two embryo donors to its bank. She asks her best friend and her sister to do this for her. They do not want to, but they know how she suffers. If they refuse, they feel, they will be denying her a child. She feels this way too. She would be angry at them and not at the embryo transfer industry. So, feeling violated, the woman's friend and sister lay on gynecological tables, feet in stirrups, and allow doctors to artificially inseminate them and later flush embryos out of their bodies.

Asked about Seed's idea, Buster said in 1983 that he and his team thought it could be done and they might put the plan into effect once the clinics are started.

At some point, the embryo transfer pioneers hired a California public relations firm that, in its press releases, gave out a telephone number for women interested in giving or receiving eggs. The last four digits of the exchange spelled B-A-B-Y. Presumably that number, too, will bring in more embryo donors.

"We would expect in five to ten years' time to have a potential donor bank of several thousand women," Seed told me in 1984. "That's exactly what we're looking for."

Once the UCLA group had its donors, it began work. It paid donors (or more accurately in this case, egg vendors) $5 to $10 for a blood sample, $50 for an insemination and $50 per lavage. From January 1983 to February 1984, it inseminated 10 donor women a total of 46 times with sperm from the husbands of 13 infertile recipients. In 42 attempts at uterine lavage, they flushed out 18 embryos. Two recipient women had apparently normal pregnancies (Press briefing remarks, 1984, Feb. 3).

But two women were impaired in the experiment. One recipient suffered an ectopic pregnancy, an embryo lodged in her right tube. Doctors operated on her to remove the embryo. She lost her tube as well. Another woman, a donor, was left with an embryo inside her when it could not be flushed out. She spontaneously aborted nine days after her expected period.

These failures point out some of the risks of the experimental technology to women. The risks include these:

—The embryo may not be washed out with the fluid, leaving the donor pregnant as happened in the very first round of experiments. "The donors simply have to agree to an abortion," Michael Eberhard, senior vice-president of Memorial Health Technologies, said. "If they won't, if that would not be emotionally or ethically acceptable to them, then we've got to screen them out. They don't belong as part of the donor program." Buster plans to deal with the problem at an earlier stage by using a new class of drugs to cause the embryo to be reabsorbed into the donor's body. He has applied to the Food and Drug Administration (FDA) to use these as yet unapproved research drugs for this purpose. So the women would be subjected to another level of experimentation with these new drugs.*

* It may appear that if the FDA approves the use of the drug for research purposes, then its use is not improper. But the fact that the FDA approves certain kinds of experimentation on women does not mean that it is right. An example from my first book, *The Hidden Malpractice:* The FDA approved the Pill on a basis of a study involving only 132 Puerto Rican women who had taken the Pill for one year or longer, and 718 other women who had taken the drug for less than a year. Five of the women died during the study, three with symptoms suggesting blood clots. No autopsies on the women were performed. At Senate hearings on the Pill in 1970, the FDA admitted that it had approved the Pill on the basis of "rather superficial" data, some of which was "little more than testimonial or opinionative in character"

—During the lavage, the embryo may be flushed up the oviduct, leaving the donor woman with an ectopic pregnancy. "That's one of the major hazards," comments Dr. Jaroslav Hulka, one of only two ob/gyn members of the International Embryo Transfer Society. "So far, I think it's uniquely human. I don't think the cow has ectopic pregnancies.... That's one of the worrisome aspects of trying to take a technology developed in one species and apply it to another."

Hulka, of the Department of Obstetrics and Gynecology at the University of North Carolina, said that if he flushed a woman's uterus and got nothing, he would have to tell her: "Golly, lady, I can't find the egg. You might have an ectopic. Come back in two weeks and we'll do an ultrasound to see if there's an ectopic in your tube."

If, upon examining her tubes with ultrasonic radiation, he found an ectopic pregnancy, he would have to operate on her. He might be able to save the tube. If the embryo ruptures the tube, the donor woman, in the process of trying to give an egg to an infertile woman, may be transformed into an infertile woman herself. An ectopic pregnancy that is never detected and removed could threaten the woman's life.

The recipient also risks an ectopic pregnancy when the embryo is transfered into her uterus. This, too, happened in the first round of human experiments. She may also be at a slightly greater risk of acquiring a pelvic infection from the donor via the transfer procedure (Walters, LeRoy, 1983).

—In the future, Buster plans to synchronize the cycles of donor and recipient artificially. So the women will be exposed to the risks of hormones used for that purpose.

—As Dr. Maria Pia Platia and Dr. Gary D. Hodgen, researchers with the National Institutes of Child Health and Development (NICHD) observe, there is a risk to the donor of venereal disease through artificial insemination with the sperm of the recipient's husband.

—The donor risks pelvic infection as a result of the uterine lavage. Like an ectopic pregnancy, this could destroy her reproductive potential. (Not entirely, of course. She could then switch roles and become an egg *recipient,* rather than donor.)

(Corea, 1985). So the FDA approved the Pill but, in my opinion, the experimentation it allowed on women was, while legal, improper. The FDA operates within a culture where women are devalued and it would be surprising if it in no way shared that devaluation. The devaluation of women is what makes it possible to look at experimentation on women and not see anything wrong.

—The recipient undergoes the unknown risk of carrying an embryo whose genetic makeup is totally foreign to her own, as opposed to a normal pregnancy where half the genes are hers. Doctors Platia and Hodgen point out this risk.

Researchers often assert that embryo transfer is analogous to artificial insemination by donor. In fact, one of the first terms the Seeds used for the procedure was "artificial embryonation," a term chosen in order to emphasize the procedure's similarity to artificial insemination.

"The genes are donated by a female to the infertile couple instead of by a male," Randolph Seed told the ethics board. "Another variation is that the fertilization takes place in vivo," i.e., in her body. Since AID is accepted by the medical profession, the Seeds "see no reason why the other [embryo transfer] should not be," *The Boston Globe* reported (Snider, 1980).

But there *are* reasons, as we have just seen. Fertilization of the eggs in a woman's body, minimized as a mere "variation" on AID, is partially what makes embryo transfer so much more hazardous than artificial insemination. AID poses no risk to the sperm donor nor does it violate his bodily integrity. An egg donor, however, risks infection, abortion, the hazards of experimental drugs, surgery for ectopic pregnancy, the impairment or loss of her fertility, and, in the event of further complications, even death.

The price Memorial Health Technologies will charge for embryo transfer has not yet been set, but senior vice-president Eberhard told me in March 1984: "We think it will be competitive to the in vitro [fertilization procedure]." That, he added, was somewhere in the range of five thousand to seven thousand dollars per attempt.

Eberhard is considering a two-tiered price structure with a lower charge to women who do not get pregnant through embryo transfer. Most of the women and families who come to MHT, he explained, "have really been through the medical wringer. They've been going back and forth to these clinics for multiple surgeries and hormone treatments and drug treatments. They bring in files eight inches thick. They're discouraged. They feel that they're paying an awful lot of money and what have they got? I'd like to have a pricing system that said: If we don't get you pregnant with ovum transfer, we lose. And if we get you pregnant, we come out fine."

He added: "If everyone came through and we didn't get anyone pregnant, we'd go bankrupt. And I think that is the just reward for those that can't produce the product."

Even a lower price, of course, could still be thousands of dollars.

People have got to be understanding of MHT at the start, Eberhard said, because the success rate in the first year will not be as high as in the second. Asked if he didn't feel it necessary to wait until the success rate was higher before opening the business, he replied: "No. Someone's got to have the courage and the willingness to take the risk to start trying it. You have got to start sometime. There are no more research funds. It's hard raising research money." The doctors feel they are ready right now, he added, after their enormously successful research, and there are patients who want to begin.

What *is* the success rate? When I asked Buster in December 1983, he replied that it was really too early to tell yet.

Embryo transfer technology makes embryo evaluation possible. This would be useful in exercising selection in child production. By the year 2000, it may be possible to flush the embryos out of every single woman in the obstetrician's office as part of routine prenatal care, test it for every known genetic and metabolic defect and then, if—and only if—the embryo is perfect, return that embryo to the woman's womb. This, according to Richard Seed, would eliminate most birth defects.

"We've got enough work ahead of us for the next three years," he said in 1980, referring to himself and his brother. "But if we get everything organized, we'll start research in that area. We could expand the animal embryo work and try to apply it to humans. We would be replacing amniocentesis with embryo evaluation."

Sex selection would be a part of embryo evaluation, he explained. "You can snip out some cells from an embryo at certain stages of development and determine the sex of the embryo. That's been done now in cattle, horses and, I think, pigs."

This embryo biopsy technique "might be extended considerably" in the future, wrote two contributors to the *Western Journal of Medicine* in 1976. They too, like Richard Seed, believe embryos could be screened for various genetic diseases. Perhaps, they speculate further, researchers may someday find that certain birth defects like cleft palate are associated with a recognizable abnormality in the embryo. On the shaky basis of their speculation, they conclude: "Therefore, one day, in vitro fertilization and embryo culture could become the preferred mode of reproduction, with transfer to the uterus of only genetically-healthy embryos" (Karp and Donahue, 1976).

Preferred by whom? The woman? Or the doctor? I am reminded of speculation in obstetrical journals that cesarean section may become the preferred mode of delivery. Again, *who* prefers it? The woman expected to undergo major surgery for a natural process, or the men wielding the knife?[3]

Embryo evaluation does not arouse universal enthusiasm. Dr. Hulka comments: "I think most women would just as soon run the risk of genetic abnormality as the risk of killing off that pregnancy or having it end up as ectopic. The technology of embryo flushing and reimplantation is so fraught with hazard, even in animals."

Will these technologies—embryo transfer and embryo evaluation—presented as beneficent "options," become, as is the tendency with obstetrical intervention, mandatory? Will women be allowed to refuse them?

These questions concern Roz Richter, a physically disabled attorney working in women's and civil rights. She can foresee a stigma attaching to the woman who learns that she carries "defective" genes or an imperfect embryo and chooses not to substitute another's egg or discard the embryo. A stigma may also attach to the child subsequently born.

If society selects for totally healthy embryos, it is making a statement that there would be no circumstances under which a "normal" person would choose to bear a child who is not healthy, Richter observes. Women who do make that choice may be viewed as irresponsible or as emotionally unsound.

"I think there might be a serious question as to their ability to judge the situation," Richter said.

The tendency for an "option" to become mandatory is evident now in obstetrics. Already, physicians have appealed for court intervention in several cases where women resisted cesarean sections and other obstetrical procedures or where, declining to enter a hospital at all, they attempted to give birth at home. In early 1978, three home-birth couples—in Louisiana, Idaho and North Carolina—were accused of child abuse. In the North Carolina case, police, acting on an obstetrician's complaint, forcibly took the woman from her home while she was in labor and transported her to a hospital (Corea, 1979). Several women have been ordered by courts to submit to cesareans against their will provided their physicians deemed the surgery necessary for the baby. In one case in Georgia, a pregnant woman was escorted to a county hospital by deputies from the Butts County sheriff's department following such a court ruling.[4] If physicians, using the law, can attempt to force women to submit their bodies to obstetrical intervention, then they can conceivably

also attempt to make various prenatal diagnostic procedures compulsory—probably only for select women at first. Dr. Howard W.
Jones, Jr., co-director of the nation's first test-tube baby program,
has already suggested that it may be "unethical" for certain women
to refuse prenatal diagnosis. In attempting to refute the argument
that in vitro fertilization is unethical because it entails unknown
risks to a potential child who cannot give consent, Jones maintained
that this argument could equally well be applied to pregnant women
over 35 and their mates. These women, he stated, have a greater
likelihood of bearing a Down's syndrome child. "The ethics of such
a couple could be ever so much more questionable [than the ethics
of IVF teams], especially if they were unwilling to use contemporary
methods of diagnosis with abortion in the event an affected fetus
was discovered" (Jones, 1982, p. 148).

Referring, again, to embryo evaluation and transfer, Richter
said: "I think that pressure is going to grow to the point where it
becomes not only ethically irresponsible but legally presumed to be
incompetent if you don't make the choice to have the embryo
flushed away or the egg substituted."

Quite possibly, the state may force women in certain high risk
groups to undergo amniocentesis, Richter observes. Arguing that it
may have to pay for facilities or treatment for a physically or
mentally disabled child, the state could maintain that it has an
overwhelming interest in the matter.

What if the prenatal diagnostic procedure—whether amniocentesis, embryo evaluation or something other—reveals a "defective"
embryo or fetus? Would the woman be forced to abort?

Richter thinks not. This is the way it will begin, she believes:
If the results are "x," the woman will be advised of the options
technology provides her. (Today, almost the only options are to
deliver the child or abort it. Increasingly, various unproven therapies
for the fetus, all of which involve invasion of the woman's body, are
being devised.) If the pressure of one's adviser is severe enough,
Richter adds, being "advised of your option" may mean being told
what you want to do.

Another factor operates here: The woman's possible feelings of
inferiority after being told that she has a genetic defect. Advised,
then, of her option to end the pregnancy, told by a medical/ethical
establishment that the right choice is indeed to end it, she may
swing toward the doctor's choice. Though legally she may have an
option, she may not, in reality, exercise it.

Richter raises another issue. There are a wide range of capabilities within a particular class of disability. For example, some with cerebral palsy can become brilliant teachers or physicians; others will experience severe mental limitations. After such children are born, many factors determine what kind of life they can lead: access to rehabilitation services; motivation; emotional support; degree of physical impairment.

Richter comments: "The medical establishment cannot look at a child one month after birth and say: 'This child will do x, y and z. It will walk. It will have no problems.' It can't do that. It can't look at a thirty-year-old adult and say: 'Given your medical history, you will live for the next ten years and only the following five things will happen.' So I'm unconvinced that even with the new technology, it will be able to predict what the life of a particular embryo will be like. Therefore I wonder how you assess which group gets to go on and which doesn't."

And I wonder this: When babies are turned into consumer products, who oversees quality control? Who does decide which potential defects the public should judge acceptable and which not? Will those searching for perfect babies begin first by socially outlawing major (though variable) birth defects like cerebral palsy and then, when we have accepted the principle of selection, move on to ever lesser defects such as asthma? As early as 1978, Randolph Seed was already listing genetic asthma among the "severe genetic defects."

It is not just Seed who gives a therapeutic rationale for suggesting that certain people use the sperm and eggs of other, genetically "healthier," people to produce children for themselves. This is a mainstream view among reproductive technologists and their supporters. Among those you will see quoted in this book espousing that view are: Dr. Arthur Levin, Dr. Cecil Jacobson, Marcus Pembrey, Joseph Fletcher, Patrick Steptoe, Dr. Margery Shaw, Dr. Carl Wood, Dr. R. G. Edwards and the late Dr. Pierre Soupart.

What does FGR see as the potential market for its embryo transfer service now? 1. Women who are infertile due to untreatable tubal obstruction or ovarian failure; 2. Women who cannot use in vitro fertilization (IVF) because their ovaries are inaccessible for laparoscopic retrieval of eggs; 3. Couples with unexplained infertility who have unsuccessfully been through both AID and IVF programs; 4. Women who are "carriers of undesirable genetic traits" or diseases such as polycystic kidneys, Tay-Sachs disease, cystic fibrosis, hemophilia, sickle cell anemia. At a press conference, the embryo transfer pioneers added: "These women should now be able to bear their husband's children without the worry of producing a child with the same genetic affliction."[5]

Women who have no ovaries but an intact uterus should also be able to bear children by embryo transfer, Buster stated. "This is possible because the steroid hormones usually made by the ovary and required to support the pregnancy could be provided by the physician," he added.

Building on the research of Dr. Gary Hodgen, Buster's team has begun experiments on women with no ovaries or premature menopause. (A very small percentage of women run out of eggs early in life either because they had a small number deposited in their ovaries in the first place or because they lost eggs at a faster than normal rate.) While Dr. Hodgen was chief of the Pregnancy Research Branch of the National Institutes of Child Health and Development in 1983, he conducted experiments in which monkeys whose ovaries had been removed gave birth to normal offspring. Hodgen transferred embryos into the uteri of the monkeys and then treated the monkeys with two hormones necessary for pregnancy—estrogen and progesterone. The hormones were implanted in the monkeys in silastic packages so they would diffuse slowly into the circulation (Hodgen, 1983).

Hodgen, who now works for a human in vitro fertilization team in Norfolk, Virginia, suggests that the method he devised might extend the childbearing age-range of women. (The babies they bore would not be their own, of course, since the eggs would be donated.)

"Let's assume a woman is fifty and in good health," Hodgen said to me. "I know of no biological reason why that woman couldn't carry a good pregnancy."

In the future, Richard Seed told me, FGR will offer another service: "prenatal adoption." Where both the woman and her partner are infertile, a donor egg will be fertilized with donor sperm and the woman will "adopt" the resulting embryo and take it into her womb.

In the next five to ten years, FGR may also consider offering a "substitute uterine carrier" service. This would be combining surrogate motherhood with embryo transfer.

"Suppose a woman were fertile but had high blood pressure or heart disease and it was not a genetic problem," Seed said. "Suppose she was advised not to get pregnant. We could wash an egg out of her at five days [after insemination] and have her sister be the substitute uterine carrier."

Human embryo transfer is a business. Any business has a strong motivation to create and continually expand a market for its product or service.

"The embryo transfer industry is going to do just what the baby formula companies did," said Jeremy Rifkin, director of the Foundation for Economic Trends, a group that is legally challenging FGR's patent applications. "Those companies talked millions of women all over the world into the conviction that they had to have formula as a substitute for breast milk."[6] This led to disease and death in thousands of babies, particularly in the Third World, where conditions necessary for formula use often did not exist. "I think we will see the same thing with the corporations that patent and own reproductive and genetic engineering processes. They will try to convince us that we are best off not to risk a natural reproductive process. If there is the least likelihood of a problem with an individual's egg or sperm or with the reproductive process itself, we are going to be talked into not taking the risk and instead relying on a 'safer,' planned process where we know in advance what we're going to get."

It worked for baby formula, Rifkin notes. There is no reason to believe it will not work for embryo transfer.

Richard Seed plans to win international recognition for his work by 1988.

"I don't mind telling you that I expect to get a Nobel Prize," Richard Seed said in our 1980 interview.

To win the prize, he continued, he must do two things: Get the first human pregnancy through embryo transfer (he did it three years later) and make a postmenopausal woman pregnant (he's working on it).

Seed recalls that after he had once given a conference paper on embryo transfer, a colleague came up to him. "He said something like: 'You son of a bitch. I worked twenty-five years on AI and you are going to get one pregnancy and get a Nobel Prize.'" His colleague had not realized that with his work on AI he had done nothing new, Seed pointed out. "He wasn't creating a new industry, a new technology, which is what I am doing."

Seed leaned back in his chair. "People used to laugh at me when I would say I was going to win a Nobel Prize," he said. "People don't laugh anymore. None of them laugh."

Notes

1. Instrumentation could be patented, B. J. Anderson of the AMA said. But there is a question as to whether the law gives authority to patent an actual medical procedure and thereby to license a technique, which is FGR's intent.

Michael Eberhard, senior vice-president of Memorial Health Technologies, maintains that medical procedures can and have been patented and there is nothing alarming about it. "If it weren't for the private funding in this case, there would be no ovum transfer method," he said, noting that government funding had not been available. Patent law, he explained, protects the inventor-genius from having his ideas stolen and protects the investor who finances the research. "The only way private sources would invest and take that risk would be if there was some potential return. So the patent process permitted the investors to take the chance and put out the dollars."

Pointing to the great suffering infertility causes ("It breaks up marriages"), Eberhard compared objections to FGR's patent applications to protests against a drug company's patent on a smallpox vaccine. "If you had seen children wiped out by smallpox, you'd find it strange that on the introduction of a vaccine to cure that, someone found it worthy to focus a lot of attention on the drug company's patent."

George Annas, professor of health law at Boston University Schools of Medicine and Public Health, is one who opposes the patent. Speaking at a conference in Boston in April 1984, he termed the attempt to patent a reproductive process "ludicrous" and probably unconstitutional. "It's like patenting a position in [sexual] intercourse," he said.

At its annual meeting in 1984, the American College of Obstetricians and Gynecologists (ACOG) released a statement condemning as unethical and unprofessional the patenting of medical procedures and/or intentional delay or partial reporting of medical research findings. According to Dr. Myron Gordon, outgoing chairman of ACOG's committee on bioethics, the statement had been prompted by concern expressed by ACOG members and by information the committee received about potential patenting applications for the embryo transfer process (Callahan, 1984, July 1).

American Fertility Society president Edwin P. Peterson told a press conference at the society's 1984 annual meeting that the majority of physicians in the fertility field are opposed to the concept of patenting scientific procedures. There should be a way to protect the investors who put research and development money into human embryo transfer and yet keep the information open, he said.

Giving an address at the meeting, Dr. Robert Edwards, the British IVF pioneer, criticized the patent attempt and said he and Steptoe would never do such a thing.

When I asked Dr. Marie Bustillo, a member of UCLA's embryo transfer team, to comment on the patenting attempt, she replied: "It's a problem. But the company that sponsored research spent over $2 million without charging patients. It did this by forming a limited partnership. It needs to pay the investors back. In order to get the money back, it's necessary to serve as many patients as possible."

Asked to comment on Edwards' criticism of the patent attempt, she said: "I don't know who financed Steptoe and Edwards' research but I suspect it was their patients. The question is: Was that ethical?"

I asked her if she thought it was ethical for her team to charge women for embryo transfer at this very early stage in the development of the technique. She replied: "I'm not so sure it *is* ethical to charge patients at this point but we have no choice because there's no money. Patients are begging for it. There is no federal money available."

Many patients contacted the team wanting the procedure, she said, particularly after the blitz of publicity in February 1984, when the birth of the first embryo transfer baby was announced.

A pattern emerges in the development of many new reproductive technologies—not just embryo transfer: Experimentation on women is presented through the media as a "medical breakthrough." There is much hoopla and many cries of "new hope for the infertile." Infertile women begin clamoring for what they think of as a "new" rather than "experimental" procedure. The demand for the procedure created by the researchers through the media is then used to justify further experimentation on women.

2. "The interview was designed to ascertain compliancy and ability to manage project-related stresses, demands and risks," the researchers wrote (Bustillo et al., 1984).

3. In one ob/gyn journal, physicians wrote: "it may well be that during the next 40 years the allowing of a vaginal delivery or attempted vaginal delivery may need to be justified in each particular instance. Perhaps it is not altogether too provocative to suggest that vaginal delivery may yet become the exception rather than the rule" (Southerst and Case, 1975, p. 259).

Elsewhere, Dr. William F. Kroener stated: "The long-held concept of vaginal delivery if at all possible is rapidly giving way. The new growing principle seems to be, *vaginal delivery only of selected patients*" (his emphasis) (Hibbard, 1976, p. 804).

4. See "Court orders cesarean if needed to save baby," *Boston Sunday Globe,* Jan. 25, 1981, p. 11. For additional information on women forced to undergo cesareans, see Hubbard, 1979.

5. That a man's issue be reproduced in the world is a patriarchal ethic. Biotechnology now makes it more possible for "barren" or genetically "defective" women to fulfill this ethic. (See discussion of this in Chapter 11.)

6. Women were not just "convinced" to use baby formula. Once birth was moved into hospitals, women's efforts to breast-feed their babies were sabotaged by medical practices, including the prescription of antiseptic "care" of the woman's breasts. This involved washing breasts with hexachlorophene or soap and water three or four times a day—a treatment that could lead to dried, cracked and bleeding nipples. Nursing became painful. (See Chapter 16 for other details.) There were cases in which it was quite important for women to have baby formula available to them. But the market was expanded far beyond the need.

Part Three

IN VITRO
FERTILIZATION

7

Man-Made Ovulation:
The State of the Art

On July 25, 1978, British gynecologist Patrick Steptoe surgically extracted from an unconscious woman the world's first "test-tube" baby, Louise Brown. Steptoe had retrieved an egg from the woman in an operation nine months earlier. Then his partner or "co-lab-parent," Dr. Robert Edwards, fertilized that egg in the laboratory using the sperm of the woman's husband. Finally, Steptoe transferred the embryo into the woman's womb where it developed into baby Louise.

The procedure is called "in vitro" (literally, "in glass") fertilization as opposed to "in vivo" (within the body). Eminent North American embryologist Dr. Clifford Grobstein prefers to call the procedure "external human fertilization." His term, he writes, more accurately characterizes the main point, which is that "the process has been externalized, thereby rendering it more accessible and susceptible to manipulation, including intervention" (Grobstein, 1981, pp. 1–2). (I use both terms interchangeably.)

Louise Brown's birth culminated work begun a hundred years earlier when a Viennese embryologist first tried to fertilize an egg outside a female body. This first attempt, made in 1879, came only one year after the role of semen in procreation was demonstrated. In the century that followed, men made many further attempts at in vitro fertilization (IVF), most often using the eggs of rabbits (as the embryologist had) and women.

Pharmacrats needed to overcome technical problems before they could fertilize an egg in a petri dish, and they had to have subjects with which to perform their experiments. From the 1940s through the 1970s, women undergoing gynecological surgery in the United

States and elsewhere were the experimental subjects. Pharmacrats attempted to recover eggs from the women and sometimes to study or fertilize those eggs in the lab. They published their studies. I have read *none* in which it was stated that the woman's consent to the search for eggs in her body and/or to experimentation with those eggs was sought and obtained. It is impossible to tell from the reports if the women—sometimes referred to as "the material"—were told anything at all about the planned research on their eggs.[1]

Most scientific reports on human embryo experimentation, biologist Leon Kass has noted, are "strangely silent on the nature of the egg donors, on their understanding of what was to be done with their eggs, and on the manner of obtaining consent." He added: "The researchers owe us an account of how consent was obtained and of what the couples [sic] were in fact told."

In 1970, two researchers wrote: "Much of our knowledge of mammalian fertilization is relatively recent and the time is now ripe for increasing concentration of research effort on the primate—with special attention to the human primate. The role of the obstetrician-gynecologists in this endeavor will be increasingly apparent" (Mastroianni and Noriega, 1970).

Indeed it is. Women undergoing laparoscopy as part of an infertility exam or for sterilization; women undergoing hysterectomies for uterine fibroids or for cervical cancer or for "premalignant diseases"; women operated on for endometriosis and for polycystic ovaries; and women undergoing unspecified "gynecological surgery" in the United States and other countries have had eggs taken from their bodies.[2]

In a fifteen-year project they began in 1938 and termed the "egg hunt," gynecologist Dr. John Rock and pathologist Dr. Arthur T. Hertig took hundreds of eggs from poor women receiving charity medical care at the Free Hospital for Women in Brookline, Massachusetts.* Though they received no fees from the women, prestigious physicians sought appointments to the hospital and journalist Loretta McLaughlin gives some indication why. One advantage of an appointment was that the charity hospital "provided almost absolute research freedom, far less interference than at the larger, Harvard-affiliated hospitals in Boston proper," McLaughlin wrote in a laudatory biography of Dr. Rock. "During Rock's scientifically bountiful

---

* In their papers on this work (Rock and Menkin, 1944; Menkin and Rock, 1948; and Rock and Hertig, 1948), the researchers do not mention if or how they obtained the consent of the women. But according to one reporter, Rock's assistant, Miriam Menkin, explained the research to the women and asked them if they were willing to participate (McLaughlin, 1982, p. 76).

years there, the Free became something of a private research preserve for its principal staffers."[3]

The hysterectomies performed on women whose wombs and oviducts would be searched for eggs were all medically necessary, the researchers assert. We can hope so, although studies have appeared periodically over the years indicating that many of the hysterectomies physicians judge to be "necessary" are, in fact, not so. (None of the studies deal specifically with the practices at the Free Hospital for Women.)[4]

Because Rock and Hertig wanted to maximize their chance of obtaining *fertilized* eggs from the women's extirpated organs, they tried to perform the operation around the time of the woman's fertile period—ovulation. Hertig and Rock maintain that the women were not *instructed* to engage in intercourse during the fertile period immediately preceding the operation but were simply told to record the dates when they did. However, their assistant, Miriam Menkin, said she did indeed encourage the women to have unprotected intercourse at that time to increase the chance of getting an embryo (McLaughlin, 1983, p. 75).

Rather than performing the operation at just the time physicians diagnosed a need for it, Rock had the women spend several months taking their temperatures daily and charting their ovulatory cycles so the researchers could predict a date for the operation when they were most likely to find an embryo. Week after week, the charity patients brought their charts to the hospital until a surgical date optimal for the research could be determined.

Hertig and Rock collected 34 fertilized eggs from 211 women who were unknowingly pregnant at the time of surgery. Out of loyalty to their university, the men named the first egg they found the "Harvard egg." They named another the "Dominic egg" for Boston Red Sox centerfielder Dominic DiMaggio who hit a crucial long double during a 1946 World Series game as Hertig was looking at the egg under a microscope.

The women in this experiment belonged to a lower economic, social and gender class than the doctors who asked them to participate. Most were Catholic. Did they truly understand the nature of the experiment? Did they understand that embryos might be taken from their bodies? Would they have considered that an abortion? Menkin told journalist McLaughlin that she was a "nervous wreck" during the experiments, afraid that if something happened to prevent the scheduled surgery from taking place—such as the patient coming down with a cold—the woman might miss a period and know she was pregnant (McLaughlin, 1983, p. 77). Menkin does not explain her worry further but presumably if the patient knew she was pregnant, she would either experience the anguish of undergoing what she might consider a sinful abortion (through the hysterectomy), or she—a woman judged to need surgery—would instead go through with the pregnancy and raise an unexpected child.

These women were not paying for their operations. As charity patients, did they feel free to withhold their consent to the experiment? Were they confident that if they did refuse to do what the doctor asked of them, they could still receive health care and be treated decently?

Rock and his colleagues were generous with the ovaries they removed from women at the Free Hospital as this acknowledgment in a paper on maturing human eggs in the laboratory indicates: "We acknowledge with gratitude the kind cooperation of Doctor Pemberton, Dr. G. V. Smith and Dr. John Rock and their associates at the Free Hospital for Women in making the specimens used in this study available to us" (Pincus and Saunders).

Others were experimenting with women's eggs as well. Dr. Landrum Shettles, a gynecologist whose attempts to fertilize eggs externally caused a furor in the 1950s, recalls that "nice, little old ladies" frequently asked him then where he got the human eggs he used in his experiments. "Most of them I just poached," he would say.[5]

One account reported: "In the course of performing various operations requiring abdominal incision into the peritoneal cavity of the female, Dr. Shettles pierced the ovaries of his patients with a syringe and aspirated ... some of the eggs from their follicles ... without harming the patient in any way" (Rorvik, 1971, p. 83). The question, as Princeton theologian Paul Ramsey points out, "is not whether Dr. Shettles *harmed* these patients in any way, but whether they *consented* in any way to have a procedure done to them that was wholly unrelated to the condition that called for the abdominal incision to be made."[6]

While some researchers speak of "fishing for eggs" in women and others of "recruiting," "harvesting" or "capturing" them, the most vivid image in the scientific journals is that of men hunting for eggs in the bodies of women: "Miller, Engel, and Reiman, searching operative specimens from 24 patients, found 5 ... ova." "Ova were sought in the washings of the excised reproductive tracts of 48 patients after they had ovulated."[7]

In Melbourne, Australia, from 1970 to 1972, a research team

attempting to fertilize eggs in the lab "collected eggs when operating on ovaries and also when using the technique of laparoscopy," according to the team leader, a gynecologist. He does not mention whether the women being operated on knew that men were taking their eggs for research (Wood and Westmore, 1983, p. 44).

Sometimes pharmacrats culture eggs from healthy ovaries which had been excised from women with the rationale that castrated women will never develop ovarian cancer. (The rarity of this disease is seldom mentioned when these "prophylactic" operations are being justified.)

Before pharmacrats could fertilize an egg outside a woman's body, they had to: concoct a culture medium in which eggs could mature; find a way—in human experiments—to obtain eggs from a woman's body; "capacitate" sperm, that is, condition the sperm surface (something that normally occurs within the female genital tract) so that it acquires the ability to penetrate the egg's outer layer.

Progress came rapidly. Reviewing the scientific literature in 1970, two researchers wrote that, if strict criteria were used, complete external fertilization of an egg had not yet been convincingly accomplished in the human. Yet a short eight years later, the first "test-tube" baby was born in England.

The experiments on in vitro fertilization (IVF) became serious only about fifty years ago when Gregory Pincus and E. V. Enzman showed that if rabbit eggs were placed in culture, they would complete the maturation process outside the body. While another team soon repeated the experiment—this time with mouse eggs— researchers made little progress for a good twenty-five years thereafter.[8]

During those years, various researchers claimed to have fertilized eggs in the lab, but they failed to use a stringent criteria to prove that fertilization had indeed occurred.[9] Eggs that the investigators thought were dividing because they had been fertilized might, in fact, have been disintegrating because they were dying. Or they might have been undergoing parthenogenic cleavage, that is, egg development *not* initiated by sperm, but by some chemical or mechanical stimulation.

In 1959, when M. C. Chang of the Worcester Foundation in Massachusetts said he had fertilized a mammalian egg in vitro, his claim could not be dismissed. His criteria for fertilization were so stringent that many scientists accepted his work as the first incontestable evidence of the external fertilization of a mammal's eggs.

So, success at in vitro fertilization was rare. As late as 1979, one researcher reviewing the published studies wrote that there were only four species in which it had been unequivocally attained: rabbit; mouse; rat and—as of the previous year—woman (Whittingham, 1979).

Here was one of the difficulties: Eggs extracted from the ovaries of female animals are not fully developed. Before researchers could attempt to fertilize them, they needed to support the maturation of the eggs in an artificial culture. This has proved difficult. Pincus and a colleague reported the first instance of human eggs matured externally in 1939. There was not another success with human eggs until R. G. Edwards achieved it in 1965. Edwards was the major early worker in egg maturation, testing various culture media. Between 1960 and 1965, he published studies on the external maturation of eggs of many species. He outlined the time sequence of the maturation of women's eggs in 1965.

A great difficulty he encountered, and one he repeatedly refers to in his book, *A Matter of Life,* was that of getting women's eggs.

First, as a graduate student, he had worked with mice. After he had "bombed" their ovaries with hormones, he had learned a good deal about the way eggs ripen. Later, while researching in another field, "the eggs were always there in the background beckoning me on to my real work." Occasionally, he dreamed of eggs.

He arranged for various gynecologists to call him when they thought they might have ovarian tissues to "bequeath" him. He would go to the hospital. While the physician cut into the woman's body, he would stand, masked and gowned, holding his sterile glass pot, "the receptacle for the precious bit of superfluous ovarian tissue."

Dr. Edwards needed more eggs. He never had enough. He "scouted around" for them and "tried to rally more doctors to my cause." He "came away empty-handed." His sources "dried up."

"Human eggs were still slow coming my way," he wrote, "despite the fact that I had struck up friendly relations with some of the gynecologists at Cambridge's Addenbrooke's Hospital."

So he worked more often with the eggs of cows, sheep and monkeys. Now and then, a lab threw a monkey ovary his way. He would get the ovaries of cows and sheep from the local slaughterhouse. He found his visits there unpleasant. It was "sad," he reports, to see the cows lining up, to hear the crack of the gun and then the soft thud of the creature falling.

At Cambridge, he wrote, "I would have been more content if

only human eggs had come my way more freely."

In 1966, he set off for Johns Hopkins in Baltimore. There, he would share human ovaries with the pathologists.

In Baltimore, Edwards, working with his American colleague Dr. Howard Jones, tried to fertilize human eggs that had been matured in culture. Suspecting—but not knowing—that human sperm, like that of other species, had to be capacitated or conditioned before it could fertilize an egg, Edwards tried to achieve that capacitation in various ways.

He placed the human sperm in rabbit uteri and tubes, thinking the secretions in the reproductive tract of another animal might be able to condition human sperm; he asked female patients at Johns Hopkins Hospital—where he was then conducting his experiments— to have intercourse with their husbands so that sperm from the cervical mucus in the women could be collected some hours after the act; or he cultured sperm samples with small pieces of human oviduct. After these attempts at capacitation, he placed the sperm in culture with the eggs. None of these 104 eggs were fertilized.

He placed twenty more eggs of women in the reproductive tracts of rabbits, and sixty-seven others in monkeys, in attempts to fertilize them there. But he could retrieve few of the eggs. None were fertilized. "Species other than rabbit or monkey will have to be tested for as hosts for human fertilization," he and his colleagues concluded (Edwards, 1966).

The next year, Edwards traveled to Chapel Hill, North Carolina, to work again with American gynecologists and pick up his experiments where he had left them off in Baltimore. Because he wanted to use capacitated sperm in attempting to fertilize human eggs, he needed to collect sperm that had come into contact with the secretions of the female reproductive tract. This time, rather than persuading women to have intercourse with their husbands so his colleagues could go in afterward and collect the sperm, he constructed a tiny chamber that he could fill with sperm and insert into the womb of a female patient whom he had persuaded to volunteer for this experiment. The chamber was lined with a porous membrane that would theoretically allow secretions from the womb to pass into it but would not let sperm escape, possibly impregnating the women.

Edwards' wife Ruth asked him if he were certain the sperm would not escape. He assured her he was (Edwards and Steptoe, 1980).

So, with the collaboration of the American gynecologists, he collected bits of human ovarian tissue, extracted eggs from the tissue, ripened the eggs, collected sperm (from whom he does not say, but in other experiments, he had used his own), put them into the porous chambers, and found women volunteers who would allow the chamber to be inserted into them at night and removed in the morning.

"I must confess that I had many a sleepless night fearing the chamber would burst inside the uterus, releasing the spermatozoa with disasterous results," Edwards recalled.

" 'You said you were sure they couldn't escape,' Ruth said.

" 'I am sure,' I replied." (He was not.)

" 'Then go to sleep, for heaven's sake,' Ruth said.

"Fortunately," Edwards continued, "the membrane held."

Again he failed to fertilize any eggs but it was "a pleasant summer interlude for me and my family," Edwards wrote.[10]

Since the porous chambers had not worked, Edwards needed another way of getting sperm that had been capacitated within a woman's body. One day in 1967, he read an article by Patrick Steptoe, a gynecologist who had been pioneering the use of the laparoscope in operative gynecology since 1959 in Oldham, Lancashire. That instrument—a miniature telescope—might provide a way of collecting sperm from a woman's fallopian tubes after she had had intercourse, Edwards thought. Later, it would also provide a way to extract ripened eggs from women's bodies.

Edwards called Steptoe. They subsequently met at a British Fertility Society meeting. Steptoe was useful to Edwards not only because he could wield a laparoscope, but also because he could provide Edwards with pieces of ovary for experiments. As they discussed their possible collaboration at that meeting, Steptoe said to Edwards: "All the clinical material [i.e., women] is centered in Oldham. Cambridge is a long way away" (Edwards and Steptoe, 1980, p. 77). They figured they could set up a research laboratory for Edwards in Oldham and he could drive down from Cambridge whenever necessary.

Thus was launched the collaboration between Steptoe and Edwards in 1968. Steptoe began sending Edwards eggs from ovaries he removed from women during gynecological operations at Oldham.[11]

Edwards took another shot at fertilizing human eggs. This time he tested a culture medium for the capacitation of sperm rather than the reproductive tract secretions of rabbits, monkeys or women. After maturing the eggs in the lab, he fertilized them in a new culture medium refined by one of his Ph.D. students, Barry Bavister. Edwards and Bavister placed their own sperm in what Edwards called "Barry's magic culture fluid," along with eggs cultured from ovaries either removed from Steptoe's patients or, in one case, provided by a friendly local gynecologist.

The results caused a great stir in England. For the first time, it was reported in 1969, human eggs had been fertilized outside a woman's body.[12] But the outcome of the experiment was not entirely pleasing. Only thirty-four of fifty-six eggs matured. Only seven eggs appeared to have been fertilized. Some were abnormal. As a control for his experiment, Edwards observed eggs which he did not expose to sperm. Five percent of these underwent cleavage-like parthenogenic development, suggesting that the eggs he thought were fertilized might be undergoing other changes instead.[13]

Maturing eggs totally outside the female body did not seem to be working well. Edwards and his colleagues were concerned about the poor maturation rate and possible abnormality of eggs matured externally. "Problems of embryonic development seemed likely to accompany the use of human eggs that had been ripened in vitro— all the animal work confirmed that," Edwards wrote.

So they changed their experimental course. They began trying to fertilize eggs that had been matured in the ovary itself, inside the woman's body, rather than in culture fluid. To induce the eggs to mature inside the body, they needed to "impose some control over the menstrual cycle," Edwards wrote, by giving the women hormones, "rather as I had done with those mice in Edinburgh a decade or so earlier" (Edwards and Steptoe, 1980, p. 88).

At that time, Edwards had had to work night shifts because the mice ovulated at night. This irritated him, especially because he was then dating the woman he would marry. He knew that a colleague had been stimulating the ovaries of baby mice with hormones to induce them to ovulate and it occurred to him that the ovaries of adult mice might "be persuaded to ripen their eggs during office hours," from 9 to 5. That would be "marvellously convenient," he wrote.

His colleague agreed to work with him on the project, preparing a hormonal concoction (a "witch's brew") containing serum from a pregnant mare and a pregnant woman. Edwards injected adult mice with hormones and produced what he termed "ovulation to order." The mice "could be made to ovulate by day or by night, four times successfully within a few days." Other researchers conducted the same experiments on women. "What was true for mice was true for women," Edwards reported (Edwards and Steptoe, 1980, pp. 27–31). The result was those multiple pregnancies that began making the headlines: quadruplets, quintuplets, even sextuplets.

I will describe human ovulation here so that we can understand how men like Edwards can control it. The ovaries contain hundreds of thousands of follicles—balls of cells with an immature egg in the center. Each month, at the beginning of the menstrual cycle, one follicle in either of the two ovaries begins to enlarge. Its accessory cells proliferate and fluid accumulates to form a cavity in the mass of cells. The egg within matures. As the blisterlike follicle enlarges, it moves closer to the ovarian surface. On about the fourteenth day of the menstrual cycle, the follicular mass bursts and the egg is set free. This is ovulation. Some women can feel this as a cramp (mittelschmerz) on either side of the abdomen or lower back.

What causes that one follicle (occasionally more) to enlarge and release an egg? Hormones produced in the pituitary gland, at the base of the brain, do. One, follicle-stimulating hormone or FSH, stimulates the growth of the follicle in the ovary. The second, luteinizing hormone or LH, later induces ovulation and transforms the follicle into the corpus luteum, a structure that, emitting hormones itself, helps maintain pregnancy. The hypothalmus, the floor of the brain, controls the cyclic release of these pituitary hormones. When the level of estrogen produced by the ovaries drops below a certain point, the hypothalmus sends out the releasing hormone for FSH. This stimulates the pituitary to release FSH, thus triggering the growth of ten to twenty follicles in the ovary.

One of these follicles will mature. During its two-week growth and maturation period, the follicle secretes increasing amounts of estrogen. As it approaches maturity, it secretes progesterone as well. This combination of estrogen and progesterone probably triggers the hypothalmus to secrete the releasing factors for FSH and LH simultaneously. The subsequent FSH–LH peak probably triggers ovulation, the release of the egg from the follicle.[14]

Now, a decade after "bombing" the ovaries of mice to produce "ovulation to order," Edwards wanted the same control over women's ovaries. The hormones, in this case, were called "fertility drugs." He and Steptoe began by injecting one hormone into the women to stimulate the growth of egg follicles. This was Pergonal, a human menopausal gonadotrophin or hMG. It contained approximately equal FSH and LH activity. Then they injected a hormone that appears to be chemically identical to LH (human chorionic gonadotrophin or hCG). This induces the ripening process and ovulation.

Based on his experience in the culture of human eggs, Edwards estimated the ripening process would take about thirty-six hours. The women were to be given four injections of hormones over eight to ten days.

Through these powerful hormones, men controlled the ovulation of women. They had "taken over the first part of the menstrual cycle of our patients," Edwards wrote (Edwards and Steptoe, 1980, p. 123). In 1970, he and Steptoe declared: "Fine control has been imposed on the initiation of maturation and the timing of ovulation in cyclic women by injecting gonadotropins" (Steptoe and Edwards, 1970).

During a scientific symposium, another researcher reviewed what he and his colleagues were accomplishing by using human gonadotropins (substances that stimulate the gonads—ovaries in women, testes in men). He explained that they were trying to cause the maturation of several follicles. They would then track the growth of the follicles by measuring the rise of estrogen in the blood. When, studying their laboratory data, they believed the estrogen level had reached a critical point, they stopped the egg-ripening hormone (hMG) and gave an ovulation-inducing preparation, either LH or hCG. Using their lab data as a source of feedback information, he explained: "We have assumed the role of the hypothalmus" (COG, 1979 April).

Here are men taking over one function of a woman's brain.

When men assumed the role of the woman's hypothalmus, researchers agreed, ovulation became much less sloppy, much more efficient. Australian pioneers in human IVF "could induce the production of oocytes to a timetable. This procedure allows doctors to arrange the time of ovulation and fertilisation in advance" (Lee, 1980 Dec.). Other Australian doctors would investigate "methods of programing the ovarian cycle to control the time of ovulation, allowing for more efficient case preparation and handling within the routine hospital organization" (Gair, 1981). Still other researchers could "make ovulation more precise and more productive" (*The Age*, 7/25/81).

Steptoe and Edwards kept other women on a natural cycle. Since these women would produce only one egg each, the researchers needed some signal to tell them when to go in and catch that lone egg. That signal was the surge of LH in the urine. Usually about day 13 of the menstrual cycle, the pituitary suddenly discharges LH. An hour or so after LH is released into the bloodstream, it spills over into the urine. Edwards measured the LH in the urine so he could give Steptoe an idea of when to do the laparoscopy.

The question then became: Could Steptoe, using laparoscopy, withdraw the ripened eggs directly from the woman's ovaries, without damaging the eggs? No one had ever done it.

Steptoe thought he could. By 1968, he had had much experience with the instrument whose use he was pioneering. During the preceding decade, he had inserted the laparoscope into 40 percent of the women admitted to his gynecology department (Biggers, 1979).

This is what happens during the operation: The physician places the woman under general anesthesia. Then he pumps inert gas into her to distend her abdomen and provide room for him to view and work on the internal organs. He tilts her head down 20 degrees so the intestines fall back by gravity. He makes small incisions in the abdominal wall to allow the insertion of instruments among which is the laparoscope, a slender optical device. The instrument contains a bundle of quartz fibers able to transmit light in irregular paths and produce images by means of lenses and mirrors. Light is passed from one end of the device to the other inside the woman's body.

For the operation, Edwards and his research assistant Jean Purdy designed equipment that could be used to collect eggs by sucking them with a vacuum from the ovarian follicles, the small, cystlike structures in which the eggs matured. This puncturing of the follicle and sucking out of the egg is "man-made ovulation," as a leading researcher in IVF terms it (*JRM*, 1973).

The egg had to be removed just before ovulation. Timing was crucial. If they went in too soon, the egg would not yet be mature enough; if they went in too late, the egg would have burst out of the follicle and, traveling down the oviduct, been lost forever to their suction device.

While Steptoe told Edwards the operation "makes few demands on the patient," and could be used repeatedly on the same woman (Edwards and Steptoe, 1980, p. 87) and while Edwards described laparoscopy as a "relatively minor operation," Britain's Medical Research Council viewed it differently. In 1971, the Council had turned down a request by Steptoe and Edwards for support of their research in women because—among other reasons—it had reservations "about the justifiability of employing the procedure of laparoscopy for purely experimental purposes" (Edwards and Steptoe, 1980, pp. 106–107).

In turning down the funding request, the Council had written Edwards that it "had serious doubts about ethical aspects of the proposed investigations in humans, especially those relating to the implantation in women of oocytes fertilized in vitro, which were considered premature in view of the lack of preliminary studies on primates and the present deficiency of detailed knowledge of the possible hazards involved." The Council would consider funding experimentation in primates, but not in women, it informed Edwards. Steptoe and Edwards continued working in women, without funding from the Council.

At this stage, they needed women on whom to experiment with the egg suction procedures and hormonal brews they were developing. "Our patients were childless couples who hoped that our research might enable them to have children," Edwards wrote (Edwards and Fowler, 1970). Commenting on this sentence—the solitary reference in the whole article touching on how consent was obtained from the women for experimentation, biologist Kass wrote: "From the report that they had hopes, we can surmise that they considered themselves to be patients. But as far as these experiments are concerned, they are only experimental subjects" (Kass, 1971).

Only one other scientific article reveals anything more about the women used and how they were informed. Steptoe and Edwards wrote: "The object of the investigations was fully discussed with the patients, including the possible clinical application to relieve their infertility" (cited by Kass, 1971).

Were the women (or "couples," as Kass inaccurately refers to the experimental subjects) told that the much more likely possibility was that the surgery performed on them would be applied to *other* infertile women in the future and not they themselves? Kass wonders. If not, he concludes, such a false generation of hope would be both cruel and unethical.

Steptoe and Edwards agreed that the hopes of the women "must not be raised unjustifiably and that they fully understood the situation—the opportunities and dangers and how they would be involved," Edwards wrote. (As we will see in Chapter 9, there is evidence from women in the English, Australian and American IVF programs that they did not understand the situation.)

In beginning the human trials, Steptoe and Edwards were taking an extraordinary departure from scientific procedures: *They (and subsequent researchers) had not verified the safety of in vitro fertilization in primates before attempting it in women.*

As a federal ethics board which held hearings on IVF noted in 1979: "Experts appearing before the Board agreed that there has been insufficient controlled animal research designed to determine the long-range effects of in vitro fertilization and embryo transfer. The lack of primate work is particularly noteworthy in view of the opportunity provided by primate models for assessing subtle neurological, cognitive and developmental effects on such procedures" (DHEW, 1979).

Before the birth of Louise Brown in 1978, the number of animal species and the total number of animals born following IVF and embryo transfer was extremely low: fewer than 200 rabbits, 200 mice and 50 rats. Most of those test-tube animals were accounted for in only 22 published reports (Walters, 1979). Between 1971 and 1973, ethicists and researchers including Leon Kass, Marc Lappe, Benjamin Brackett and Luigi Mastroianni argued that further animal research should be conducted before attempting IVF and embryo transfer in women.[15]

Others involved in experimentation on women—Robert Edwards of Cambridge and Dr. Mason Andrews of Norfolk General Hospital among them—denied the need or relevance of animal studies, arguing that they would be too expensive (chimpanzees cost a lot of money) and, if required, would forfeit for many infertile couples a chance for a baby (Walters, 1979; Edwards, 1974).

In 1970, Professor Carl Wood, chair of Monash University's Department of Obstetrics and Gynecology, reported that "using human volunteers would be more efficient and far more likely to bring results" (The Age, 7/25/81).*

In late December 1971, Steptoe and Edwards decided to implant the first embryo in a woman. From 1971 to 1977, they used almost eighty women in their research. They were unsuccessful. The problem came in transfering the embryo into the uterus. The pregnancies did not "take."

To understand one explanation for the failure, we go back to the woman's cycle. The functions of the ovaries and uterus in that cycle are coordinated by a complex hormonal system. This system regulates the production of the egg in the ovary and preparation of the uterus for the embryo.

At ovulation, the follicle bursts, ejecting the egg into the oviduct. The collapsed follicle is transformed into the corpus luteum (yellow body).[16] If pregnancy occurs, the corpus luteum persists, producing

---

* During an ABC television discussion of IVF following Louise Brown's birth, the late Dr. Andre Hellegers, professor of gynecology at Georgetown University, said he thought it was imprudent to go straight "from mice to women." He added: "I personally would have advocated going through the monkey stage." Dr. Joseph Fletcher, medical ethicist from University of Virginia Medical School, cheerfully responded, "There must always be a first time with human runs" (ABC, 7/13/78).

hormones—estrogens and progesterone—that stimulate the endometrium (the lining of the uterus). Under hormonal stimulation, the cells of the endometrium proliferate and the vascular supply increases. The uterus is preparing for the implantation of the embryo and formation of the placenta. The early embryo also produces a hormone (chorionic gonadotropin) that keeps the corpus luteum functioning during the first third of pregnancy.

There are many possible reasons for the failure of embryo transfer.[17] Steptoe and Edwards, however, felt their failures had been caused by the hormones they had given to induce artificial ovulation in women who had normal cycles. Their treatment with gonadotropin hormones had upset the normal rhythm of the ovary and uterus, they believed, distorting the second phase of the cycle during which the embryo should have implanted. First, they attempted to correct the abnormal conditions they had created in the womb through the administration of yet more hormones to sustain the embryo's growth in the mother. In addition to steroid supplements, they gave hCG to some women, bromocriptine to others, clomiphene to still others.

Nothing worked. "It appears difficult to maintain the correct uterine conditions to establish and sustain pregnancy after the disorders caused by the treatment with gonadotropins," Edwards and Steptoe wrote (1980).

Several researchers doubted that the failures had really been caused by the hormones used in superovulation. They pointed out that many pregnancies had occurred in women given these same hormones as a fertility drug. But, having had no success with women whose cycles they had hormonally regulated, Steptoe and Edwards abandoned superovulation.

They did so reluctantly. "We'd be no longer controlling the menstrual cycle, merely observing it—and we would be tied mercilessly to the patient's menstrual and ovulation cycle," Edwards complained to his research assistant Jean Purdy (Edwards and Steptoe, 1980, pp. 134–135). In November 1977, they began a new series of experiments that did not include hormonal regulation.

Steptoe performed laparoscopies on sixty-eight women to recover eggs. He grasped each ovary with forceps, rolling it around in order to get at all the follicles. He held the ovary while the eggs were aspirated. After attempting to fertilize the egg and support the embryo's growth in culture, they transferred the embryos. While in three cases they operated on women again in order to place the embryos in their uteri, in most cases they transferred the embryos nonsurgically. They placed the embryo into a plastic tube, inserted that into a metal tube, and then, placing the tube through the cervix, deposited the embryo.

Two of the first three women into whom they transferred embryos became pregnant. Steptoe and Edwards thought they had the system cracked. So early in 1978, in quick succession, they transferred embryos into eight more women. None "took." They did not know why.

While world attention focused on what was to be the birth of the first "test-tube" baby, Louise Brown, Steptoe and Edwards were keeping a secret. One Englishwoman pregnant through in vitro fertilization aborted. The fetus was abnormal. It had an extra set of chromosomes, suggesting that more than one sperm might have fertilized the egg in the petri dish.* (In the dish, the egg is exposed to large numbers of sperm relative to those found in the oviducts during natural fertilization. So there may well be an increased risk of such abnormal fertilizations, researcher R. V. Short has noted.)

Medical World News reported:

> It was the eight failures plus an aborted fetus with genetic abnormality that led Dr. Steptoe and his collaborator, physiologist Robert Edwards to withhold the details of their initial success for so long despite worldwide clamor for the information. "Lesley Brown was pregnant," says Dr. Steptoe, "and we realized we didn't know exactly why. We thought we'd done exactly the same with the others as with Mrs. Brown—but we kept failing."

When Steptoe finally revealed that one of the women in his experiments had aborted an abnormal fetus, he said that if he had disclosed it at the time it happened—during Lesley Brown's pregnancy—it would have resulted in "serious misunderstandings from the press," and he was afraid that his experiments with women (clinical investigations) would have had to have been halted (MWN, 1979).

Subsequently, another woman who had undergone three operations for the recovery of an egg aborted at twenty weeks. The infant was born alive but died after two hours.

In July 1978, Steptoe delivered Louise Brown by cesarean section. Six months later, the second such baby, Alistair Montgomery, was born in Glasgow. So of the sixty-eight women who had undergone laparoscopy, two bore normal babies.

* "The woman aborted at 10 weeks, according to one report (Short, 1979b); at seven weeks, according to another (MWN, 1979). The genetic abnormality of the fetus was incompatible with life."

After Louise Brown's birth, test-tube birth technology was still primitive. By December 1980, of all the 278 women who had participated in known experiments with human in vitro fertilization, three had given birth to test-tube babies. So the live birth success rate for human IVF was .04 percent—less than 1 percent.[18]

Despite that, premature claims for IVF came thick and fast. For example, Richard B. Payne, president and chair of the Executive Committee of Medical Center Hospitals in Norfolk, Virginia, testifying in support of the Norfolk IVF clinic in 1979, stated that "the medical [IVF] program has been *amply* [my emphasis] demonstrated by the physicians in England."[19]

Producing the world's first test-tube baby was like landing on the moon and stirred a similar public response of wild excitement and enthusiasm. Just as men had conquered outer space, now were they taming "inner space." In fact, embryologist Dr. Clifford Grobstein noted that nine years before the unusual test-tube birth, "the first human footprint was set in lunar sand." Linking the two events, he wrote, was the new array of options each opens up for the human species, "the footprint pointing toward extraterrestrial migration, the baby toward new interventions and procedures for procreation." Taking the two events together, one could spin scenarios of colonization beyond the solar system, he wrote (Grobstein, 1981, pp. 1–2). One experimental biologist, Dr. E. S. E. Hafez, already had envisioned sending frozen human embryos into space—embryos that would later grow and take over other planets (*Life*, 1965, Sept. 10).

There was still another link: Each crowned a race for glory.[20] At a symposium on IVF held several years before the birth of Louise Brown, embryologist Dr. Anne McLaren of Edinburgh University expressed concern about the competitive nature of the work: "I fear Dr. Edwards will go too far, too fast. I am worried by the possibility that the desire to be first in the field will bias the judgement of those in a position to carry out egg transfer."

The late Dr. Pierre Soupart, who had also conducted experiments on the in vitro fertilization of human eggs, thought Steptoe and Edwards had bypassed a crucial step in their research by failing to test whether an embryo might be subtly damaged by the IVF process. When asked by CBS television reporter Jay McMullen, "Were you or your colleagues ... concerned that they might be cutting some scientific corners in order to win the race?" Soupart replied, "Well, quite obviously they have already cut one.... Short of that, there isn't much more corner that they could cut" (McMullen, 1979).

After the birth of the two test-tube babies, Steptoe and Edwards were celebrated worldwide. They presented their results at a meeting of the Royal College of Obstetricians in January 1979 and left the hall to a standing ovation. Reporting on that meeting, Professor R. V. Short of the MRC Unit of Reproductive Biology in Edinburgh commented: "It is interesting that there was no comment or questioning about risks, and absolutely no adverse criticism of the investigators. . . . In retrospect, one wonders how it was possible to justify this procedure to women initially, without any assurance that it would work. Was it reasonable to carry out the surgical procedures involved in the absence of any knowledge about the normality of any embryos that might result from it? Has the woman who had the twenty-week abortion benefitted from such an experience?"

He added: "We must applaud the perseverance of the investigators and their technical achievement, even if we have misgivings about their ethical approach to their patients. In the wave of professional euphoria that follows, and spurred on by the potential financial rewards in return for a relatively minor outlay in expenditure, many people will try to follow in Edwards' and Steptoe's footsteps."[21]

Indeed, the British "feat" as it is often termed, both culminated the race to be first and set off a scramble among teams of gynecologists and physiologists around the world to repeat and then outdo the feat.[22]

In Australia, a team formed in 1970 and headed by Professor Carl Wood of Monash University in Melbourne (a former collaborator with Steptoe and Edwards) reorganized and accepted 101 women for "treatment" in 1979. It successfully grew seventeen embryos from these women and transferred them into wombs. Only two pregnancies developed, both at Royal Women's Hospital.

On June 23, 1980, one of these women, Linda Reed, gave birth to Candice, Australia's first and the world's third test-tube baby. She was "one of the most expensive babies in the world," costing more than $1,500,000, New Zealand's Evening Post reported (7/5/80). The excited staff of the hospital's maternity ward pinned a notice on the ward door congratulating the head of the IVF team. Team member Dr. Alexander Lopata said after the birth: "What happened today is extremely important for our team" (DT, 6/24/80).

By early 1982, fourteen test-tube babies had been born in Australia, twelve of them "produced" by the Monash group headed by Wood and Dr. Alan Trounson. Australia had become the top contender in the IVF race and Australian newspapers reported this scramble as a sports event. "More Join Test-Tube Baby Race," proclaimed *The Australian.* Declared *The Bulletin:* "Australian scientists have taken the lead in the race to perfect the 'test tube' baby technique with the announcement in Melbourne of eight pregnancies including two sets of twins—a world first."[23]

Melbourne's Monash University took to issuing bulletins with birth scores such as: "Monash, 8, Rest of the World, 2" (*The Age,* 6/25/81).

By 1984, nine additional IVF teams were operating in Australia. The most successful team, Monash, had modified the techniques of Steptoe and Edwards. The main reason for the team's increased success rate, it believed, was its return to the techniques Steptoe and Edwards had abandoned. It superovulated women and controlled the timing of ovulation.[24] It also used ultrasound (high frequency sound waves) to help determine when ovulation was imminent. Through the use of an ultrasound scanner, it was able to see the ovary and watch the follicles ripen.

The Monash group added another variation to the IVF technique. Since 1976, it had been working on a technique, developed after research on cattle, to freeze human embryos. In early 1981, Trounson revealed that for more than a year his team had been freezing 3-day-old human embryos, thawing, and implanting them. Some embryos, on thawing, were seen to have been damaged by ice or chemicals. But one embryo, stored for four months before being thawed, did "take" when implanted in a woman. Excitement at what was believed to be the world's first pregnancy resulting from a previously frozen embryo proved premature. Twenty-five weeks into the pregnancy, in July 1983, the woman endured a miscarriage. True success came to the Monash team a year later. The world's first frozen-thawed baby, a blue-eyed girl, was born March 28, 1984, by cesarean section.

This was one reason the team gave for freezing embryos: The hormones administered to women to control ovulation may interfere with the condition of the uterus so that it is not able to hold on to a transferred embryo. By freezing the embryo, they can transfer it during a later cycle, allowing the woman to recover from surgery and hormones in the meantime.

If parents consented, Trounson said, the normal excess embryos would be frozen for possible later reimplantation rather than discarded. Trounson said he hoped someday that women who produce eggs might be able to give them to women who do not. (That "someday," as we will see, arrived about one year later.)

The United States came onto the scene late. Because of the ethical questions raised by in vitro fertilization research, the government had essentially placed a moratorium on this research by prohibiting the use of federal funds until the issues were aired. The Department of Health, Education and Welfare (now Department of Health and Human Services) appointed an Ethics Advisory Board (EAB), which held hearings in 1978.

One of the arguments presented for federal support of in vitro fertilization research was that the United States should lead the world in pioneering this technology, not take a second place to other nations. A witness testifying before the EAB deplored the fact that the first test-tube baby was British rather than American. He complained that the moratorium on federal support had led, in effect, to an "in vitro fertilization gap" (quoted in Kass, 1979).

On the day Louise Brown was born in Britain, doctors Howard and Georgeanna Jones, former associates of Edwards, moved to Norfolk, Virginia, to begin work at the Eastern Virginia Medical School. When asked by reporters if they could set up a test-tube baby program in Norfolk, the Joneses replied yes—if the money were forthcoming.

It was. An anonymous benefactor donated funds to launch the program. The clinic obtained a certificate from Virginia's commissioner of health after stormy public hearings during which anti-abortion forces protested the potential wastage of embryos in the procedures, and some charged the doctors with experimentation on women. The Joneses survived the hearings and opened the clinic on March 1, 1980.

They began by allowing women to ovulate naturally, as Steptoe and Edwards recommended, but switched to "controlled ovulation" after ten unsuccessful months, when news of the Australians' success using hormones reached them.

On December 28, 1981, America's first test-tube baby, Elizabeth Jordan Carr, was born, as many of her predecessors had been, by cesarean section.

By 1984, well over a hundred IVF teams had set up clinics, largely in the industrialized world. The countries in which clinics operate include France, Austria, Sweden, Italy, Germany, Holland, Switzerland, Australia, Israel, Japan, Yugoslavia, Belgium, Finland and Canada. (Pharmacrats at Toronto East General Hospital named their in vitro program LIFE—Laboratory Initiated Fetal Emplacement.) In England, Steptoe and Edwards had launched a private IVF clinic at Bourne Hall, Cambridgeshire, in September 1980. Other clinics had opened in a number of Britain's leading public hospitals. In the United States, following Norfolk's lead, at least sixty-one clinics sprouted up in cities across the country.[25] The directors of three of these clinics predicted that every American university and city hospital, and perhaps even every group of doctors, would open test-tube baby clinics (McManus, 1982).

According to *Contemporary Ob/Gyn*, as of February 1984 the hundred-plus clinics around the world had produced approximately two hundred test-tube babies. There were scarcely more test-tube babies, then, than test-tube baby teams.* There is, moreover, some question as to whether all those designated as test-tube babies actually are. Some of the women who reportedly delivered IVF babies still had intact oviducts so there is the possibility that they conceived their babies naturally. Pointing this out in a letter to the *American Journal of Obstetrics and Gynecology* (1982), Dr. Leonard B. Greentree of Columbus, Ohio also noted that the very first supposedly sterile patient who had requested IVF at the Norfolk clinic had become pregnant the natural way while waiting to be admitted to the clinic for the IVF procedure. "If this event had occurred only a few weeks later, this normal pregnancy would have been heralded throughout the world as a feat for 'test-tube' babies as a whole," he wrote. "Instead, this particular birth was literally swept under the carpet with no fanfare whatsoever."

While test-tube baby teams are popping up everywhere, there are even more forming than have been publicly announced. Some American medical centers conducting or planning IVF programs are avoiding publicity because of possible opposition in their communities (Sullivan, 1981; Klemesrud, 1983).

Most of us think IVF has been developed to help women with blocked oviducts, but expansion of the medical indications for IVF beyond this condition began early.[26] From the start, pharmacratic teams in Britain, the United States and Australia used IVF on a variety of women: on women who had antibodies against sperm (despite the fact that the relationship between sperm antibodies and infertility is unclear); on women with infertility due to "hostile cervical mucus" (the "hostility" of the woman's body being directed against the sperm); on women in whom the cause of infertility was unknown and might, in fact, reside in her male partner. Use of external fertilization for this purpose was "obviously a gamble,"

---

* By September 1984, *Time* was reporting that 700 test-tube babies had been born, and that there were approximately 200 IVF clinics around the world (Wallis, 1984).

researcher Dr. Roger V. Short has commented.* Today, IVF is used on healthy, fertile women in order to enable their infertile male partners to have children. Women with bad tubes will be a very small percentage of the people for whom IVF will be useful, said Dr. Cecil Jacobson, chief of the Reproductive Genetics Unit at Fairfax Hospital, in an interview in 1980, only two years after Louise Brown's birth. "The biggest population [for external fertilization] are going to be men with low sperm counts," he said.

These men are often infertile because too few of their sperm reach the fallopian tubes to fertilize an egg. But if the sperm is placed in a lab dish with an egg, it can—unless it is defective— fertilize that egg. (Evidence suggests that the fertility of these men is depressed, not just because their sperm count is low, but because the few sperm they do produce may be abnormal in some way, Dr. Roger Short has pointed out [Short, 1979b].)

"With test-tube babies, we can help men who only produce a thousand sperm," Jacobson explained. "We can help men whose testicular development is not normal: they make sperm but they don't come out." IVF can also help men who were exposed to diethylstilbestrol (DES); men who are paralyzed; men with war injuries, he added.

At the American Fertility Society meeting in 1982, a panel of IVF experts—Patrick Steptoe of Britain, Howard Jones of the United States and Alexander Lopata of Australia—agreed that there was no reason why IVF should not be used to help men with low sperm counts. (This was, according to Dr. Jones, perhaps the most exciting new indication.)

I did find a reason and this is it: The procedures are not performed on such a man but rather on the woman he married. She, rather than he, would bear the burden of hospitalization and exposure to the risks of repeated general anesthesia, repeated surgery, trauma to the ovaries and uterus, amniocentesis, ultrasonic radiation, and the unknown long-term effects of hormones administered her. (It might be argued that this woman, wanting a child herself, would willingly, even eagerly, seek IVF "therapy" on her own body to deal with her husband's condition. For a discussion relating to this point, see Chapter 9.) "Since the procedure would not be to correct any

* At the 1984 meeting of the American Fertility Society attended by leading IVF researchers including Steptoe and Edwards, Dr. M. C. Chang, an elderly man who, twenty-five years earlier, had been the first to fertilize a mammalian egg in vitro, rose to his feet to complain emphatically that physicians were using IVF much too often in treating women. His position was not a popular one.

defect in her but rather that of her husband, it would be one step further from the usual medical criterion that intervention is for the benefit of the immediately afflicted," Grobstein wrote (1979).

Externalizing fertilization opens up many options for researchers besides that of helping men with low sperm counts. Pharmacrats do not necessarily have to transfer the fertilized eggs into a woman's uterus. Instead, for example, they could test new drugs and chemicals on embryos (Mastroianni, 1979, p. 5). Or they could take cells from embryos to repair defects in other human organisms, thus using embryos to "therapeutic advantage," as Edwards phrased it (Edwards and Steptoe, 1980, p. 187). Embryos could be left to grow in the laboratory until nervous tissue formed and then transplanted into adults suffering from various forms of nervous disorders, including paralysis. It is possible, though unlikely, that the nervous tissue of an early fetus might be capable of overcoming paralysis by bridging a gap in the nervous system of the sufferer, wrote Professor Carl Wood, head of an Australian test-tube baby team (Wood and Westmore, 1982). In 1981, Professor Wood stated that some scientists were approaching his team at the Queen Victoria Medical Center in Melbourne with proposals for just this kind of "extremely imaginative" research. "You can see that using the human embryo not for itself but for what it can do to help others presents a whole new field of medicine," Wood said (Baker, 1981). Elsewhere he commented: "I am facing increasing demands from very imaginative and capable people who don't see any ethical problem in developing research in the test-tube field" (SHM, 1981, Oct. 28).

"Imaginative" applications of IVF technology include attempts to fertilize human eggs with gorilla sperm. This kind of experiment, Dr. Roger Short told a federal ethics board in 1979, might give insight into man's evolutionary origins. The sperm of man and gorilla are almost indistinguishable, he said. If the sperm of the four great apes could fertilize a woman's eggs in vitro, this would suggest that man and gorilla are more closely related than has been thought.

"The obvious fear would be that if fertilization occurred in vitro, somebody would be tempted to implant the human/great ape hybrid embryo back into the uterus of an ape, or even a human, or more simply, to inseminate a female great ape with human semen," Short told the board. "Someday, no doubt, such experiments would be attempted, and it is impossible to forecast their outcome." He suggested several safeguards including performance of the experiments on "dead human oocytes recovered from a cadaver at postmortem" (Short, 1979, p. 7).

Attempts to create chimeras (man/animal hybrids) also become possible with external fertilization, as Edwards wrote in 1971. Animal sperm would fertilize human eggs and a novel creature would subsequently be born. In 1981, Professor William Walters, a leading figure in an IVF program at Australia's Monash University, said the possibility of such hybrids horrified him. The human component within the hybrid or "parahuman" would be condemned to a demeaning situation, he said.[27]

Another possible variation: Human sperm might fertilize the egg of an animal. Researchers showed in 1978 that it was possible to get human sperm to fertilize hamster eggs in vitro. This provided a technique for examining the genetic makeup of human sperm. "It is probable that experiments will be proposed that will call for the use of human embryos obtained by means of in vitro fertilization," Dr. Barton Childs told a federal ethics board, "and which have nothing to do with infertile couples or even the reproduction process, and some decision will have to be made as to the ethics of the employment of such embryos for these purposes" (Childs, 1978).

While pharmacrats are keenly aware of these and other uses of IVF, public discussion of the technology focuses on it as a form of therapy and a means of expanding options. The objective of Steptoe and Edwards' work, Dr. Grobstein wrote, "was to give new hope for children of their own to couples suffering from forms of infertility" (1979, p. 1). This is a typical presentation of the technology. Dr. Arthur Levin's is slightly different. With the "spectacular advance" of external fertilization and embryo freezing, he wrote in *Parents* magazine, couples might have children at the precise intervals they wished. Such child spacing might save babies' lives: "It has been shown ... that when women have children spaced too closely together, there is a higher risk of conceiving babies with genetic defects. They might be able to avoid the risk if, when they are young, an egg is extracted from the wife, fertilized in the lab with her husband's sperm, and frozen for use years later" (Levin, 1978).

This language of therapy used in describing IVF obscures the fact that medicine is not just a healing art but is also an institution of social control. IVF gives the power structure potent tools for such control. It makes a certain scenario possible: the application of animal husbandry to human beings in processes that will reduce women to breeders and offer a centralized group of white men control over who is born into the world. This would not necessarily be a conspiracy or even a conscious policy. The efforts of diverse men to create technologies that will increase male control over women and reproduction may be unformalized and intuitive, but nonetheless effective.

External fertilization does make "human husbandry" possible, as embryologist Grobstein terms it. Once an embryo is formed in a petri dish, there is no technical necessity for the embryo to go into the uterus of the woman who produced the egg.

Because fetal tissue apparently does not trigger the rejection reactions that occur when organs are transferred between children and adults, any woman capable of bearing a child may be able to receive the embryo. "The surrogate mother could act as a deputy for the genetic mother, *being no more than a vehicle for bearing somebody else's baby, as is common with farm animals*" (my emphasis) (Scott, 1981, p. 217). A leading Australian researcher in human external fertilization points out that in such cases, the maternal role would be divided between the ovarian and uterine mothers (Walters, 1976). The identity of the woman entitled to be called "mother" could then become a matter of legal dispute.[28] In separating genetic parentage from gestational maternity, Grobstein notes, offspring could be born who, given social constraints and the individual choices of lovers, otherwise never would have been. "As an example," he wrote, "controlled inbreeding could be practiced, as with domestic animals, to emphasize particular traits judged to be desirable. This might lead to 'breeds' of people comparable to those of cats and dogs."[29]

Of course, benevolent rationales would be given for using certain women in the same way animals are now used. Surrogates could be employed in instances where an infertile wife has normal and accessible ovaries but no uterus. The wife's eggs could be surgically removed and fertilized in vitro with her husband's sperm. The embryo could then be implanted in a "deputy or surrogate mother," who would bear the child and then turn it over to the genetic mother.

Professor Carl Wood pointed out that in addition to cases where a woman's health would be threatened by pregnancy, "fear of pregnancy or conflicting career interests (perhaps in the case of a professional model) might also lead to consideration of the surrogate option" (Wood and Westmore, 1983). Obviously in these cases "the surrogate option" would be a class-related phenomenon. No cleaning woman or factory worker with "conflicting career interests" will be hiring the wife of a doctor or a businessman to bear her babies for her. Quite the reverse. Those of her class will be the breeders.

While pharmacrats emphasize the therapeutic uses of the technologies, these technologies do make tools available for a eugenic program. Consider the tools:

Egg Donation

Australia's National Health and Medical Research Council issued guidelines on IVF research approving egg donation in 1982. The first birth of a child conceived with a donated egg occurred in Australia in November 1983. The mother was a woman in her midtwenties who was infertile because of an abnormally early menopause. The IVF team at Monash University in Melbourne fertilized the donated egg in the laboratory with the sperm of the woman's husband.

Beginning their work only four years after Louise Brown's birth, the Australian team made at least fifteen unsuccessful attempts using eggs donated by women in their IVF program before they achieved a birth. Transfers had been attempted in women with genetic disease, or without ovaries, or with ovaries from which eggs could not be obtained, Dr. Alan Trounson reported. Professor Carl Wood, head of the Monash team and Trounson's colleague, said that more than three hundred couples enrolled in his IVF program had expressed a willingness to accept a donated embryo. Forty couples were asked if they would donate an embryo and only two or three objected, he said. He added that sisters and friends of infertile couples had expressed a desire to donate eggs for IVF (SMH, 1982, May 5).

Pregnancy was achieved in one of the early transfers in a woman who received a donated egg fertilized by donor sperm. At ten weeks' gestation, the woman had a spontaneous abortion of an abnormal fetus.

The work of Trounson and Wood was briefly interrupted when the government placed a moratorium on use of donor sperm and eggs in the state's two IVF programs. (The moratorium was requested in October 1982; but on the advice of the IVF team's hospital ethics committee, the team continued using donor eggs until March 1983 on women already in the program. It then ceased all such work.) Dr. Trounson threatened to resign, saying his work was being frustrated by the moratorium. It was "unfair and discriminatory," he said (Wright, 1983). The moratorium was lifted on December 16,

1983, following a report by a government-appointed committee favorable to the research.

In 1984, Professor Wood announced that he, other IVF researchers, and an ethics committee were discussing the future of "genetic breeding," the selection of sperm and ova for the production of a child to desired specifications.

"Already we have had couples come and ask us if a male other than the husband could donate sperm because they were not happy with the husband's appearance or personality," Wood said. "Similarly women have been asking for donor eggs because they're not happy with some aspect of themselves."

Among those aspects were appearance and intellectual capacity.

Wood's team has not complied with these requests but if it received many more it might make a submission to the State Government committee examining the ethics and social implications of in-vitro procedures. The exact nature of the submission was not specified (Schauble, 1984; Whitlock, 1984, May 17; Milliner, 1984).

Given the low opinion we women very often have of ourselves, that internalized oppression that makes us feel a deep sense of inadequacy, one would expect that the use of donor eggs could, in time, become fairly common. This possibility will be heightened should authority figures act as if it were perfectly reasonable for us not to want to use our imperfect genes to produce our imperfect children. It appears likely that they will.

While Australia has led in the use of donor eggs, Dr. Joseph D. Schulman, a member of the IVF program at George Washington School of Medicine in Washington, D.C., predicted in 1983 that research using donor eggs could be expected in the U.S. in the future (OGN, 1983, July 1).

Dr. Cecil Jacobson of George Washington University is enthusiastic about the use of donor eggs. If donor eggs were used, he told me, many women—not just the infertile—could be helped by IVF, including those with genetic diseases, endometriosis, hyperthyroid, and a history of miscarriage. It could also help older women, perhaps in their 50s, who have been "scared off" maternity, afraid that if they bore a child of their own, it would be defective. Finally, Jacobson said, it could help women who do not produce good eggs, possibly because their eggs were damaged by exposure to toxins in the workplace. This is a large group of women and will expand as our knowledge of the effects of workplace toxins on eggs grows, Jacobson believes.

Dr. Jacobson's suggestion that donor eggs be used as a treatment for women with defective genes is one that appears frequently in the literature on, and in discussions of, in vitro fertilization. For example, a physician in the Paediatric Genetics Unit at the Institute of Child Health in London argued in 1979 (only one year after Louise Brown's birth) that the prevention of genetic disease was one of the most compelling reasons for the development of egg donation and embryo transfer techniques. Sperm donation (AID) could be considered for genetic defects on the father's side and egg donation for defects on the mother's side, he wrote.[30]

Dr. Jacobson believes that the "very large group of people" who produce poor eggs or have genetic diseases will use the eggs of other women and will not mind doing so. "The process of pregnancy is much more important to a woman than is the origin of the sperm and egg," he said. (Women I talked with questioned Jacobson's assertion.) This would mean that a large number of women would not reproduce themselves.

Egg donation can be used with IVF and with the Seeds' embryo transfer technique. In both procedures, donors for eggs must be selected. This allows pharmacrats to make eugenic decisions about who is fit to be reproduced. Seed himself is fussy about the quality of women he uses in his embryo transfer program. He has used some women in his research on egg flushing whom he would not use for an actual transfer, he said during our interview in Chicago. He added that they were "very nice girls but I would not use them as donors mostly because they are a little crazy as far as I am concerned. They are kooky. And I'm not interested in transferring eggs from kooky people."

The new reproductive technologies, Seed told me, "are basically techniques that have all been developed and will come to be developed to cure or treat certain infertility problems. But they're all capable of eugenic manipulation. I believe they will be used for that and I believe it is desirable and I'm not interested in the negative aspects being discussed. As a matter of fact, I don't think there are any negative aspects but in order to make it interesting, everybody wants to jazz it up and make some horror story out of it."

In talking openly about eugenics, Dr. Seed is unusual. Most pharmacrats present the technologies solely in therapeutic terms.

"We're not using donor ova yet," Dr. Robert Edwards of Britain told the press at the American Fertility Society meeting in New Orleans in April 1984. "We're about to start this." Pointing out that sperm donation was an accepted practice, he added: "We think it is unfair to a woman not to be able to give a donated egg."

Donor eggs, he explained would be useful for women with genetic defects. "Many couples are responsible," he said. "They are to be commended that they don't want to bring an abnormal child into the world."

Sperm Donation

Sperm donation could also be used with in vitro fertilization. In cases where the husband has a low sperm count and his wife has blocked tubes "we have extended the technique of in vitro fertilization by utilising donor sperm," wrote doctors Ian Craft and John Yovick in 1979 after setting up an IVF program in London's Royal Free Hospital (Craft, 1979, Sept. 22). That was only one year after the birth of the first test-tube baby.[31] Further, sperm donation could be used as a means of sex predetermination by placing the egg in culture with only male-producing or only female-producing sperm. Researchers are now working on developing methods for separating the two types of sperm.

"Embryo Adoption"

Sperm *and* egg—in other words, the entire embryo—could be donated as well in cases where both husband and wife are infertile or have "defective" genetic material. "In the future, it may be possible for the test-tube baby procedure to reduce the incidence of, or eliminate, certain defects from the population," wrote Professor Wood. "For example, where both partners are carriers of recessive genes that in combination would result in a major birth defect, it may be possible to select eggs and sperm cells that would avoid such a situation." Embryo donation, he writes, can be seen as prenatal adoption.[32] The embryos would be conceived in the laboratory using the eggs and sperm of genetically "healthy" strangers and implanted in women labeled genetically diseased.

Sterilization

A common scenario in science fiction involves a world where everyone is sterilized, frozen eggs and sperm are stored in banks, and a scientific elite determines who may reproduce. Real-life pharmacrats are also quite aware that laboratory reproduction could be linked with sterilization, though they usually present the linkage in benevolent terms. For example, the late geneticist Dr. Hermann J. Muller wrote that in places like India where (allegedly) voluntary male sterilization was prevalent, sperm banks should be established: "For when vasectomy is complemented by stores of sperm kept in vitro, the process of procreation thereby achieves its highest degree of control" (Muller, 1961, p. 648). Muller has made the object of the persistent linkage between reproductive technology and sterilization clear: control.

Researchers also link the use of embryo transfer and of in vitro fertilization to sterilization. When the federal ethics board held hearings on IVF, Dr. Robert Edwards wrote the board that while he and Steptoe would continue their work "to help the infertile" with IVF: "We equally intend to develop our methods for the reversal of sterilization. Tubal occlusion [i.e., sterilization] could then be used by women to limit their fertility, relieving them of years of steroidal contraception [the Pill, etc.] in the knowledge that they could conceive another child in the event of remarriage or the death of their family" (Edwards, 1979).

Dr. Carl Djerassi, who helped develop the Pill (a steroidal contraceptive women might well yearn to be relieved of, considering its multiple adverse effects), had a similar notion: If women think they can always use IVF to bear a child, they will more readily agree to be sterilized. In a discussion of techniques to sterilize women, Djerassi wrote: "If this currently controversial procedure [IVF] ever becomes a routine, widely used method of conception, it could have a major impact on the acceptability of sterilization among women."[33]

Sterilization and gamete storage may at first be presented as "insurance," a new option enhancing people's lives. That could change. We are already seeing rationales for compulsory sterilization and laboratory reproduction. The rationales are "overpopulation" and genetic deficiencies. "It would easily come about that overpopulation would force us to put a stop to general fecundity, and then, to avoid discrimination, to resort to laboratory reproduction from unidentified cell sources," ethicist Dr. Joseph Fletcher wrote (Fletcher, 1976, p. 335). Elsewhere, he had stated: "As things stand now, such is the moral lag between medical science and popular attitudes, there is no law requiring genetically unfortunate people to give up 'normal' sexual reproduction and turn to adoption or artificial insemination or egg transfer" (Fletcher, 1974, p. 49).

Embryo Freezing

Before sterilization could be combined with in vitro fertilization, pharmacrats would need a way to freeze and store the eggs extracted from women. In 1982, Steptoe and Edwards announced plans to freeze newly fertilized human eggs and store them in a bank for use by the natural mother or for donation to infertile women. On a television program in England, Edwards said that spare embryos could be donated, with the permission of the genetic mothers, to women who were unable to conceive a child (NYT, 1982, Jan. 29). Plans to transfer the embryos were temporarily abandoned in the controversy that followed the researchers' announcement. The team is indeed freezing the embryos but is awaiting a go-ahead from the Warnock Committee, a British ethics commission, before thawing and transferring those embryos. The Warnock Committee report is expected sometime in 1984.

Australian researchers also established an embryo bank and, as we have seen, produced the world's first "freeze-thaw" baby in 1984.

Dr. Richard Seed of Chicago plans to freeze human embryos in the future. He knows of three groups in the United States now working on freezing embryos but when asked to name them, declined. "They're being very quiet about it," he explained.

One group that has made its work on freezing embryos public is the University of Southern California Medical Center in Los Angeles (OGN, 1983, Aug. 15).

When the egg freezing technology is perfected, the American Association of Tissue Banks will be ready. In its provisional guidelines for sperm banks published in 1980, it stated: "Guidelines for cryobanking human eggs and embryos also will be devised, as the state of the art dictates" (AATB, 1980, p. 37).

Would the human embryos frozen in banks be considered persons or property? If the embryo were property, it might remain in the bank and change hands as adoption became less frequent, observed Alan Rassaby of Australia's Monash University Bioethics Centre. "It may well be that a person could mortgage or sell an embryo," he said. Another issue that needs clarification, he stated, is whether the embryo could be passed on in a will when both parents died or whether the state would take over ownership of the embryo (Baker, 1981).*

* At the time this paragraph was written, the situation described in it had actually occurred though that fact had not yet come to light. In the spring of 1984, the IVF team at

So it may become possible to surgically remove eggs from a woman and freeze them. Later, a single egg could be thawed, fertilized in a dish, and then transferred to a woman's womb. "If such a procedure were perfected," Randolph Seed, the embryo transfer pioneer, said in 1978, "it could permit a woman, before undergoing irreversible sterilization, to put some mature oocytes 'in the bank,' so to speak, as insurance against a later change in circumstances under which she elects to have an additional child or children."

Suppose a woman puts her eggs in cold storage as Randolph Seed envisions. Once the eggs are banked, they need not be transferred into the uterus of the woman from whom they were taken. It would be most difficult for a woman to control the use of her extracted eggs. The control would pass into the hands of those who do the extracting and freezing.

Already the egg of at least one woman in an in vitro fertilization program has been lost. The woman, Nancy, who underwent surgery four times in Australia for egg harvesting, wondered if doctors had used her egg for someone else or had performed tests on it. No one would tell her at the time what had happened to her egg; she found out accidently that it had been lost.

"I could understand that a dish may have been tipped or something like that," Nancy said. "I found it difficult psychologically—and this is just me—hoping that they hadn't used it for someone else rather than me. But I know they wouldn't have, looking at it very logically. But that was just me and my mind playing tricks and you have to guard against that a bit" (ABS, 1981).

If certain frozen eggs—say, those belonging to women of color—were being thawed and returned to the bank lifeless so they

---

Australia's Queen Victoria Medical Center revealed that the previous year a couple who had supplied two human embryos frozen for transfer procedures had been killed in a plane crash. The couple were Mario Rios, 57, a California property developer who was a millionaire, and his wife Elsa, 40. Their embryos are in storage at the medical center. The question has been raised as to whether the embryos should be destroyed or implanted in some woman's body and raised to maturity, whereupon they would receive a share of the millionaire's estate. One anti-abortion group that wants legal guardians appointed for the embryos strongly opposes the thawing of those embryos. Thawing would be tantamount to abortion, it contends. The issue is unresolved. A legal committee set up by the Victoria state government in Australia is reviewing it (NYT, 1984, June 18; NYT, 1984, June 23).

After resigning as chair of the committee coordinating social/psychological research into donor programs at Queen Victoria because she was in moral conflict over the speed of the test-tube baby team's advances in reproductive technology, social psychologist Dr. Robyn Rowland commented: "We've not even considered that we are going to have frozen embryo banks and suddenly we have got them and we're talking about their ownership" (Whitlock, 1984, May 25). (For more on Rowland's resignation, see the Afterword.)

could never engender a child; if eggs were mixed up accidently or were purposely transferred into others without the "donor's" knowledge, we would not know it. (Some of us might suspect but then dismiss our suspicions as tricks our minds were playing on us.) There would be as few whistle-blowers in the clinics as there are now in industry, medicine and government. On rare occasions, some clinic employee would talk. There would be a scandal. But after the storm, business would continue as usual. There are periodic storms now over the unjustifiably high hysterectomy rate in this country, but gynecologists ride them out and go on operating, decade after decade.

Problems could arise even with unfrozen embryos. In 1983, IVF pioneers expressed concern about the commercial exploitation of IVF. Private gynecologists could present themselves as IVF specialists and pay central laboratories to do the fertilizations for them. Under such circumstances, there was considerable danger that a woman might be given the wrong embryo, Dr. Robert Edwards said (Veitch, 1983, June 6).

Embryo Screening

Embryo screening is another of the methods external fertilization provides for controlling the nature of the child born through the process. (This method is also available in the Seed brothers' embryo transfer process as we saw in Chapter 6.) The embryo can be screened for "defects" (that category capable of infinite expansion) and for gender before a decision is made as to whether to transfer it. In 1982, the directors of three IVF clinics—Dr. Richard P. Marrs of Los Angeles, Dr. Martin Quigley of Houston and Dr. Anne Colston Wentz of Nashville—predicted that in the future test-tube embryos will likely be screened to eliminate those with birth defects or those of a sex their parents do not want.

First, screening for defects: "Pieces of tissue can be removed from blastocysts and used to type certain characteristics of the embryo and one method of alleviating the birth of children with inherited disorders would be to place *an embryo of the correct genotype* [my emphasis] into the uterus," wrote Steptoe and Edwards a year before Louise Brown's birth (Edwards and Steptoe, 1977). This is embryo evaluation, the practice used now in cattle. The late Dr. Pierre Soupart had applied for a grant to evaluate the health and sex of human embryos, a procedure that, he maintained, was "a matter of practicing preventive medicine" (McMullen, 1979).

Second, screening for gender: The fact that studies on sex preference consistently show a stronger preference for sons than daughters should make this procedure worrisome. The child's sex could be selected by snipping off a piece of the embryo, examining its chromosomes and discarding embryos of the undesired sex. In a 1970 article, Edwards and his wife and colleague, Ruth Fowler, suggested that several embryos could probably be "grown" for each couple. "The embryos replaced in the mother could be chosen for various characteristics," they wrote. One of those characteristics was gender.

One method of evaluating embryos would be dividing them to identify their sex and detect genetic diseases, a procedure already carried out with animal embryos. Both halves of the embryo can grow to become complete entities. Pharmacrats can check one half for defects and, if it is found acceptable, implant the other. Speaking before reporters at the 1984 American Fertility Society meeting, Dr. Robert Edwards predicted that IVF teams would begin dividing human embryos. "We could select the most healthy embryo to put back in the mother," he said.

Genetic Engineering

Finally, external fertilization offers pharmacrats this option in controlling the quality of human beings produced through women: genetic engineering. "The earliest procedure in genetic engineering ... is artificial insemination," the *Journal of the American Medical Association* noted in 1972. "Next ... artificial fertilization ... next artificial implantation ... in the future, corporeal gestation ... and finally, what is popularly meant by genetic engineering, the production—or better, the biological manufacture—of a human being to desired specification."

Here is how IVF makes genetic engineering feasible: The period between the fertilization of an egg in a dish and the transfer of that egg into the uterus is what Dr. Grobstein calls the "open window." During this period, he notes, the embryo is accessible for observation "or for various manipulations." Once pharmacrats develop techniques for genetic engineering, they could adjust the embryo's genetic makeup before transferring that embryo.

"The procedures leading to replacement and implantation open the way to further work on human embryos in the laboratory," Edwards and a colleague wrote (Edwards and Sharpe, 1971). In 1981, Professor Wood, leader of an Australian IVF team, said it might be possible to produce a "superbaby" with all the undesirable qualities removed by genetic engineering, the Sydney *Telegraph* reported (Kaplan, 1981). In 1983, the late Dr. Raymond Vande Wiele, co-director of an IVF clinic in New York City, told *The New York Times* that within ten years, doctors should be able to reach "the ultimate goal": correcting a family's genetic defects outside the womb (Klemesrud, 1983).

A contributor to a nursing journal, jubilant over the birth of Louise Brown, ridiculed fears some may have that, with external fertilization, the genetic engineering of embryos becomes possible. Experiments with genetic engineering are kept under strict governmental control, the article inaccurately maintained. One can be reasonably sure that "no 'devil' will be allowed to be born," it stated. Presumably to reassure those who still feared the manufacture of a "devil," it added chillingly: "Medical and genetic science is advanced enough to control possible behavioural disorders" (NJI, 1978).

Such are the implications of "human husbandry." The burden of this human husbandry will fall on women but researchers will present the burden as a boon, a gift to women, "therapy," "preventive medicine," an expansion of options allowing women richer lives, lives free of the "risk" of producing defective children. The technology will enable women to exercise their "right" to bear babies. It will eliminate inherited diseases and birth defects by controlling which particular eggs and sperm meet in the petri dish; it will expand the choices and "options" open to parents as to the sex of their child and the timing of its birth; and it will improve the species by upgrading the gene pool. In short, the technology will improve life for all human beings but specifically for mothers and babies. Through the control of consciousness—always more efficient than force—women will be grateful for the animal breeding techniques applied to them and will, in fact, pay for them.

Notes

1. "The *material* consisted of 17 *patients* . . ." (my emphasis) (Rannevik, 1980, p. 92). The Nuremberg Code on human experimentation states: "The voluntary consent of the human subject is absolutely essential. This means that the person

involved should ... be so situated as to be able to exercise free power of choice, without the intervention of any element of force, fraud, deceit, duress, overreaching, or other ulterior form of constraint or coercion; and should have sufficient knowledge and comprehension of the elements of the subject matter involved as to enable him to make an understanding and enlightened decision.... There should be made known to him the nature, duration, and purpose of the experiment" (United States v. Karl Brandt et al., 1946–1949).

2. In the studies researchers published on their attempts to recover, study and/or fertilize women's eggs, there is, in almost every case, no indication that the women consented to the extraction of their eggs or even knew that their eggs had been taken. (That consent may possibly have been obtained from women in one study is hinted at by the use of the adjective "volunteer" in the following sentence: "The ovum donors, who were volunteer women of infertile married couples ..." [Soupart and Morgenstern, 1973].) It is impossible to tell from the reports if the women were told anything at all about the planned research on their eggs. I am referring to the following articles, all of which report on attempts to recover women's eggs or to experiment with them:

—Noyes, 1965
—Clewe, 1971
—Soupart and Strong, 1974
—Edwards, 1966
—Rock and Menkin, 1944 ("Utilizing the surgical material available at the Free Hospital for Women ...")
—Menkin and Rock, 1948
—Rock and Hertig, 1948
—Shettles, 1955 ("The ovum was aspirated, with a 20-gauge needle and syringe, from a mature follicle of a normal ovary in a patient undergoing laparotomy about the middle of her menstrual cycle.")
—Shettles, 1958
—Shettles, 1953
—Pincus and Saunders, vol. 75, no. 4
—Mastroianni and Noriega, 1970 ("Ovarian tissue was removed at laparotomy from patients in the reproductive age group and placed immediately in warm culture medium.")
—Edwards, Bavister and Steptoe, 1969 ("We thank Professor N. Morris and Drs. M. Rose, J. Bottomley and S. Markham for ovarian tissue.")
—McMaster, 1978 ("Immature oocytes were collected at laparoscopy ...")
—Kennedy and Donahue, 1969
—Taymor, 1980 ("The majority of workers carrying out oocyte harvest and in vitro fertilization ...")
—Mettler and Semm, vol. 5, no. 1 ("Over the last 10 years we have become accustomed to pelviscopy as a diagnostic and surgical procedure. It was, therefore, a natural extension of this research that led us to adapt the technique to include ovum recovery.")
—Jaszczak and Hafez, vol. 5, no. 1 (This study, the ultimate objective of which was to improve egg recovery rates in primates, was conducted on five monkeys and on forty-one women. The monkeys were injected with hormones. Their uteri and oviducts were flushed and their ovaries removed for study. The

women scheduled for hysterectomies were injected with hormones. The uteri and oviducts of some women were flushed, either while those organs were in the women's bodies or after they had been removed to the laboratory. The ovaries of other women were removed or biopsies were taken from them for study.)

—Liedholm, Sundström and Wramsky, vol. 5, no. 1 (These researchers in Sweden were trying to improve on Steptoe and Edwards' technique for transferring human embryos. Their subjects were five women scheduled for hysterectomy for "premalignant diseases." They placed a sham egg in a medium in a straw and then placed the straw in a syringe. The straw was small enough to be inserted into the uterus without dilating the cervix, the entrance to the uterine body. They injected the sham eggs into the women. After removing the uteri from the women, they cleaved the uterus through the uterine cavity and noted where the sham eggs had landed. They found that they had landed very close to where they had estimated they would land. "We thus feel that we have an instrument and technique suitable for transplantation of a human embryo.")

—Persson, vol. 5, no. 1

—Sundström, Liedholm and Nilsson, vol. 5, no. 1

In the following study, consent for injection was apparently obtained but the authors do not mention if they obtained consent for disposal of the eggs: Lopata et al., 1978 ("Eggs for in vitro insemination were collected only from women who agreed to have an injection of 3000 i.u. hCG 36–38 hours before the operation.")

Only three documents address the issue of consent to the use of gametes (sperm and eggs) for in vitro fertilization and subsequent laboratory studies of resulting embryos, ethicist Dr. LeRoy Walters found in a study of the literature on IVF. Walters quotes IVF pioneer R. G. Edwards who, in an early essay on ethical issues in IVF research, wrote: "When we first considered asking patients to help us, the early stages of fertilization had been accomplished in the laboratory by ourselves and our colleague, B. D. Bavister, using eggs taken from ovaries excised for clinical reasons unconnected with our studies. The clinical application of our work demanded that eggs be removed just before ovulation directly from the patients. They had to be given hormones—four injections over 8–10 days—followed by a minor operation (known as laparoscopy) in order to remove the eggs. The husband had to provide an ejaculate." Edwards then describes how he and his colleagues obtained informed consent from sperm and egg donors. Whether consent standards in effect in Great Britain at the time of Edwards' earlier studies (using eggs from surgically removed ovarian tissue) would have required the consent of women from whom the ovarian tissue had been removed is not clear from Edwards' statement, Walters comments. (See Walters, 1979, p. 37.)

3. McLaughlin, 1983, p. 41. Rock and Hertig, as well as their colleague Gregory Pincus, who also conducted experiments on human eggs, were partly inspired in their reproductive research by a novel which had been published a few years earlier, Aldous Huxley's Brave New World. Journalist Loretta McLaughlin, who interviewed both Rock and Hertig, reports this in her 1983 biography of Rock (p. 62). In Huxley's futuristic novel, pharmacrats fertilized, grew and hatched human eggs in the laboratory. Some of the eggs were preselected to develop into workers, others into rulers.

4. See Morgan, 1982, for a discussion of this research.

5. Rorvik, 1979, p. 94. In one of his papers, Shettles reported: "Follicular ova were obtained from ovaries prior to or immediately after their removal from patients undergoing gynecological surgery" (Shettles, 1953).

6. Ramsey, 1972. Can physicians legally remove eggs from a woman and experiment upon them without asking her consent? Perhaps. Under the terms of the federal government's guide to institutions on the protection of human subjects, a subject's informed consent to the use of her tissue is required only when she is at risk. "The regulations are silent as to the need for informed consent where the subject is determined not to be at risk," two attorneys have written. They surveyed seven hospitals in the Boston area to determine hospital policies. Only one clearly required the women's consent to use of her tissue. In the other hospitals, either no consent was required or hospital policy was silent on the issue. For example, at Boston University Medical Center, the lawyers wrote: "No consent is required to be obtained for the use in research of tissues discarded following routine clinical use" (Weiner and Levine, 1979).

7. Grobstein writes of "fishing for eggs" (1981, p. 21) and Steptoe of "harvesting" them (COG, Oct. 1977). The first egg hunting passage appears in Clewe, 1971. Also see Taymor, 1980. The second passage appears in Noyes, 1965.

8. A breakthrough in in vitro fertilization research came in 1951 when two researchers discovered, independently, that in a number of animal species sperm had to be "capacitated" before it could fertilize an egg. The secretions within the female genital tract, where capacitation usually took place, probably conditioned the sperm. The fluid available to early researchers as a culture medium for maturing and fertilizing eggs had been inadequate. Major improvements in that culture medium in 1956 and 1963 opened up the field of embryo culture. Sources for the section on the history of IVF researches are: Rock and Menkin, 1944; Menkin and Rock, 1948; Whittingham, 1979; Mastroianni and Noriega, 1970; Karp and Donahue, 1976; Soupart and Strong, 1974; Rock and Hertig, 1948; Biggers, 1979.

9. Claims were made in 1944 and 1948 by John Rock and Miriam Menkin; by Landrum Shettles in 1955; and by R. G. Edwards in 1966 to have fertilized human eggs in vitro. All claims were challenged on the grounds that criteria for fertilization were lax. The first egg Rock and Menkin claimed to have fertilized came from the ovarian tissue of a 38-year-old woman undergoing a hysterectomy for a prolapsed uterus (that is, one which had dropped down into the vagina) with an eroded, lacerated neck. Rock removed the woman's right oviduct and ovary along with her uterus though there is no indication these organs were diseased (Menkin and Rock, 1948). "The woman never knew it," journalist Loretta McLaughlin later reported, "but she was to become the mother-in-absentia of the first conception in a test tube" (McLaughlin, 1982, p. 82). For his experiments, Rock obtained sperm from interns. He had these men masturbate in cubicles on which he had hung large posters of nude women he had obtained in Sweden (McLaughlin, 1983, p. 78).

10. Edwards, 1980, p. 59. In 1969, two other investigators obtained ovaries that had been surgically removed from women. They tried to culture eggs from the ovaries in various media but only 45 percent of the eggs matured to any reasonable degree. Since that time, other attempts have been made to culture human eggs externally but with no greater success than earlier attempts. (See Kennedy and Donahue, 1969.)

11. Steptoe and Edwards began collaborating in 1968 "when Dr. Edwards was already working at Cambridge on the in vitro fertilization of mice and hamster ova and was anxious to test the method on human ova. He had been unable to obtain a steady supply of suitable *material* [my emphasis] until Mr. Steptoe began sending ova from ovaries removed during routine gynecologic operations at Oldham" (Lister, 1978).

12. As usual in this field, the results are contestable. Dr. Pierre Soupart has also been credited with having been the first to externally fertilize human eggs.

13. Edwards, Bavister and Steptoe, 1969. As Dr. Luigi Mastroianni pointed out during a course for physicians in 1981 (a course I attended), experiments with in vitro fertilization have been much talked about but there is a common misapprehension that these experiments are easy and have been accomplished many times. In fact, he said, they have been successful very rarely indeed. "The fact that it's been carried out so rarely in animals makes its success in humans all the more spectacular," he told his physician-students.

14. See the Boston Women's Health Book Collective's *Our Bodies, Ourselves,* one of my sources here, for a more complete description of the menstrual cycle.

15. In pointing out the lack of primate research, I am not arguing that my sister animals, whose lives I value, should have been violated before those of my own kind were. I am simply calling attention to the highly experimental nature of IVF technology in women.

16. If the egg is not fertilized, the corpus luteum remains about ten days, transforms again to form the scarlike corpus albicans (white body). Bleeding and tissue sloughing occur in the uterus. That is menstruation. The endometrial walls, thickened in preparation for the embryo, thin again.

17. Among possible reasons for the failure of embryo transfer are these:

—Since embryos develop more slowly in the dish than in the womb, the physiological state of the uterus might advance beyond that of the embryo.
—An embryo cultured in a dish may not release certain humoral or hormonal factors an embryo developed in a woman does. As a result, the endometrium may not be receptive to that embryo.
—The egg follicle may be damaged when physicians suck out the egg ("man-made ovulation") during surgery. When the damaged follicle is then transformed into the corpus luteum, it may malfunction, failing to produce enough hormones to stimulate the endometrium.
—The corpus luteum, lacking a hormonal signal from the cultured embryo, may not persist.
—Trauma to the ovaries during laparoscopy, or to the uterus during embryo transfer, may contribute to the failure.

18. Lopata, 1980. Lopata points out that Edwards and Steptoe monitored 78 women in their IVF research; the Melbourne group monitored 132 for a total of 210. But in an earlier series, during which they administered hormones to control the menstrual cycles of their subjects, Steptoe and Edwards had used additional subjects. Since I could not find, in any published report, the number of women involved in that first series of experiments, I asked Steptoe for the number during

an interview. He replied that, oddly enough, there were almost the same number as in the second series. So I have added 77 women to Lopata's figure, for a total of 287 subjects.

19. Prepared comments of Richard B. Payne presented at the public hearing on the Norfolk IVF clinic, Oct. 31, 1979.

20. The triumph for the British team culminated a race during which various participants would periodically shout that they had done it—had fertilized human eggs in vitro; had transferred those eggs to a woman's womb; had, in one case, produced live babies from the eggs—and the others, speeding on for the prize, would shout back that the victory claimants had *not* done it. I am referring here specifically to claims made by Dr. Douglas Bevis of Leeds University, England; Dr. Landrum Shettles in the United States; Dr. Subhas Mukherjee in India; and Steptoe and Edwards in England. Shettles, for example, said in an interview that he did not accept Steptoe and Edwards' claim to have produced the first test-tube baby because—among other reasons—they failed to document that claim. Steptoe and Edwards, for their part, cast doubt on the claims made by Douglas Bevis in 1974 that he had produced three test-tube babies. He had not documented his work, they pointed out.

In 1973, Shettles attempted human in vitro fertilization using Doris Del Zio as the subject. He had failed to clear his work with any board protecting the subjects of experimentation. His superior at Columbia Presbyterian, Dr. Raymond Vande Wiele, stopped the project after the egg had been exposed to sperm. In speculating on why Vande Wiele took this action, Shettles gives us a glimpse of the competitive atmosphere in which, in his view, he conducted his experiments: "The real problem, in my view, had to do with his resentment of the publicity I was getting.... He was the head of the department. I guess he felt upstaged" (Rorvik, 1981; for an account of the competition, also see Packard, 1977, pp. 245–249 and 241–242).

21. Short, 1979. Short, who had been on Britain's Research Council when it refused financial support to Steptoe and Edwards in 1971, had softened toward the researchers a decade later. Asked how he now felt about the Council decision, he replied: "It would have been impossible, I think, for any governmental organization ... to say intuitively, 'I think the process is going to be safe, we give it our blessing, go ahead and do it.' ... But, as so often happens, I think private enterprise has paid off and Edwards and Steptoe have got the practical results while those of us who have played it a bit more cautiously are still fiddling around" (Williams and Stevens, 1982). And what of the women "private enterprise" used?

22. Three months after the birth of Louise Brown, pharmacrats in Calcutta announced the birth of another test-tube baby. This baby, they claimed, had been frozen as an embryo for fifty-three days by a biochemical engineer who, while getting a master's degree in nutrition at Cornell University, had learned to freeze food. He joined the Indian team at the invitation of gynecologist and physiologist Dr. Subhas Mukherjee. Mukherjee had worked with animal embryos at Edinburgh University. Then he took a post at a public hospital in Calcutta where he was to conduct research on contraception. Instead, keeping his experiments secret, he worked on human embryos. After the birth announcement, the Indian government said it had known nothing of Mukherjee's experiments.

CBS reporter Jay McMullen interviewed Mukherjee after the birth: "Were you afraid then, that the publicity might result in a termination of your research?"

"That's right," Mukherjee replied. "We didn't want anybody to know about this, because we wanted to work."

When it achieved a pregnancy, the Calcutta team decided not to conduct amniocentesis, which, while detecting fetal abnormalities, also poses some risk of abortion. "Because particularly the pregnancy was so valuable in this case," Mukherjee explained to McMullen. "So, I [not necessarily the parents] would rather have an abnormal baby than no baby at all. You see, this is exactly what we tried to prove, that one can freeze and transfer human embryos producing a viable fetus" (McMullen, 1979).

Some researchers doubted Mukherjee's claim, calling it a hoax. The Indian Medical Association appointed a committee to examine his data—data Mukherjee could not authenticate. Describing his claim as "incredible," the committee said that the mother of the "test-tube" baby had conceived naturally. In June 1981, the humiliated Mukherjee hung himself from the ceiling of his home (Gupta, 6/26/81). A noted Delhi doctor who had known Mukherjee well said there was "intense jealousy" in the profession at Dr. Mukherjee's earlier success, the *Sydney Morning Herald* reported.

23. The race is on: "More Join Test-Tube Baby Race," *The Australian,* Jill Baker, 3/31/81. "Australian doctors and scientists are leading the world in the research race with test-tube baby programs." "Australia Leads World in 'Test-Tube' Baby Techniques," Ron Hicks, *The Bulletin,* 12/23/80. "Landmark Baby Is One Today," *The Western Australian,* 6/23/81. This newspaper boasted that the IVF team from Melbourne's Monash University "have put Australia well in the lead in the test-tube baby field."

One more example of the sportscasting mentality: "Babes on Ice in Test Tube 'World First,' " *Sunday Independent* (Australia), 5/6/81: "Human embryos are now being frozen and preserved in another world first for the test tube baby team at Melbourne's Queen Victoria Hospital."

24. The Monash team superovulated the women for reasons of cost efficiency. "If you're going to follow the woman's own natural ovulatory cycle and let her do the whole thing alone, you need to have operating theatres available at your beck and call," Dr. Trounson, Monash's "egg man" explained. "You need to have staff that are on call all the time to obtain the eggs. And of course if you admit a number of patients at once, they can all go [i.e., ovulate] together. So nobody really knows what's happening so if you can take over all that [unintelligible word] by just giving the girls an injection, you've really achieved something in terms of the cost of the procedure" (ABS, 4/4/81).

Cost efficiency was also the motive for an ovulation-induction procedure in an IVF program in London's Royal Free Hospital. *Medical World News,* referring to Dr. David H. Smith, a gynecologist with Royal's IVF program, reports: "But, adds Dr. Smith, the major reason for inducing ovulation with drugs rather than adopting Dr. Steptoe's technique of using a urinalysis kit to detect the onset of LH surge, is economics. In addition to having staff members on call to time the cycle, it cost $143 per person each month, he says" (MWN, 1980, Nov. 24).

25. COG, 1984, Jan., pp. 127–142; SPN, 1983, 1 (1–6). The U.S. IVF clinics are:

ARIZONA. *Phoenix:* Arizona Fertility Institute; Good Samaritan Medical Center

CALIFORNIA. *Los Angeles:* University of Southern California–Los Angeles County Women's Hospital. *Northridge:* Northridge Hospital Medical Center. *San Diego:* University of California, San Diego, Medical Center. *San Francisco:* University of California, San Francisco, School of Medicine.

COLORADO. *Denver:* University of Colorado Health Sciences Center; Reproductive Genetics In Vitro

CONNECTICUT. *Farmington:* University of Connecticut Health Center–John N. Dempsey Hospital. *New Haven:* Yale University Medical School

DISTRICT OF COLUMBIA. George Washington Hospital

FLORIDA. *Miami:* Jackson Memorial Hospital

GEORGIA. *Atlanta:* Georgia Baptist Medical Center; Reproduction Biology Associates

ILLINOIS. *Chicago:* Michael Reese Hospital; Mount Sinai Hospital; Rush–Presbyterian–St. Luke's Medical Center; Northwestern Memorial

KANSAS. *Kansas City:* University of Kansas Medical Center

KENTUCKY. *Louisville:* Norton Hospital

LOUISIANA. *New Orleans:* Tulane School of Medicine; Pendleton Memorial Hospital

MARYLAND. *Baltimore:* Johns Hopkins Hospital; Union Memorial Hospital

MASSACHUSETTS. *Boston:* Beth Israel Hospital; Brigham & Women's Hospital; New England Medical Center

MICHIGAN. *Ann Arbor:* University of Michigan's Women's Hospital. *Detroit:* Hutzel Hospital. *Grand Rapids:* Blodgett Memorial Medical Center. *Royal Oak:* William Beaumont Hospital

MINNESOTA. *Minneapolis:* University of Minnesota Medical School

MISSOURI. *St. Louis:* Jewish Hospital

NEVADA. *Reno:* Northern Nevada Fertility Clinic

NEW JERSEY. *New Brunswick:* University of Medicine and Dentistry of New Jersey

NEW YORK. *Manhasset:* North Shore University Hospital. *New York City:* Columbia–Presbyterian Medical Center; Mount Sinai Medical Center. *Rochester:* Childbearing by Alternative Reproduction (CARE) Clinic at University of Rochester Medical Center

NORTH CAROLINA. *Chapel Hill:* North Carolina Memorial Hospital. *Durham:* Duke University Medical Center

OHIO. *Cleveland:* Mount Sinai Medical Center. *Columbus:* Grant Hospital; Ohio State University College of Medicine. *Dayton:* Miami Valley Hospital

OKLAHOMA. *Tulsa:* University of Oklahoma, Tulsa, Hillcrest Infertility Center

OREGON. *Portland:* University of Oregon Health Sciences Center

PENNSYLVANIA. *Philadelphia:* Hospital of the University of Pennsylvania; The Pennsylvania Hospital. *Pittsburgh:* Magee–Women's Hospital

TENNESSEE. *Nashville:* Vanderbilt University Medical Center

TEXAS. *Carrollton:* Carrollton Community Hospital. *Dallas:* Presbyterian Hospital. *Houston:* Baylor College of Medicine; University of Texas Health Sciences Center. *San Antonio:* University of Texas Health Sciences Center

UTAH. *Salt Lake City:* University of Utah

VIRGINIA. *Norfolk:* Eastern Virginia Medical School

WASHINGTON. *Seattle:* Swedish Hospital Medical Center

WISCONSIN. *Madison:* University of Wisconsin Center for Health Sciences

26. *Australia:* At Monash University, of the 103 women Professor Carl Wood and Dr. Alan Trounson treated with IVF as of December 1980, 60 percent were

women with blocked tubes; 25 percent were women with unknown fertility problems; and 15 percent were women whose husbands had low sperm counts.

Dr. Alexander Lopata's group at Royal Women's Hospital and the University of Melbourne performed IVF on women with tubal disease; sperm antibody problems; intractable endometriosis; infertility of unknown cause; and on women whose husbands had semen abnormalities.

In Australia, IVF has also been used as a diagnostic tool to indicate whether the infertility problem resides with the sperm or the egg. Operating on the woman under general anesthesia, doctors remove two eggs from her. They place one egg in a petri dish with the husband's sperm and the other egg in another dish with sperm from a donor of known fertility. If the donor's sperm fertilizes the egg and the husband's does not, the researchers would suspect that the husband's sperm was defective. (In neither case would they know for certain.)

United States: In a paper delivered before a meeting of the American College of Obstetricians and Gynecologists in Washington, D.C., and dated September 29, 1980, Dr. Howard Jones of the Norfolk (Virginia) IVF clinic said that IVF should be applicable in four situations: low sperm production; hostile cervix; "infertility in the 'normal infertile couple' "; and tubal disease.

Britain: Steptoe and Edwards listed these indications for IVF in 1979: tubal damage; low sperm count; prolonged infertility of unknown origin (idiopathic); presence of sperm antibodies; the control of sex-linked diseases (Short, 1979b).

27. (SMH, 6/5/81.) This is a speciesist comment, which considers only the consequences to the human being important and not those to the other animal involved. Philosopher Peter Singer defines "speciesism" as "a prejudice or attitude of bias toward the interests of members of one's own species and against those of members of other species." He compares speciesism to racism and sexism (Singer, 1975, p. 7).

28. One law professor cites a series of possible cases involving Mrs. A., "the biological mother" who provides the egg, and Mrs. B., "the hostess mother" who carries the pregnancy: Mrs. B. fails to register the child's birth in the agreed-upon manner; she requires an abortion; she refuses to hand the child over to Mrs. A; Mrs. A refuses to accept the child. The question involved in all these cases, the law professor writes, is: "Who is the mother of the child?" (Cusine, 1979).

29. Medical ethicist Dr. Janice Raymond thinks an important factor is left out in discussions on the genetic determination of traits. People who cared about developing certain traits in children enough to actually breed for those traits would probably take great pains to ensure that they also got the social conditions necessary for the emergence of those traits. They would control the social context. That social context (not solely the genes) would be an influential factor in whatever happened.

30. Marcus Pembrey, letter to *Lancet*, 10/13/79. "It was encouraging to note that about half of [Ian] Craft's patients who undergo elective sterilization would allow ova to be donated to an infertile couple," Pembrey wrote. "Perhaps a similar proportion would donate ova to couples facing a high risk of transmitting a serious genetic disease." Ethicist Joseph Fletcher agreed that IVF could be used not only as therapy for infertility but to improve "quality of life." One legitimate purpose of IVF would be "to avoid passing on a woman's genetic defects by substituting a donor's egg for implant. In short, it [IVF] may be done for reasons of either

pathology or quality of life" (Fletcher, *Journal of Reproductive Medicine,* 1973).

In 1979, Steptoe told a meeting of the British Association for the Advancement of Science in Edinburgh he saw no reason why a donor egg should not be fertilized in a petri dish and then implanted in the womb of a woman who had a genetic disease ([Sydney] *Sun,* 8/7/79). Margery W. Shaw, a physician and lawyer with the Medical Genetics Center at the University of Texas, approves such a procedure. Artificial insemination by donor has been accepted for use in avoiding genetic disease or defect, she pointed out, adding: "In vitro fertilization by egg donor is the flip side of the same coin." Access to IVF should not be restricted to infertile married couples, she argued. Such a restriction might even open up a hospital to a lawsuit. If a hospital offering both IVF and AID denies a request for IVF by an egg donor for genetic reasons while offering AID for those same reasons, then an equal protection argument could be made for the couple who are refused as patients, she noted (Shaw, 1980, p. 4).

31. In the Monash IVF program, in cases where sperm cells may be contributing to infertility, the couple may be asked if they want the wife's eggs to be fertilized with the husband's sperm only or with those from a donor, or with both. If embryos develop from both the husband's and donor's sperm, the couple must then decide if one or both embryos should be transferred into the wife's womb (Wood and Westmore, 1983).

32. The British medical journal *The Lancet* calls it "embryo adoption." In an editorial, it asked: "And where infertility has both male and female contributory factors, what about embryo adoption, as a means of offering the fulfillment of pregnancy, childbirth and parenthood?" (12/5/81, vol. 11, no. 8258).

33. Djerassi, 1979, pp. 150–151. Djerassi and Edwards are not the only researchers in the field to have linked sterilization with this new technology. Dr. Landrum Shettles has noted that IVF's potential for bypassing blocked uterine tubes "might have the greatest impact in the reversal of the effects of voluntary sterilization by tubal interruption, which is increasingly the method of choice for 'permanent' fertility control in the human female" (JRM, Nov. 1979). Steptoe has also observed that a woman who was sterilized could give several eggs that could be fertilized by her husband's sperm at a later date and be implanted into her uterus (SMT, Jan. 1980).

8

Doctor-Induced Infertility and Other Risks

Pharmacrats often claim that their experimentation on women with IVF is justified by the natural right women have to bear babies. This "right" is pulled out when it is useful in an argument justifying IVF but shoved aside when it interferes with control over a woman's reproduction. A woman has a "right" to bear babies unless, that is, her nation needs fewer workers or she is the wrong color or the wrong class and it's necessary to forcibly sterilize her or inject her with hazardous contraceptives.

ITEM: One reason for treating infertility, wrote Professor Carl Wood, head of a Melbourne IVF team, "is in the interests of a particular nation. For example, where government policies rely on population growth and where 10 to 15 percent of the population is infertile, it would seem compatible with national interest to treat infertility." Many policies of the Australian state, he added, were based on a predicted population increase. In other countries where state policies relied on keeping population growth down, it may not be in the national interest to treat infertility, he stated (Wood and Westmore, 1983, p. 16). Yet when Wood is justifying his IVF program, he cites the United Nations Declaration of Human Rights, which includes a right to establish a family.[1] Apparently that basic human right is void for a woman who lives in a Third World country judged to be overpopulated.

ITEM: At the same time physicians are proclaiming the right of women to reproduce, sterilization abuse continues. In the United States, the abusers are physicians and the abused are predominantly poor women and women of color. In several lawsuits, such women have charged that they were sterilized against their will; that they were pressured into signing a consent form to the operation while they were in labor in maternity wards; that they were led to believe the operation was reversible; that, to their confusion, they were addressed in English when their language was Spanish. Such sterilization abuse has been amply documented by reports from the Health Research Group in Washington, D.C.; the Centers for Disease Control, and the General Accounting Office; and in testimony before the House Subcommittee on Oversight and Investigations.[2]

In a survey reported in the January 1972 *Family Planning Digest*, 94 percent of physicians who responded favored compulsory sterilization of welfare mothers with three "illegitimate" children or withdrawal of benefits if they refused. These were obstetrician-gynecologists, the very professionals who are proclaiming themselves defenders of woman's right to reproduce.

ITEM: In justifying IVF programs, pharmacrats loudly cite the right of women to bear babies while occasionally acknowledging, in quieter tones, that not all their patients are childless. In the Melbourne IVF program, according to Wood, it makes no difference to the priority given to couples if they already have children (Wood and Westmore, 1983, p. 56).

Many women who enrolled in IVF programs were indeed parents. A few examples: At the time she gave birth to Australia's first test-tube baby, Linda Reed had a son, Daniel, born to her four years earlier. The mother of Australia's seventh test-tube baby had a 3-year-old son, Jared. The mother of the eighth had three children from a previous marriage. Catherine Rankin, mother of the first test-tube twins born in North America, had two teen-age children from an earlier marriage.[3]

ITEM: Woman's "right" to bear a child evaporates if she fails to do so under the conditions prescribed by the patriarchy. The basic condition is that she be legally bound to a man. Physicians and other pharmacrats, the vast majority of whom are white, male and middle to upper class, choose which women are endowed with the right to bear test-tube babies. They choose "deserving and appropriate patients," as a Norfolk clinic physician terms them (Andrews, 1979). These patients tend to be white married members of a heterosexual, two-parent family. After studying the morality of IVF research, the federal Ethics Advisory Board recommended in 1979 "that embryo transfer be attempted only with gametes obtained from lawfully married couples" (DHEW, 1979). The Norfolk clinic and most others have indeed refused access to the technology to independent women.

ITEM: In at least one Australian IVF program, "deserving and appropriate patients" must be able to speak English "to facilitate communication" (Johnston, 1981). There are millions of immigrants in Australia—Italians, Turks, Greeks, Yugoslavs, Lebanese and Indochinese—and, depending on the proficiency of their English, this requirement would help bar them from the program. At the same time non-English-speaking women are barred from the IVF program, other women of low status are allegedly being injected with a hazardous contraceptive. The women's health movement in Australia has often alleged that tribal Aboriginals, the poor and mentally handicapped, have been special targets for use of Depo-Provera, an injectable contraceptive associated with cancer in two animal species and with other serious, debilitating "side" effects, including impairment of fertility beyond the anticipated period (NT, 1981; RTC, 1981; Corea, 1981).

How did "deserving and appropriate" women in IVF programs become infertile in the first place? There are at least 4.3 million married women in the United States, or somewhat under 15 percent of married couples, who are infertile though some feel those figures vastly underestimate the extent of the problem.[4] Some women have reproductive tract or hormonal abnormalities they were born with or developed due to natural events.

The fertility of others may have been impaired by herbicides, by pesticides and by hazardous wastes dumped in their neighborhoods (Barlow and Sullivan, 1982; CEQ, 1981; Van Strum, 1983). This worries Barbara Menning, founder of Resolve, an organization that counsels infertile couples. "I think the reproductive organs are the miner's canary of the human species," she says. "When our miscarriage rate approaches 40 percent in some areas near illegal chemical waste dumps and nuclear reactors; when our children are born defective, not in the 5 percent range, but in the range of 25 percent where Dioxin has been used; when our infertility rate approaches 20 percent as it will be in the 1980s—then I think we as a species are in deep trouble" (Menning, 1981).

Still other women became infertile as a result of excessive surgery or of earlier experimentation on them with contraceptive drugs and devices. The patriarchal mentality that views nature (and "nature" includes women) as a force to be controlled and mastered has created the pesticides, contraceptives and herbicides now jeopardizing human fertility (Corea, 1984). Women then "need" the further experimental drugs, devices and surgery involved in external fertilization. The fertility-saving technology is, in many cases, being delivered by the same men who brought women the earlier fertility-destroying technologies. So physicians, who have contributed to the impaired procreative capacity of some women, now plan to make (certain) women (partially) fertile again.

These are some of the medically induced ways in which women have lost their fertility:

—Through infection (PID, or pelvic inflammatory disease) caused by: an intrauterine device (IUD); sexually transmitted diseases, which the medical profession makes only a token effort to prevent; or cesarean sections performed for questionable reasons
—As a consequence of taking the Pill or Depo-Provera
—As a result of reproductive tract abnormalities induced by diethylstilbestrol (DES)

When physicians are diagnosing pelvic pain, doing an infertility work-up, handling certain obstetric problems, or otherwise treating women, they sometimes use procedures that can impair the woman's fertility. At a district meeting of the American College of Obstetricians and Gynecologists in 1981, Dr. William R. Keye urged his fellow physicians to stop doing this. Alternative, nondestructive procedures are often available, Dr. Keye of Salt Lake City pointed out.

"We may cause more infertility than we care to believe," he later wrote in a magazine for ob/gyns. Noting the 36 percent rate of iatrogenic (doctor-caused) illness reported on a certain hospital service, he added, "Our experience also suggests that iatrogenic infertility is common." He reported that of sixty-five women with pelvic disease who were evaluated for infertility at the University of Utah Medical Center, twenty-five (38.5 percent) had previously undergone obstetric or gynecologic procedures that may have contributed to the disorder.[5]

Pelvic infection is the leading cause of infertility in women because it can damage the reproductive organs. In an interview in August 1984, director of the national VD hotline, Remy Lazarowicz, estimated that one million women in the United States suffer from pelvic inflammatory disease (PID) and its consequences annually (1982 statistics). More than 60,000 women become infertile due to PID each year. In women who have had PID, the risk of ectopic pregnancy, which could destroy their oviducts, is seven to ten times higher than in women who have not had the disease (OGN, 1980, June 1). Among the causes of PID are gonorrhea,[6] obstetrical surgery,[7] and the IUD.[8]

The doctor-inserted IUD has caused infertility; so has doctor-prescribed DES, a synthetic hormone. Despite the fact that there has never been any clear evidence that DES could prevent miscarriage, physicians gave the drug to women in the 1940s through the 1970s for that purpose. DES has since been associated with impaired fertility in daughters born to those women.[9] (Also, a small percentage of the DES daughters—as they have come to be called—developed vaginal cancer or cervical clear-cell adenocarcinoma.) On the unsubstantiated theory that DES would ensure a strong pregnancy, many obstetricians had also routinely prescribed the drug to women without a history of miscarriage. When one woman asked a doctor just what drug he was giving her, her doctor replied: "This is a hold-the-baby-in pill" (Corea, 1985).

DES daughters who have difficulty "holding the baby in" may look upon that phrase with bitterness. They have a high incidence of upper-genital-tract abnormalities and impaired reproductive outcomes, investigators have found. Dr. Charles Mangan, head of the DES clinic at the University of Pennsylvania School of Medicine and one of those investigators, said: "This will probably turn out to be more of a problem than the adenocarcinoma associated with diethylstilbestrol (DES) exposure." Reliable data suggests that these daughters have an increased risk of ectopic pregnancies.[10] Such pregnancies could damage the woman's oviducts, thus making her a candidate for more intervention: in vitro fertilization.

The Pill, too, may be linked with infertility in some women. It has been found to halt ovulation in certain women. Those who have had irregular menstrual periods or impaired ovulation are at particular risk (Kleiman, 1979). Some doctors believe Pill-induced sterility may be caused by damage to the ovaries or endometrium (Seaman, 1980, pp. 100–107).

That pharmacrats opt for an invasive, unreliable, expensive cure for infertility such as IVF rather than establish practices to prevent infertility appears at first strange. But it is strange only if curing infertility is what IVF is all about. As I argued in Chapter 7, it is not.

Infertile women, who have often been injured by previous medical treatment, the risks of which had been downplayed to them, enter IVF programs, the risks of which are being downplayed to them. There is a terrible consistency in this.

Reviewing the ethical literature on IVF, Dr. LeRoy Walters, director of the Center for Bioethics at Georgetown University, notes that "relatively little attention has been devoted to risks to the

would-be mother" (Walters, 1979, p. 18). But as with DES, the Pill
and the IUD, risks exist. They include:

—Hormonal treatment to superovulate her. A major complication
is hyperstimulation of the ovary. The overstimulated ovaries enlarge
greatly and form many cysts. Severe hyperstimulation, though rare,
is life-threatening. In one study of 101 women, four experienced
severe hyperstimulation requiring hospitalization (Jewelewicz et al.,
1973). "Hyperstimulation with powerful fertility drugs can literally
blow them [the ovaries] up or burn them out" (Menning, 1977, p.
134).[10] In the settings in which IVF is now carried out, careful
monitoring has greatly reduced, though not eliminated, the risks of
hyperstimulation. But if human IVF becomes an industry, as one
pioneer in the technology has speculated it may (DeCherney, 1983),
and if thousands of for-profit clinics pop up around the world
operated by physicians without the requisite training, hyperstimulation could become a more serious problem.

—Possible adverse effects of hormones.[12] The long-term effect
of these hormones on women are not known and may never be
known. These women may have subsequent health problems which,
if they are common enough, may not be attributed to the hormones
given them years earlier. At a conference on reproductive technology,
Dr. Maureen Flannery, a family physician in rural Kentucky, said
that this was what frightened her about the DES story: The only
reason DES was discovered to be a cause of cancer was that it caused
a *rare* cancer, vaginal adenocarcinoma. If it had caused an increase
in more common diseases such as breast or uterine cancer, its
carcinogenicity would not have been discovered. Doctors might still
be prescribing it to pregnant women. If the hormones administered
to women in IVF programs turn out to cause *common* cancers or
other diseases, the diseases may never be traced back to the IVF
programs.

—Possible trauma to the ovary caused by sucking out the egg.
We do not know whether the surgical manipulation involved in IVF
procedures adversely affects the ovary's secretion of hormones and
all the bodily processes affected by those hormones. Pharmacrats
puncture the follicle in order to aspirate the egg. That follicle is
transformed into the corpus luteum, which secretes hormones that
help maintain the pregnancy. The full effects of the manipulation of
the follicle are unknown.[13]

—Repeated operations, with attendant risks of anesthesia.
Women in IVF programs have undergone up to seven operations

under general anesthesia for "egg recruitment."

Dr. James Schlesselman has noted the possibility that, while IVF may in itself not induce abnormalities in embryos, the medical treatments used to establish an implantation and maintain a pregnancy may enable defective embryos to survive. If this were true, there would be more spontaneous abortions of IVF embryos than of those conceived in a woman's body. (In fact, the spontaneous abortion rate *is* higher for IVF fetuses than for those conceived naturally [COG, 1984, Jan.; Jansen, 1982].) So more attempts would be needed to achieve a live birth through IVF.

"Because of this, the implications of in vitro fertilization appear to be much greater for the mother than for the child," he wrote, "in that the mother would be repeatedly subjected to the costs and risks associated with the surgical procedure for the collection of mature ova and the hormonal treatment to induce superovulation and achieve implantation" (Schlesselman, 1979, p. 146).

—Risks accompanying the tools and procedures for monitoring an IVF pregnancy. These include ultrasound radiation, amniocentesis (the withdrawal and study of amniotic fluid from the uterus), and endometrial biopsy.

—Potential damage to the uterus during embryo transfer.

—Infection introduced into the uterus during the embryo transfer.

—Ectopic pregnancy. This complication, in which the embryo fails to implant in the uterus, is potentially life-threatening. The ectopic rate for IVF pregnancies is higher than that for normally conceived pregnancies—5 to 10 percent compared to .5 to 1 percent. (The rate for normal pregnancies used to be even lower, .5 percent, but it has been rising in the last decade, probably because of increasing gonorrhea, use of IUDs and pelvic infections.)

Ethical discussions of external fertilization have focused not on risks to the woman, but on possible damage to the fetus. This concern was expressed at a 1979 hearing to determine whether the first IVF clinic in the United States should be certified. Dr. Howard Jones, clinic director, was asked then whether it was possible to predict the possibility that IVF would result in a malformed fetus. "Dr. Jones stated that, while this was an area of concern, it was not one of alarm," the minutes of the project review committee report. "He explained that there were no human data available but that, on the basis of a large amount of animal data, this did not appear to be a problem" (EVHSA, 1979, Sept. 20).

While Jones, and Steptoe as well, argued that the animal work was reassuring, not everyone agreed. Embryologist Dr. Richard Blandau of Washington State University, Dr. Luigi Mastroianni, Dr. Pierre Soupart of Vanderbilt University, Dr. John Biggers of Harvard and Dr. Gene Sackett of the University of Washington all questioned this.

The statement is frequently made that hundreds of thousands of cows and sheep have been produced by IVF and embryo transfer without evidence of congenital abnormalities. That statement is incorrect, Dr. Blandau maintains. The vast majority of such cow and sheep embryos transferred were not fertilized externally. They were fertilized inside the animal's body and flushed out, using embryo transfer technology. Gross congenital abnormalities have seldom been recorded as a result of these transplants, he noted. But he asked: "Who would be concerned over any deficiency in creative ability in a cow or sheep?" (Blandau, 1980).

Just a year before Jones reassured the project review committee, Dr. Pierre Soupart questioned whether the data obtained from lab animals could be extrapolated (applied) to human beings "especially when the extrapolation concerns chromosomes, which are very specific for every single mammalian species." Soupart disapproved of his British colleagues trying to transfer externally fertilized human eggs *"without having studied systematically the possibility of chromosome aberration(s) which could possibly result from the IVF procedure itself"* (his emphasis).[14]

A further source of concern: Since 1973 several reports had indicated an increased level of chromosomal abnormalities in the aborted fetuses of rabbits, mice and women who had been chemically induced to ovulate (Whittingham, 1979).

In fact, there are several ways in which IVF could lead to the formation of defective fetuses.[15]

Some researchers worry about the effects of ultrasound—high frequency sound waves—on the IVF child. During the complicated IVF procedure, physicians repeatedly use ultrasound on a woman's ovaries to visualize the developing egg follicle. Such pictures give pharmacrats a rough guide to the likely time of ovulation. No one knows what that ultrasound is doing to the eggs in the ovaries. These eggs contain half the genes of a potential child. If ultrasound is injuring the eggs, this has ominous implications for the children born of those eggs.

Dr. Arthur D. Bloom, professor of pediatrics and human genetics and development, and director of clinical genetics at Columbia University College of Physicians and Surgeons in New York, worries about ultrasound. Despite the suggestions of some workers in the field that ultrasound is innocuous, its effects on human beings and experimental animals have not been well documented, he said during a seminar at the New Jersey Medical School in Newark in 1981. Citing several studies, Bloom said: "It's clear that ultrasound may prove teratogenic" (i.e., capable of producing deformity in the developing embryo).[16]

Embryologist Dr. Richard Blandau, a lean, alert man in his sixties, is worried too. During discussions on the use of ultrasound in IVF programs, he forcefully told physicians at the American Fertility Society meeting in 1981 how serious his concern was. His audience was cool to him. Perhaps sensing this, Blandau said before one of his presentations: "I'm going to tell you things a lot of you won't like." And later: "I'm not trying to be an S.O.B. but I think it's important to recognize that there's room for more investigation in this field."

A baby is born with all the eggs she is ever going to have, he explained. Egg precursors—the oogonia—are transformed into eggs by reducing their number of chromosomes to half. What happens if, during this process, ultrasound radiation hits the eggs? No one fully understands the biophysical effects of ultrasound. There is not enough scientific evidence to assure that the radiation will not injure these eggs, he said.

"But how many people are looking at this?" he asked the fertility specialists. "I become significantly worried when young people talk about following the growth of the follicles [with ultrasound]." (Young men had been doing just that during an earlier presentation.) The cytogeneticists at the University of Washington, he added, "are beginning to have discomfort about this."

Blandau pointed out that the ultrasound equipment is not that good and is not well standardized. The machines do not show exactly how much energy they are giving out so physicians cannot control the radiation levels exactly.

"We can't forget the damaging effects of diagnostic X-rays on children," he reminded the physicians. "Diagnostic ultrasound is similarly being used before its full effects are known."

During a later panel discussion, Dr. Joseph D. Shulman, chief of the section of human genetics of the National Institutes of Child Health and Human Development, was asked about ultrasound's potential effects on genetic material. Noting that the issue has been "of some concern," and that the data on this point were incomplete,

Shulman replied: "So far the data are unconvincing for any genetic damage. The data suggest that the benefits of ultrasound outweigh the risks as we now understand them. This doesn't mean that assessment won't change with new information."

Blandau, a fellow panelist, leaned forward. "What *are* the data?" he asked Shulman.

"The data concern ultrasound used in prenatal diagnosis," he responded. "I'm not able to cite data on the effects of ultrasound on fetal oocytes."

"Exactly," Blandau said. "There *are* no data on the effects of ultrasound on the oocytes."

I sat in the audience, surrounded by physicians, thinking: These are the men who brought us the Pill, the IUD and DES and who thought the benefit/risk ratio for each was just fine. I recalled the questions nursing instructor Denise Connors raised about such phrases as "benefit/risk analysis": Whose benefit? Whose risk? Whose analysis? In the case of in vitro fertilization, it is the patriarchs who make the analysis, the patriarchs who reap the benefits in terms of increased control over reproduction, and women who take the risks.

As Blandau urgently voiced his concerns about what physicians were doing to women with those ultrasound rays, world experts on IVF sat in the audience and on various panels with him. None had information to reassure him. At the close of Blandau's most compelling presentation, after the sparse applause had petered off, a physician sitting directly behind me turned to one of those world experts beside him and said of Blandau: "He's getting old."

The expert laughed.

The possible risks to women involved in IVF experimentation never became an issue in the early years of the developing technology, so pharmacrats were not obliged to justify their treatment of women. (As we will see, their use of benevolent terms to describe their work and obscure its experimental nature, probably helped to ensure that this never became an issue.) But potential harm to the IVF child *was* an issue. Pharmacrats had to address it if they wanted to do their research on IVF and do it with a minimum of public protest.

In the years preceding and immediately following Louise Brown's birth in England, experts knew that there were potential risks to the child born of externally fertilized eggs. Some wrote of the risks in their scientific journals. But in public, proponents of IVF employed their status as experts and misused language to minimize those risks. They assured the world that it need not worry about the birth of abnormal babies through external fertilization.

Testifying in support of Norfolk General Hospital's application to open its IVF clinic in 1979, Dr. Roy Parker, chair of the Duke University Medical Center department of ob/gyn, stated at a public hearing: "This proposal [for] in vitro fertilization is scientifically sound and safe for mother and baby. Experimental and clinical data show that the embryo and the baby are at no greater risk for abnormal development than occurs in the usual in-life fertilization and migration of the egg to the uterus."[17]

Earlier, Steptoe had been equally reassuring at his first meeting with Lesley and John Brown in 1976. He and Edwards believed, he explained to them, that if they ever successfully fertilized eggs in the lab, the abnormality rate among the resulting offspring would be no greater than that following natural conception. If pregnancy occurred, he added, they could detect any serious abnormality through prenatal diagnostic techniques and abort the fetus. " 'Such an event, however, is unlikely,' I told them" (Edwards and Steptoe, 1980, p. 143).

How could he know that? At the time he was reassuring the Browns, no test-tube babies had ever been born and there were only a handful of test-tube mice, rats and rabbits. And in a paper published in 1970, he had stated that "the normality of embryonic development and the efficiency of embryo transfer cannot be assessed" (Edwards, Steptoe and Purdy, 1970). That same year, Steptoe and Edwards wrote that the eggs are retrieved from a woman's body during a stage of egg cell division that could be a sensitive one for the induction of chromosomal abnormalities.[18] One potential abnormality could result in Down's syndrome (mongolism). Furthermore, when an interviewer from Contemporary Ob/Gyn asked Steptoe: "If a woman became pregnant by this method [IVF], would her baby be normal?" Steptoe had replied in 1977, one year after he had reassured the Browns: "We don't yet have enough experience with humans to answer with confidence that all-important question."[19]

But two years later, Dr. Mason Andrews had managed to acquire confidence in the safety of the external fertilization "service" his Norfolk clinic was offering women. He wrote to the Virginian–Pilot in 1979: "On the basis of extensive authoritative scientific judgement those of us involved in the program are confident that the careful monitoring of pregnancies resulting from this process will detect no greater than normal incidence of problems."

Between Steptoe's comment in October 1977 and Andrews' in October 1979, only two human babies had been produced through external fertilization. Certainly those two births did not provide enough new data to justify Andrews' confidence.

Despite ignorance within the pharmacratic community as to the full risks of external human fertilization, some proponents of the technology even argued that fertilization outside a woman's body might be *less* risky than natural conception. Dr. Jack Rary of the Norfolk IVF clinic stated in 1979: "We actually believe the rate of risk might be less than with natural conception, because the egg and sperm will be kept in a much more sterile condition."[20]

A woman's body, then, is dirty?

And Dr. Mason Andrews wrote to a local newspaper: "The promptness of fertilization achieved in this program could even reduce the incidence of problems below the incidence in all naturally occurring pregnancies" (*Virginian–Pilot*, 1979, Oct. 10).

Yet these statements by Rary and Andrews are mere speculations, not backed up by any solid studies.

Dr. Howard Jones acknowledged in 1979 that no one knew what the risk of increased birth defects was with external fertilization. "At present, about 15% of pregnancies are genetically undesirable, and many of them are aborted," the *Virginian–Pilot* reported Jones as saying. "I don't want to minimize this problem; it is a concern we all have."[21]

That concern did not seem to be reflected in the consent form prepared for women in the Norfolk IVF program. Minimizing the risks, the form stated: "The risks of the development of an abnormal fetus are at this time basically unknown, although from animal experimentation and from what is known about the abortion of abnormal fetuses, it is anticipated that the risks will be no greater than the risks which are accepted by any couple who initiated pregnancy."[22]

Before opening its IVF clinic, Norfolk General Hospital applied for a "Certificate of Need" from the Eastern Virginia Health Systems Agency (EVHSA). The documents filed by the hospital with its application and reports from the EVHSA staff reveal that the proposed program, "Vital Initiation of Pregnancy" (VIP), was clearly experimental, not therapeutic. Norfolk General Hospital called the VIP program "a study" (EVHSA, Consent Form 33). And the EVHSA staff, in its report recommending approval of the clinic application, notes that the program, while viewed as a new service, "is primarily a research project" (EVHSA, 1979, Nov. 9, p. 4).

Medical language makes it easy to discuss the misuse of women without *recognizing* that misuse. For the word experimental, health professionals substituted "developmental." For research subject, "pa-tient." For experiment, "therapy," "treatment," "elective program," a "service."

By a tacit agreement to use such language, the physicians and EVHSA staff gave each other permission to conduct and approve experimentation on women. They kept up the fiction of a healing relationship with their research subjects and probably began to believe in it. If one person within this group had called the thing by its proper name, the mutual permission-giving would have been threatened.

The healing relationship was fictional because although healing was certainly intended to result, the researchers had very little reason to expect that, at this early stage, it would. The proper procedures for performing IVF were by no means established. This was little more than a year after the birth of the world's first test-tube baby. Only one other such baby had been born since then. Steptoe and Edwards, the team responsible for those two births, made so many wrong assumptions about matters, such as the best timing for uniting sperm and egg in the laboratory, that "the birth of Louise Brown now seems like a fortunate coincidence," stated Dr. Howard Jones, head of the Norfolk IVF team, looking back in 1984 (Wallis, 1984, p. 48).

The minutes of an HSA Project Review Committee for September 20, 1979 record: "Dr. Jones was asked if the controls over this program would be left to the doctor and patient. Dr. Jones stated that this procedure was viewed as additional help for the infertile couple and as such was a matter between the physician and the patient." Yet everyone involved had already acknowledged that this was a research project. In these very same minutes, Jones' project is referred to as an "experiment" and there is no record of his having protested the use of that word. Should control over an experiment be a matter between the experimenter and his clinical material ("The clinical material is located in Oldham," Steptoe had said of women) or should some mechanism have been set up to protect those women?

Note the juxtaposing of the words "patients" and "research" in these sentences from the EVHSA staff report: "the charges for this elective program will be paid for by the *patients* in the program. The program will take advantage of the presence on the Eastern Virginia Medical School of the highly qualified professionals needed to conduct this type of *research*" (my emphasis) (EVHSA, 1979, Nov. 9, p. 11).

Three women on the EVHSA board voted to disapprove the project. One was Irene Walsh, a Virginia Beach nurse. The *Virginian-*

Pilot reported: "Mrs. Walsh expressed confusion about the term 'research.' 'Is this a health-care service? Are we ready to determine it as a health care service?' T. Melvin Butler, a board member from Hampton, said he looked at it as 'applied research' " (Lockamy, 1979).

Both the researchers and the HSA staff claimed that the VIP program was, in addition to research, a "service" to couples. (In an understatement, the HSA staff did acknowledge that "the success rate is uncertain.") By calling the research a service, they could require women used in the research to pay the costs of the experiments, whether or not they were the beneficiaries. (The objectives of the research, the HSA staff noted, were not solely to impregnate infertile women but also to learn more about the hormonal aspects of the menstrual cycle and to time the occurrence of ovulation more precisely.)

Norfolk's *Ledger–Star* reported in 1979 that a local IVF clinic proposal "asking for about $200,000 in research money" from the U.S. Department of Health, Education and Welfare could not be submitted until HEW had decided whether it would fund IVF projects. "In the meantime," the newspaper stated, "patients undergoing preliminary tests must pay their own lab expenses," an estimated $4,000 per woman (Baksys, 1979, Nov. 24). It is unclear whether that meant that if the medical school had gotten the grant (it never did), the women would no longer have had to pay for the school's research.

Referring to Dr. Mason Andrews of the Norfolk clinic, *The Washington Post* reported: " 'Peculiarly,' he said, his pale blue eyes twinkling, 'this doesn't take much money. Because the people who want to use [the clinic], pay their own way' " (Colen, 1979).

It is highly unusual for subjects in a research project to bear the hospital charges involved in that research. These subjects, however, were not required to pay the salaries of the researchers. In an oblique acknowledgment of the experimental nature of the program at Norfolk, the HSA staff wrote: "Professional fees will be waived during the developmental stage of this project" (EVHSA, 1979, Nov. 9, p. 15). Andrews himself said: "There will be no physician charges as long as the procedure is considered experimental" (Colen, 1979).*

* In its use of medical language that renders the misuse of women invisible and in its willingness to allow "patients" to pay for its research, the Norfolk IVF team was hardly unique. Teams which followed Norfolk on the scene have generally taken the same approach. During a panel discussion on IVF at the 1984 American Fertility Society, panelist Dr. Alan DeCherney of the Yale IVF program, speaking of IVF researchers in general, commented: "Our studies are funded primarily by patient funds and that's not fair." The room was full of physicians running IVF programs but none insisted that this point was important and must be discussed. It was allowed to pass without comment.

Had the Norfolk researchers injured any of the "patients" in the experiment or any fetuses that may have resulted from the research in those early years, those "patients" would have received no compensation for their injuries or the injuries of their babies. They would not even have been entitled to free medical care from the institution that caused their injury and that benefited from the experimentation on their bodies.

Dr. Gerald Holman, dean of the Eastern Virginia Medical School, stated that the medical school did not have insurance for people injured by research, and that the medical school's test-tube baby project was "definitely" an example of research. The medical school could not afford to pay expenses of a child born with a defect because of the research, Holman said (Wallace, 1979).

Two years after Holman made his announcement, Dr. Luigi Mastroianni said during a course on in vitro fertilization held for physicians in conjunction with the 1981 American Fertility Society meeting: "I think there's a substantial risk of being sued for an abnormal child. I think it would be difficult to conjure up a defense. You'd be a sitting duck. That's O.K. We take risks when we think what we're doing is right." Dr. Alexander Lopata, another instructor of that course agreed that the possibility of being sued by a patient who had an abnormal child following IVF was a real problem.

Another physician had been trying to deal with the problem. He and a law professor drafted preliminary legislation that would absolve the doctor and hospital of legal liability for any defects in children produced through IVF. They announced the legislation at an international conference on legal medicine held in 1979. Under that proposed legislation, *Ob/Gyn News* reported, "no physician or institution would be held liable for the occurrence of genetic defects that are unpredictable on the basis of current medical knowledge" (Coren, 1979). Note that "current" knowledge concerning potential genetic damage was almost nonexistent at the time. It essentially consisted of twelve studies on mice, rats and rabbits conducted by researchers who, two scientists suspected, may not even have been systematically *looking* for abnormalities in the test-tube offspring (Biggers, 1979, pp. 32–34; Sackett, 1979, p. 3).

Dr. William J. Sweeney, II, of New York Hospital who, with a law professor, announced the recommended guidelines at the conference, told *Ob/Gyn News:* "It's important that laws come into effect before the procedures take place. God forbid anything occurs without any statutes . . . we'll be in real trouble. The Norfolk clinic really shouldn't do anything without them."

Attorney Mark E. Cohen took a different approach to the problem. In a law journal, he recommended that strict liability for birth defects attributable to their IVF experiments be imposed upon the experimenters. "Strict liability is imposed when the defendant's actions are abnormally dangerous," he wrote, "even though the defendant has taken all possible precautions to ensure the safety of the activity.... At present, IVF children are subject to abnormally dangerous risks" (Cohen, 1978).

Some years earlier, Dr. James Watson, co-discoverer of the DNA structure, had suggested an alternative method of handling the problem. The physician attending the birth of a test-tube baby should have "the right to terminate [the] baby's life should it come out grossly abnormal," he argued (cited in Walters, 1979, p. 17). No one has followed up his suggestion.

Notes

1. Dr. R. G. Edwards, the British IVF pioneer, has cited the same document. But that "right to marry and found a family" in Article 16 of the U.N. declaration surely does not imply a human right to enroll in programs set up by Wood and Edwards. It implies a right *to be allowed* to marry and found a family—against racist marriage laws, for example, or forcible sterilization (Daniel, 1982, p. 73).

How can we have a "right" to a biological feature or capability? Does everyone have a "right" to a certain IQ? To a 34-inch bustline? To blue eyes? To athletic prowess? Emily Culpepper and Ruth Hubbard raise these questions in Holmes, Hoskins and Gross, eds., *The Custom-Made Child?* (Clifton, N.J.: Humana Press, 1981).

2. "Test-tube twins born in Canada," *Daily News*, March 1982; "Boys 3, girls 7, on world test [tube] scoreboard," *Sydney Morning Herald*, June 29, 1981; "Now—it's a test tube Aussie; two babies ... race to be first," *The Sun* (Sydney), Feb. 6, 1980; Lopata et al., 1980.

Doris Del Zio, who was the subject of one of the first IVF experiments in the United States, had already given birth to a daughter. John Brown had a daughter from a previous marriage whom he and Lesley raised from the time the daughter was a child.

3. For details on these reports and accounts of cases of forced sterilization, see Corea, 1985; and contributions by Sandra Serrano Sewell and Helen Rodriquez in *Birth Control and Controlling Birth*, Holmes, Hoskins and Gross, eds., (Clifton, N.J.: Humana Press, 1980).

Dr. Rodriquez points out that sterilization abuse is not only the result of overt coercion or a lack of informed consent. "Abuse also occurs whenever an individual chooses sterilization because of his or her social and economic conditions.... The social problems which affect the poor have influenced many people ... to be sterilized. The lack of medical care, safe, effective contraception, and access to abortion create an atmosphere of subtle coercion. The present HEW policy which now reimburses 90 percent of the costs of sterilization while providing no funds for abortion is an example of the way in which options are limited and choices skewed."

4. The 15 percent figure is based on a study which is already outdated, the data having been collected from 1965 to 1976. There are no more recent studies. It is not possible to document whether the rate of infertility in the population is changing because there are no earlier studies with which to compare the most recent. However the prevalence of pelvic inflammatory disease, IUD use, and environmental toxins that impair fertility suggests to some observers that infertility is on the rise.

Roughly one in six couples at the present time are experiencing infertility problems. About half of these will overcome the problem and eventually achieve a pregnancy. Not all these infertile couples are childless. Of the 4.3 million currently married women in the U.S. aged 15 to 44 with impaired fecundity, 47.3 percent or more than two million women want to bear a first child (840,000), a second child (641,000) or an additional child (556,000) (National Center for Health Statistics figures cited in Walters, 1983).

5. "Iatrogenic factors may impede patient's fertility," *Ob/Gyn News*, May 1, 1981; Keye, 1982. Keye recommends, among other measures, that physicians use laparoscopy rather than laparotomy for diagnosing pelvic pain and that they avoid ovarian wedge resection when possible or use techniques that avoid the risk of adhesions. Among the procedures Keyes lists that can cause infertility are: cervical conization; dilation and curettage (D&C); endometrial biopsy; myomectomy; cesarean section; hysterosalpingography; tubal insufflation; oophorectomy; uterine suspension; hysteroscopy; and hydropertubation.

Barbara Menning, an R.N. and director of Resolve, an organization that counsels infertile couples, has also spoken out on doctor-caused infertility. Women with a history of infection or inflammation are at an increased risk of getting pelvic inflammatory disease (PID) after undergoing an X ray and dye study of the uterus and tubes during an infertility work-up, Menning notes. "Many doctors routinely prescribe that study even though they hear the woman say that she's had a previous history of infection or inflammation," she adds. "This shouldn't happen because there are other tests that can be substituted."

Judy Norsigian, co-author of *Our Bodies, Ourselves*, stated at a government-sponsored health seminar that the physician's lack of interest in, and/or knowledge about, prevention and treatment of diseases that may impair fertility is a major problem confronting certain women. PID, she said, was a good example. "All too often, signs of inflammation and infection are either ignored or overlooked, even when a woman herself might point out the important symptoms," she said. "Sometimes, these symptoms are passed off as psychosomatic. We have heard numerous accounts of failure to remove an IUD at the first sign of infection. . . . One wonders how long it will take before the IUD's capacity to inflame the uterine lining and the wick-like role of the IUD in spreading infection will be part of the awareness of almost all practitioners" (Norsigian, 1978).

For more information on doctor-caused infertility, see "Lower pregnancy rate seen after endometrial biopsy," *Ob/Gyn News*, Jan. 15, 1981; Milligan, 1981. Milligan states that physicians contribute to infertility by failing to deal adequately with nongonococcal urethritis (NGU) and PID. Both diseases can affect fertility. Treatment of these diseases is frequently medically mismanaged, she writes.

6. According to the Centers for Disease Control, about 273 cases of PID caused by gonorrhea occur every year in the U.S. Clearly, to preserve fertility, venereal diseases should be prevented. But the physicians who insist they must launch external fertilization programs demand no such preventive health program. They know that if condoms and vaginal contraceptives were more widely used, many venereal diseases and the PID and infertility that sometimes result from them would be prevented. They do not share this knowledge with women.

"In the area of prevention, [physician] failure to inform women about the prophylactic benefits of condoms and certain vaginal contraceptives continues to be a problem" (Norsigian, 1978). It is still a problem today, Norsigian said in an interview in 1984.

See "PID of venereal origin reaching epidemic status," *Ob/Gyn News,* June 1, 1980, p. 14. The social costs of this PID include infertility in 20 percent of cases and a sixfold to tenfold increase in the risk of developing ectopic pregnancy, Dr. James W. Curran of the Centers for Disease Control said.

7. While gonorrhea causes about 273 cases of PID every year, other factors, including obstetrical surgery, cause an equal number. The cesarean section rate has increased by 156 percent in one decade and with that increase has come a rise in fertility-threatening reproductive tract infections. Increased interventions in normal childbirth by obstetricians and an expansion of indications for cesarean section that remain unjustified by scientific studies account for the rise in birth surgery. See Marieskind, 1979; Corea, 1980. Infections are much more common among women who give birth surgically than vaginally. In one study, cesarean mothers had a 20.4 percent rate of uterine infection while women with vaginal delivery had a 1.4 percent rate (cited in Banta and Thacker, 1979, p. 14). Also see:

—F. Gary Cunningham, 1979, Sept. "Treating infections following cesarean section," *Contemporary Ob/Gyn,* 14: 77–82. Cunningham: "Ours [infection rate following cesarean] at Parkland [Memorial Hospital in Dallas] is high because we have many examinations; we have students, we have residents . . ."
—Leigh G. Donowitz and Richard P. Wenzel, 1980, "Endometritis following cesarean section," *AJOG,* 137(4): 467–469.
—John P. Elliott, 1982, June, "The case for antibiotic prophylaxis before some cesareans," *Contemporary Ob/Gyn,* 19: 117–127. Elliott writes: "Infectious morbidity following cesarean section has been reported to range from 19% to 85% with most investigators reporting a 50% to 60% range. If half the patients delivered operatively develop febrile morbidity, a section rate of 20% means that 10% of all obstetric patients will be affected."
—D. Hagen, 1975, Sept., "Maternal febrile morbidity associated with fetal monitoring and cesarean section," *Obstet. Gynecol.,* 46: 260.
—Gogoi, 1971.

8. The risk of contracting pelvic inflammatory disease is four to nine times higher in women with an IUD than in those without it (Keye, 1982). This fact should come as no surprise; from its earliest days, the IUD went hand-in-hand with infection. In the 1930s and 1940s, the devices were associated with such a high rate of infection and other complications that the medical community abandoned them.

Nothing changed to make them safer. But in the early 1960s as fear of a "population explosion" spread through the land, population control groups fixed on the discredited IUD as one device that could bring the birth rate down. These groups declared that "new data" showed how very safe IUDs were. The "new data" consisted of two studies which, in fact, added nothing to the existent knowledge of the IUD. The author of one of the papers asserted that in his study, the IUD proved to be twenty-five times as safe as the diaphragm, an assertion any physician today would find laughable (Oppenheimer, 1959). Nonetheless, population control groups, using that and another study, convinced physicians of the IUD's safety. Physicians began inserting the devices on a mass scale.

By 1981, they were acknowledging that the IUD renders some women sterile. In the last four or five years, evidence has mounted pointing to a relationship between IUDs and a certain type of pelvic infection, Dr. William J. Ledger, chair of the ob/gyn department at Cornell University Medical Center in New York, stated that year. "A growing body of clinical evidence suggests a relationship between IUD use and infection," he continued. "Serious illnesses—even death from sepsis—have been reported in nonpregnant wearers."

Dr. Raphael Jewelewicz, an ob/gyn at Columbia University, commented that he did not want to condemn IUDs but he had a certain impression about many "nulliparas" (childless women) who had been coming in for the past several years for treatment of infertility: They were wearing IUDs and they had extensive pelvic adhesions. "I don't think I would recommend an IUD to an unmarried nullipara," he added. Dr. Ledger replied: "I wouldn't argue with that" (Richart, 1981).

For more information on IUD-related infertility, see:

—William L. Faulkner and Howard W. Ory, 1976, "Intrauterine devices and acute pelvic inflammatory disease," *JAMA*, 235(17): 1851–1853.
—Katherine Roberts, 1977, July, "The intrauterine device as a health risk," *Women and Health.*
—Claudia Dreifus, 1980, March, "Intrauterine devices: A story of pain—and risk," *Redbook.*
—Use of IUD said to double risk of acute salpingitis." *Ob/Gyn News*, 1980, June 1.

9. "Reproductive complication rate high among DES-exposed women," *Ob/ Gyn News*, 1981, Dec. 15.
For more information on DES–related infertility problems, see:

—"Fertility and infertility: What's new?" *Contemporary Ob/Gyn*, 1979, June. "Structural uterine abnormalities associated with exposure to diethylstilbestrol (DES) impair reproductive function according to investigators at Harvard Medical School, Boston."
—Decherney et al., 1981. The investigators found "withered" oviducts in eleven infertile DES daughters.

10. "DES and science," 1981, *DES Action Voice*, 3(2).

11. Also see Jewelewicz et al., 1973, "Ovarian hyperstimulation syndrome—relationship between preovulatory estrogen levels and ovarian hyperstimulation in gonadotropin-treated patients." In Rosenberg, ed., *Gonadotropin Therapy in Female Infertility.*

12. Among the hormones Steptoe and Edwards gave women in their experiments were: Pergonal (human menopausal gonadotropin); human chorionic gonadotropin; clomiphene; norethindrone; and 17-hydroxyprogesterone.

13. "It has been suggested that one of the reasons for the low frequency of success with present methods of human IVF is that some trauma occurs to the ovary in the process of removing the oocyte; this may produce adverse hormonal consequences (since the ovary is the main source of the hormones that support pregnancy) which could interfere with implantation" (Shulman, 1978).

14. Soupart, 1978. Referring to experiments begun around 1970 to externally fertilize human eggs that had been chemically induced to ripen within women's bodies, and then surgically removed from the ovaries, Dr. Laurence E. Karp wrote: "Although some apparently normal preimplantational embryos have been observed, there have been no studies of chromosomal or developmental normality among these zygotes" (Karp, 1978).

15. These are the ways in which IVF could lead to the formation of defective fetuses:

There is a risk (how great, nobody knows) that the external fertilization process could select defective eggs and sperm. The egg cells that ripen under artificial hormonal stimulation may not be those that would mature normally. Some unknown factors may control the normality of ovulated eggs, one researcher hypothesized during a government ethics board hearing on IVF (Gould, 1979). An egg recovered directly from a given follicle could be abnormal, he added. Dr. John Biggers of Harvard points out another problem area. Some types of abnormal sperm appear to be eliminated during the passage through the female genital tract. But the sperm placed in the petri dish have not passed through the woman's body. So, in omitting the normal sperm screening process, IVF may present an increased risk of fertilization by abnormal sperm. "The extent of this risk is unknown," Biggers commented. "The problem needs study . . ." (Biggers, 1979, pp. 32–34).

Another risk: The way in which eggs are exposed to sperm in the lab dish may result in an increase in triploidy. In this state, the fetus has three sets of chromosomes rather than the normal two. If physicians place higher concentrations of sperm near the egg than would normally reach that egg in the woman's body, the egg's natural resistance to fertilization by more than one sperm may be overwhelmed. Two or more sperm may enter the egg. (This is polyspermic insemination.) This may already have happened. At the same time Leslie Brown was pregnant with the world's first test-tube baby, recall, another woman in the IVF program aborted a fetus with sixty-nine chromosomes—three, rather than two, sets.

Biggers has noted: "There is no information available which allows the prediction of the possible incidence of abnormal babies." All we have to go on in making such a prediction, he pointed out, is twelve studies performed on mice, rats and rabbits. Abnormalities were reported in only two of those studies. "Why congenital aberrations occurred in only two out of 12 independent studies is unknown," Biggers observed. "A major concern is whether the different investigators were concerned and actively searched for congenital aberrations."

Dr. Gene P. Sackett made the same point to the federal Ethics Advisory Board: "Although there may actually be no abnormalities [in animals produced by IVF], these negative findings could have occurred because studies have not systematically looked for abnormalities in newborns and infants using sensitive measures. This is especially true for behavior. Neither cattle, rabbit, rat or mice infants have been adequately assessed to date in any published study" (Sackett, 1979, p. 3).

Also see Gould, 1979, pp. 11–12. Gould argues that IVF research in nonhuman primates is needed before it is used in "man." From the research he cites on rates of fetal abnormality in animals produced by IVF, he writes, it is evident "that there is a potential for the development of abnormal infants subsequent to IVF and reimplantation." In the report it issued on IVF following public hearings, the EAB noted that expert witnesses "agreed that there has been insufficient controlled animal research designed to determine the long-range effects of in vitro fertilization and embryo transfer" (see DHEW, 1979, p. 35056).

There is a further possibility that IVF in itself does not induce abnormalities but rather that the hormonal treatment physicians use to establish the implantation of the embryo and the maintenance of the pregnancy may enhance the survival of naturally occurring abnormalities, one researcher has written (Schlesselman, 1979).

Another researcher noted that Steptoe and Edwards have used progestins (which are synthetic hormones) to prepare the uterine lining to receive the embryo. The use of progestins in pregnancy is associated with an increased risk of fetal abnormalities, he added, and is not recommended by the FDA (Mastroianni, 1979, p. 3).

16. "Ob. Gyns disagree over benefit/risk value of using ultrasound routinely in pregnancy," *Ob/Gyn News,* 1981, Feb. 15.

Dr. John C. Hobbins and colleagues explain that in ultrasound, "electrical energy is passed across a transducer to produce high-frequency sound waves.... The sound waves are emitted in microsecond pulses. As they pass through tissue and rebound from tissue interfaces, some of these waves return to the transducer or transducers from which they were emitted.... The reflected echoes are displayed as a constellation of spots that form an image on the screen" (Hobbins et al., 1979).

At Senate hearings on obstetrics held in 1978, Dr. Donald Kennedy, then commissioner of the U.S. Food and Drug Administration, expressed grave reservations about the use of ultrasound on pregnant women, an increasingly common obstetrical practice. He stated: "Studies of the effects of ultrasound exposure on the human fetus in utero have thus far yielded inconclusive evidence. Although no increase in infant abnormalities has yet been observed, adequate studies to detect anatomical abnormalities have yet to be performed. Neither can conclusions be drawn about delayed effects."

He later stated: "Some animal studies have demonstrated increased incidence of fetal deformities with rather low level ultrasound used earlier during development. There is every reason to believe that the fetus would be more sensitive to any of the adverse effects that might be associated with ultrasound if it was delivered early during pregnancy.... The animal studies give us some caution for concern but nothing very definitive" (Obstetrical practices in the United States, 1978, Hearing before the Subcommittee on Health and Scientific Research of the Committee on Human Resources, U.S. Senate, April 17, 1978, U.S. Government Printing Office, Washington, D.C.).

For discussions on ultrasound's safety, see:

—NIH, 1984. "Unfortunately, lack of risk [of ultrasound use in pregnancy] is only assumed rather than clearly demonstrated. Evidence dictates that a hypothetical risk must be presumed with ultrasound. For example, exposure to a large amount

of ultrasound energy for long periods of time can produce cell damage by thermal
or mechanical effects."

—Peter C. Scheidt et al., 1978. "One-year follow-up of infants exposed to
ultrasound in utero," *AJOG* 131(7): 743–781.

—Committee on Bioeffects, American Institute of Ultrasound in Medicine,
1979, "Who's afraid of a hundred milliwatts per square centim (100 mW/cm²,
SPTA)? For people who wonder about the safety of diagnostic ultrasound."
American Institute of Ultrasound in Medicine, 4405 West Highway, Suite 504,
Washington, D.C. 20014. "Many experiments have been carried out in which
ultrasound was found to cause changes in biological cells and tissues."

—*JAMA*, 1982.

17. Parker, 1979, Oct. 31. Also see Parker, 1979, Nov. 22. In his testimony at
that EVHSA hearing, Dr. Joseph R. Stanton quotes Dr. Georgeanna Seegar Jones
of the Norfolk clinic. Jones wrote to the *Virginian-Pilot* (Sept. 23, 1979): "There
have been no substantial risks in the program in England, nor do we expect any
here. It is believed that the risks to the child are no greater than they would be
with any pregnancy." That, Stanton comments, is speculation, not medical fact
(Stanton, 1979).

18. The exact quote is: "The oocytes are recovered during metaphase—I,
which could be a sensitive stage for the induction of trisomy or polysomy" (Steptoe
and Edwards, 1970).

19. *Contemporary Ob/Gyn*, October 1977. When, three months after the birth
of Louise Brown, *The Washington Star* questioned Steptoe about a possible increase
in birth defects due to external fertilization, Steptoe replied: "We do not really
know yet what the full risks are . . ." (interview in *Star*, Oct. 13, 1978).

20. Stanton, 1979. Rary's quote came in an article in the *Virginian-Pilot*, Feb.
21, 1979; Andrews, *Virginian-Pilot*, Oct. 18, 1979.

21. Stanton, 1979. Stanton is quoting from an article in the *Virginian-Pilot*,
Feb. 21, 1979.

22. Consent Form #4 entitled "Title of Study: Vital Initiation of Pregnancy,"
Norfolk General Hospital, May 23, 1979. I repeatedly asked a spokesman for the
Norfolk IVF clinic to send me a copy of the most current consent form. Despite
assurances that the form would be sent to me, I never received it.

Regarding the statement on risks in the consent form, two relevant comments:
In 1973, IVF expert Dr. Luigi Mastroianni, speaking to his colleagues, stated:
"Manipulation of the human ovum in an artificial environment might easily produce
a defective product. Such an embryo would likely be aborted early in pregnancy,
but there is no guarantee that this would happen" (*JRM*, 1973).

In 1979, Dr. Clifford Grobstein wrote of Steptoe and Edwards' experiments
with women, noting the results: 68 women underwent laparoscopy; of these, 44
yielded appropriately mature eggs; of these, 32 had eggs that were successfully
fertilized; 4 women became pregnant; two women gave birth to live babies. "Little
information is available on the causes or consequences of the failures and on how
their frequency and nature compare with the pattern in normal reproduction,"
Grobstein wrote. "Moreover, the successful products of the procedure are still in
their infancy, and it is possible that some long-term effects may yet be manifested.
Finally, a mere four pregnancies are not enough on which to base a statistical
conclusion about the level of risks to the developing fetus" (Grobstein, 1979).

9

"Informed Consent":
The Myth of Voluntarism

In vitro fertilization is a therapy developed by compassionate doctors to help humankind, according to the media presentation of it. There are no villains here, only kind doctors helping desperate patients. Pharmacrats present the compelling desire of women to bear children as a desire before which nothing must stand in the way.[1] To help women, doctors simply remove a few eggs from their ovaries, fertilize the eggs in a glass petri dish with the husbands' sperm, and return the fertilized eggs to the women's wombs.

I argue in this chapter that the situation is less benevolent than the pharmacracy portrays it. Men are experimenting on women in ways more damaging to women than anyone has publicly acknowledged. It may sound simple to just take a few eggs from a woman's ovary, fertilize them, and return them to her uterus, but in fact the manipulations of the woman's body and spirit involved in this procedure are extreme.

There are strong indications that women who were among the first IVF experimental subjects, including Lesley Brown, did not fully understand the experimental nature of the programs in which they were enrolled. While it now appears that women are clamoring for IVF, that, far from being coerced into participating in these experiments, they are crushed when doctors deny them entry, in fact the women *are* being coerced, but the coercion, which is emotional rather than physical, has been rendered invisible.

First, did the women in the clinical trials for IVF understand just how experimental these procedures were or did they believe the doctors were giving them "therapy"? IVF pioneer Dr. Robert Edwards, quoted in a 1969 *Medical World News* report, provides a clue: "We tell the women with blocked oviducts, 'Your only hope of having a child is to help us. Then maybe we can help you.' "

But Edwards and his partner, Steptoe, knew then that they could probably not help most or even any of these women have children. Did Edwards' word "maybe" adequately communicate that fact to the women? These women were clearly experimental subjects and not patients who were apt to become pregnant by the unproven techniques, Princeton ethicist Paul Ramsey points out. One way to distinguish between experiment and therapy, Ramsey noted, is to imagine the woman asking: "Doctor, are you doing this for *me* or am I doing it for you and your research?"

Ramsey added: "The answer to that question to date (1972), is that the women are undergoing surgery and other procedures for the sake of medical research and it is a cardinal principle of medical ethics that they should have knowingly consented to that, and not primarily to a therapy they hoped would relieve their own childlessness" (Ramsey, 1972).

By 1980, Edwards was writing that he and Steptoe agreed on a certain point: That the hopes of their female "patients [sic] must not be raised unjustifiably and that they fully understood the situation—the opportunities and dangers and how they would be involved" (Edwards and Steptoe, 1980).

But Lesley Brown, mother of the world's first test-tube baby, did not understand. One of Brown's nurses wrote: "It was explained to the patient that oocyte recovery and in vitro fertilization was her only chance of pregnancy. She was thoroughly briefed in the implications of the experimental techniques so that she understood what she was involved in" (Harris, 1978).

So "thoroughly briefed" was Lesley Brown that until just before the birth of Louise, she assumed hundreds of test-tube babies had already been born. Describing the first meeting she and her husband John had with Patrick Steptoe, she wrote: "I don't remember Mr. Steptoe saying his method of producing babies had ever worked, and I certainly didn't ask. I just imagined that hundreds of children had already been born through being conceived outside their mothers' wombs. Having a baby was all that mattered. It didn't seem strange that I had never read about anyone who had had a child in that way before. I could understand their mothers wanting to keep quiet afterwards about how their children had been started off. It just didn't occur to me that it would almost be a miracle if it worked with me."

After the meeting with Steptoe, she believed she would soon be pregnant (Brown, 1979, p. 106).[2]

At some point during the experiments, Steptoe did tell Brown that the in vitro fertilization method had never worked before, but not in such a way that she took in that fact. She writes of a conversation she had had with Sue, another woman in the experiment, after each of them had had embryos transferred into their wombs:

" 'Didn't you hear the nurses say it hadn't worked on anyone before?' She was carrying on again. I had been so excited after the implant, believing I was pregnant, that the nurses had reminded me of that too. 'Don't make up your mind,' one sister told me. 'Mr. Steptoe hasn't had one success so far.' She was being kind, so that I wouldn't be too disappointed, but I wouldn't listen. Mr. Steptoe had warned me in the same way, but, stupid as it sounds, I wouldn't believe him. This was my last chance. There was no other way I could become pregnant now, since Mr. Steptoe had already done an operation to remove my Fallopian tubes. This had to work" (Brown, 1979, p. 112).

Lesley did not understand until very late in her pregnancy that human in vitro fertilization and embryo transfer had never been successfully done. Neither did her husband. Soon after Louise Brown's birth, the *Daily Telegraph* reported: "The proud new father was overjoyed with his new daughter—but not too happy about being the first test-tube dad. 'I didn't know we were to be the first test-tube parents—I wish we weren't,' said Mr. Brown" (Murche, 1978).

Judith Carr, the woman who gave birth to the first test-tube baby in North America, and her husband, Roger, were equally in the dark as to the experimental nature of the therapy. "I never asked if they'd had any success," Judith Carr told a British interviewer. "I was too polite to ask that question."

She had had no idea what the odds against her becoming pregnant were, she said. "They'd done some other transfers during the week and there were a lot of happy people walking around," she recalled. "A lot of happy girls. So they had had a very successful week. So I just assumed there were lots of people floating around pregnant but quiet."

When she telephoned her doctors, Howard and Georgeanna Jones, after learning she was pregnant, she did not understand what an event her pregnancy was. "They were very excited," Carr recalled. "I thought, 'Wow, this is wonderful. It must feel good to them. . . . This is nice.' Then Dr. Garcia got on the phone and said, 'You must understand. You do know you're the first.' I went, 'You're kidding' " (Williams, 1982).

A woman who was in an Australian IVF program for four years

and who underwent four operations without a successful pregnancy, told a radio interviewer: "I really didn't realize three years ago that it was at such a beginning stage" (ABS, 1978).

Even if the women involved had fully understood that IVF was in the earliest stages of human experimentation and had knowingly consented to participate in the programs, we cannot say that they acted freely. The appearance of voluntarism is deceptive, for the control over women begins long before they can voice a "free choice."*

The patriarchy filters through all its institutions the propaganda that women are nothing unless they bear a man's children. This message comes at women from every direction: From philosophers like Arthur Schopenhauer, who argued in 1851 that "women exist, on the whole, solely for the propagation of the species" (Hays, 1964, p. 209). From psychiatrists like Dr. Bernard Rubin, who asserted that "Women have a psychobiological drive organization directed toward bearing children" (Rubin, 1965). From priests like Pope Paul VI, who declared in 1972 that true women's liberation does not lie in "formalistic or materialistic equality with the other sex, but in the recognition of that specific thing in the feminine personality— the vocation of a woman to become a mother" (quoted in Daly, 1973, p. 3). Century after century, the message seeped deeply into woman: If she cannot produce children, she is not a real woman, for producing children is the function that defines woman.

Because patriarchy has for centuries so organized society that childbearing became the main purpose of women's lives and, frequently, the only way a woman could survive and gain any status, barrenness was the greatest shame a woman could know, the greatest curse she could suffer.

The association of womanhood with childbearing remains a deeply engrained one. Not surprisingly, one study has found the psychological impact of infertility to be far greater on women than on men. In the study by Dr. William R. Keye, Jr., nearly one third of the women said they felt bad about their bodies and saw themselves as less feminine because of infertility. Only 10 percent of the men reported a negative body image (Ob/Gyn News, 1982, Jan. 15, p. 6).

In 1977, Barbara Eck Menning, who is infertile, wrote that the words "infertile woman" seemed mutually exclusive to her: "I could

* Dr. Janice Raymond, medical ethicist, has made this clear (Raymond, 1979). In my discussion of free choice, I am applying to IVF the analysis of informed consent Raymond presents in her important book, *The Transsexual Empire*.

be infertile or a woman but not both."

The propaganda Menning was subjected to—that women are nothing unless they bear children, that if they are infertile, they lose their most basic identity as women—has a coercive power. It conditions a woman's choices as well as her *motivations* to choose. Her most heartfelt desire, the pregnancy for which she so desperately yearns, has been—to varying degrees—conditioned.

Emotional coercion can be every bit as powerful as physical coercion. The law has always recognized that coercion need not involve physical force, as psychiatrist Willard Gaylin points out (Gaylin, 1974). "Economic loss, social ostracism, ridicule are all recognized by law in varying contexts as coercive forces because in a social animal the need for approval and acceptance will almost always be equated with its very survival," Gaylin wrote. To the unconscious, he continued, death can be seen as isolation, loss of love, rejection from the family group, or social humiliation.

Barren women risk all these symbolic equivalents of death.

When pharmacrats, and in some cases, husbands, speak to the unconscious of infertile women, playing on a fear of barrenness, which may signify to the women abandonment, loss of love, and nothingness, they are exercising what Gaylin calls an alternative kind of coercion.* Coercion through the manipulation of the unconscious can operate without the person's knowledge that she is being coerced, without her resentment, and with the appearance of her consent, Gaylin observed. Through a manipulation of her anxieties, she comes to want what pharmacrats compel her to want.

People may resist the notion that emotional coercion can be as powerful as physical coercion, Gaylin observed, because it threatens our belief that we are logical, autonomous and in control of our actions.

"But, of course," Raymond comments, "social controllers have been well-known for convincing the individual that she/he is in control" (Raymond, 1979).

The message comes down to women with the force of centuries-long repetition. The patriarchy gives us the message through games, stories, toys ("Sunny Suzy Suburban Doll House"). Our mothers whisper it to us. Our priests preach it. Our doctors give us treatments if our ovaries or wombs fail us. It is our cell-deep knowledge: We are here to bear the children of men. If we cannot do it, we are not real women. There is no reason for us to exist.

---

* I am applying Gaylin's insights to the situation barren women face. He does not write of this situation in his article.

Yvonne Simpson, a 29-year-old woman with two children, was refused admittance into a Melbourne test-tube baby program on the grounds that she was blind. "I am going to have this baby come hell or high water," she said, announcing that she would travel the world until she found a doctor willing to help her. An Australian newspaper reported: "Mostly Mrs. Simpson wants a baby for her fiancé, Mr. Chris Moore, 25, whom she will marry later this year." Anne-Marie Sykes enrolled in Steptoe and Edwards' IVF experiment and carried an embryo in her womb for three weeks before her body rejected it. The (Sydney) *Sun* reported in 1978: "Mrs. Sykes has three children by a previous marriage but a gynaecological problem since has prevented her from conceiving normally. 'My husband, John, doesn't have any children of his own,' she said. 'I'm doing this for him.'" Rosa Dowling, 30, entered the Norfolk IVF program. "Mrs. Dowling has two children, 11 and 7 years old, from a previous marriage but none by the 25-year-old longshoreman to whom she is married now," *The New York Times* reported.[3]

Sandra James, a 30-year-old New York woman who had undergone surgery and hormonal treatments to cure her infertility, said she used to sit in her rocking chair and cry and cry. "I felt like half a woman, not a whole woman. Sometimes I wanted to die." For a while, she tried to keep her infertility secret from her man, because she was afraid he might abandon her (Kleiman, 1979).

A 33-year-old Brooklyn woman saw more than twenty doctors and was hospitalized six times in an attempt to overcome her infertility. She suffered severe depression. *The New York Times* reported: "Her husband has no children, and said that, although he has not put pressure on her, she felt an instinctive need to give him a child" (3/19/79). (James and the Brooklyn woman are not in IVF programs but are in that group from which "test-tube mothers" emerge.)

"You'll have to find yourself a proper woman," Lesley Brown repeatedly told her husband John when, month after month, she failed to become pregnant. "I've nothing to give our marriage now that I can't have a child." John wrote: "She [Lesley] was my wife, and I wanted her to have my baby." Steptoe recalled his first meeting with Lesley and John: "She felt she was letting John down by not having a baby. Their marriage had nearly broken apart. She had even tried to persuade her husband to divorce her so that he might marry someone else who could give him a child" (Brown, 1979; Edwards and Steptoe, 1980).

So women like Brown, women "desperate" for children, "besieged" hospitals, begging physicians to experiment on their bodies. Men claimed that women demanded in vitro fertilization "services" and in doing so obscured the social reality. Given patriarchy's proscription that women must produce children for their mates, free choice is conditioned. We can say of in vitro fertilization what Raymond says of transsexual surgery: that "the concept of volunteerism has taken hold, and the coercion of a role-defined environment is not recognized as an influential factor" (Raymond, 1979, p. 135).

Physicians launching IVF programs are themselves acting out of their belief about a woman's nature and her biologically determined social role. Their work on external fertilization is designed to enable barren women to fulfill their biological destiny (Rose and Hanner, 1976, p. 216). Edwards wrote that his primary preoccupation during the 1970s was "to study human embryology and allow women, who were seemingly condemned forever to a life of infertility, to bear their own children fathered by their husbands" (Edwards and Steptoe, 1980, p. 86).

In Australia, test-tube baby team leader Professor Carl Wood was also working to help women fulfill their biological destiny. "Prof. Wood says the women in the programme are desperate to have a baby for various reasons, but behind it all is an innate wish to procreate. Many have spent a considerable part of their adult life attempting to cure their infertility. 'If I were in their position—I can't imagine being a woman anyway—I don't think that I would have that degree of endurance,' he said" (*The Age*, 7/25/81).

In pleading for government funding of their experiments, physicians used the image of hordes of desperate barren women. "Australia's 'test-tube baby' doctors have appealed to the Federal Government for money to shorten the 'heartbreak queue' of childless women," reported *The Australian*. "Thousands have besieged hospitals, operating or introducing 'in vitro' fertilisation programs, begging for help" (Webb, 6/20/81).

"Happiness of 35,000 Women at Stake," ran the paper's editorial in support of that federal funding. "For just $1 million the Federal Government could bring ecstatic joy to some 35,000 Australian women," it maintained (*The Australian*, 6/20/81).

In Norfolk, when antiabortion groups opposed the establishment of the IVF clinic, a clinic physician said he was concerned about a minority of opponents depriving their neighbors of the right to have children by the in vitro process. This is a standard approach in the defense of in vitro fertilization and other reproductive technologies. The proponents of the technology portray themselves as sensitive to the pain of suffering women, and opponents as cold and intolerant of new approaches women may choose in alleviating their pain.

But as Herbert Marcuse has shown, tolerance can become repressive. To tolerate the expansion of IVF clinics is to tolerate increased medical control over women's bodies and women's lives.

The anguish an infertile woman suffers is most real. But the pharmacracy encourages us to focus our sympathy for that woman in such a way as to increase its control over her. Feminists have a different vision of where to focus our sympathy. As Raymond has pointed out, we ask *why* she suffers and we propose ways of dealing with that pain that confront the total situation, the situation of women under patriarchy. Through feminism, we have come to see the suffering of infertile women largely (but not wholly) in political and social terms.[4] That is, we see it as the imposition on women of a definition of ourselves that leaves us, if we are not mothers, nonentities. In view of the deep-rooted source of her suffering and fear, we do not believe that encouraging an infertile woman to hand over her body to the pharmacracy for manipulation and experimentation is a truly sensitive response to her plight.

"When tolerance serves mainly to protect the fabric by which a sexist society is held together, then it neutralizes values," Raymond writes. "It is important to help break the concreteness of oppression . . . by stretching minds to think about solutions that only *appear* to be sensitive and sympathetic."

Raymond also encourages us to ask at what costs to ourselves we are channeled into reproducing. With IVF therapy, she points out, women are reduced to ultimately reproductive creatures, to medically manipulatable Matter.[5] Those enrolled in these programs have already undergone, as infertile women, many medical tests, exploratory procedures and treatments that are debilitating and destructive to them, she writes.

Infertile men endure far less. Health professionals observe that it is more frustrating to evaluate and successfully manage infertile men than women since physicians have gathered less information about control of male reproductive processes. "Often husbands seem less willing to subject themselves to the possibility of unattractive and tedious procedures necessary for adequate diagnosis," they explain (Alexander, undated, p. 4).

These are a few of the "unattractive" procedures the more "willing" women subject themselves to:

—Endometrial biopsy. The doctor scrapes the lining of the

uterus with a sharp tool and examines the tissue specimen under a microscope to determine if the woman is ovulating properly. This can be extremely painful. Katie Berry underwent the procedure. "Mrs. Berry said she received no warning of the pain, nor any means to alleviate it," *The New York Times Magazine* reported (Kleiman, 1979). The biopsy in itself may impair fertility.

—Tubal insufflation. The doctor fills a woman's oviducts with pressurized carbon dioxide to determine if the tubes are open. This is painful.

—The doctor injects a dye into the uterus and X rays the organ to see if it is structurally impaired. This exam is excruciating.

—The same test can be conducted on the oviducts. Sheila Ballantyne describes it in *Norma Jean the Termite Queen:* "A dye is being injected into Norma Jean's tubes. She has been instructed to hold her breath until the technician has taken the picture. . . . Her whole abdomen is filled with searing acid. She can't hold her breath. The picture is ruined. Now we'll have to do it again. She hears herself screaming, 'If it feels like this, I don't want children!' 'Just do it right this time; we can't afford to mess this one up.' Oh agony beyond imagining" (Ballantyne, 1975, p. 33).

—Treatment of hormonal "deficiencies" with various drugs.

—"Blowing out" the tubes of some women every one to two months to maintain an opening. The doctor forces pressurized liquid through the tubes. "When I have the therapy, I put a towel over my head and cry," said one woman (quoted in: Raymond, AAAS, 1979).

—Surgery, including: laparoscopy; procedures to remove endo-metrial tissue or adhesions; reconstructive surgery on the oviducts. Anthea Polson, mother of the world's fifth test-tube baby, underwent ten operations in vain *before* she entered an IVF program.

Barbara Eck Menning, director of *Resolve* and a proponent of IVF, recalls the four years "filled with medical and surgical mayhem" of her struggle with infertility:

> There was a year of testing on me—biopsies, dyerotubogram, post-coitals; as well as repeated tests of my husband. We had a programmed sex life keyed to a basal temperature chart. At the end of that year an acute abdominal episode, improperly handled, cost me the ovary and tube on the right side. After recovery from surgery, on to a new doctor—more tests, more programmed sex life—everything was just fine, 'relax.' Relaxing did no good. On to a new doctor. Discovery of a cyst on the left ovary—resection by surgery. Six months later, success. Pregnancy—followed by miscarriage at 13 weeks. On to

another doctor—an activist. 'We'll have you pregnant again in no time!' Emergency admission to the hospital after an acute reaction to the fertility pills he prescribed. My cycles ceased. The best effort of men and their medicine could not coax another cycle forth. At 31 I experienced menopause due to the surgical and medical assault on my ovaries (Menning, 1981).

Menning quotes another woman who went through an infertility work-up:

There is no inner recess of me left unexplored, unprobed, unmolested. It occurs to me when I have sex that what used to be beautiful and very private is now degraded and terribly public. I bring my charts to the doctor like a child bringing home a report card. Tell me, did I do well? Did I ovulate? Did I have sex at all the right times as you instructed me? (Menning, 1980).

That's what women go through before they enter an IVF program. Then the manipulations begin in earnest. Drugs are administered; blood samples taken and the hormones within measured. To prevent the embryo from lodging in an oviduct (ectopic pregnancy), some physicians close the oviducts using high frequency electric current.

Ultrasound is often used to give a rough estimate of when a woman will ovulate. The woman's bladder must be very full for this procedure so the follicle will show up on the picture. Usually, doctors instruct the women to drink a lot, but for the ultrasonogram taken right before laparoscopy, they instill sterile normal saline into her bladder through a catheter.

In another method of predicting ovulation, physicians test the women's urine to detect the LH surge. The women are instructed to urinate every three hours. Revealing the extent of medical control over women, Steptoe and Edwards wrote: "The patients were instructed to pass approximately 200 ml on each occasion." If they failed to urinate the correct amount, they were asked to adjust their fluid intake.

A researcher in one IVF program has described the scheduled urinating as "a mild form of torture for the patient."[6] A woman in an Australian program describes the procedure: "You're dehydrated. You're only allowed to have a certain amount of liquid a day. Then all of your urine is collected three-hourly. That means day *and* night. You're wakened up at 10:30, at 1:30, at 4:30, at 7:30—all night long and all day long, collecting urine. And you just sit there and wait. That might be two days. That might be four days. I've seen people wait five days. It's a very long wait and you're very thirsty" (ABS, 1981).

When the doctors decide the woman is ovulating, they rush her into the operating room for a laparoscopy to "harvest" or "capture" eggs from her ovaries. Peter Roberts, science reporter for *The Age* in Australia, observed this procedure performed on Jan Brennan, mother of the world's thirteenth test-tube baby. As we pick up Roberts' account, Brennan has been anesthetized and lies with her eyes taped closed and mouth filled with tubes carrying the anesthesia gases to her lungs. Bending over a 20-centimeter square of flesh exposed among the folds of green cloth, surgeon John Leeton made three incisions in the abdomen and inserted three instruments. Just below the navel, he inserted a laparoscope, then a hollow needle for retrieving the egg and, just below that, the holding forceps, which will search for and hold the ovaries. Leeton "uses a foot pedal to pump carbon dioxide gas into the woman's abdomen, blowing up the belly for easy access."

Leeton lets reporter Roberts look through the laparoscope: "The inner body is surprisingly pink," Roberts wrote, "with a darker red ovary clasped firmly by a harsh, inhuman-looking metal clamp."

The art of egg harvesting, he further explains, "lies in piercing the follicle with the hollow needle while at the same time using a foot-operated vaccum pump to gently suck out the egg." (This is what one ob/gyn has called "man-made ovulation.") Leeton's assistant holds a row of small test tubes. A Teflon tube begins to flow with liquid from the woman's body—the follicular fluid that may contain an egg—into the first test tube, then into another. Several tubes are taken to the lab. The follicle, "a collapsed sack, pierced by the needle," is left.

Roberts continues his description: "The intercom breaks in harshly as Leeton moves to a second follicle: 'We have an egg from tube two.' Two more eggs are announced but still the intercom demands more." Surgeon Leeton, referring to Alan Trounson, the "egg man" on the IVF team, says: "Trounson is never satisfied" (Roberts, 1981).

Woman, once deified as the life-creating Goddess, is now lying on a table with her mouth taped shut, having the eggs sucked out of her body.

Lesley Brown, mother of the first test-tube baby, underwent the operation in Oldham. Steptoe wanted her to stay in the hospital one more day to recuperate but she and her husband could not afford the expense. Lesley's wound began bleeding as soon as they got on the train home. The train continually jolted her, "and I was in agony at every jolt," she recalled. "Blood began to soak through my underclothes. It felt as if the wound had opened right up, and the thought of that frightened me half to death."

An old woman sitting nearby asked John if Lesley were all right. "She looks so white," she said, offering to revive her with her fan.

"The blood started to seep through my thick woolen dress," Lesley wrote. "I held my coat tightly around me, so no one would see. We changed trains four times on the journey to Bristol, and at one station, I was crying so much that John picked me up and carried me in his arms from one end of the platform to the next. . . . John was so upset about the state I was in that he was crying too."

They reached home. John placed Lesley on the settee and opened her coat. Lesley recalled: "Tears poured down his face at the sight of all that blood. . . . 'That's it. No more,' John said. 'You're not going back to that hospital again' " (Brown, 1979, pp. 108–109).

During that laparoscopy, Steptoe had managed to get an egg from Lesley. He did not always succeed. Two other women, Sue and Jean, were also in the program and went for laparoscopies before Lesley. Lesley recalls: "Sue had a smile all over her face when she came back from the theatre. I didn't have to ask her if it had been a success. But when Jean returned, she was breaking her heart. 'They can't do anything for me,' she cried. 'They couldn't get an egg.' "

Following the laparoscopy, the recovered eggs are fertilized. To provide sperm for this, the husband must masturbate in some hospital cubicle. Knowing that an entire hospital team is outside waiting for him to produce the sperm and that if he fails, the operation will have been in vain, the "harvested" egg useless, he often finds this difficult to do. Professor Wood suggests that one way to improve "masturbation performance" in this anxiety-producing situation, is to view "exciting and beautiful pictures of women," presumably pornography. When the husbands are having trouble masturbating, Wood wrote, "wives are asked to assist." He acknowledges that this may be difficult because the wife has just had an operation. Some women, he notes, feel sick, drowsy or uncomfortable a few hours after the laparoscopy. But asking the sick, drowsy, uncomfortable wife to arouse the husband sexually, Wood feels, has the advantage of involving both spouses in a critical step of conception (Wood, 1983, p. 69).

Once the eggs are fertilized, the women wait. "You're recovering still from surgery," one woman recalls of this time. "You're lying there because you can't get up because you're awfully sore" (ABS, 1981).

When the fertilized egg has reached a certain stage of cell division, physicians transfer the embryo into the woman's womb. On the night an embryo was transferred into Anthea Polson of Australia, her husband was more nervous than she. He explains why: "Mainly because for the three days prior to that [Dr.] Alan Trounson would come in and say, 'Well, we've got two cells, four cells, eight cells and we're ready to go.' It was like a count-down to a lunar launch" (Heron, 1981).

To transfer the embryo, the physician inserts a cannula into the uterus. The womb may be traumatized during this procedure, as David Smith, a gynecologist in an IVF program at London's Royal Free Hospital, acknowledged in 1980 (MWN, 11/24/80).

When, using many sources, I pieced together a picture of what women endure in IVF programs, their suffering overwhelmed me. Yet that suffering is never mentioned in the ethical literature on in vitro fertilization. It is the embryo, and later the fetus, ethicists worry about. The federal Ethics Advisory Board, in its report on IVF, stated: "The most frequently articulated argument against federal funding of in vitro fertilization was based on the moral status of the fertilized egg and embryo. Proponents of this argument believed that human life should be respected from the moment of fertilization" (DHEW, 1979).

The debate on IVF has been a debate among men, and embryos and fetuses—seen as a man's sperm personified—appear to be real to these men in a way women are not. The Ethics Advisory Board itself was composed of thirteen men and only two women. In his comprehensive review of the ethical literature on IVF for this Board, Dr. LeRoy Walters cites the views of twenty-nine persons and every one of them is male. Walters lists, in descending order of prevalence in the literature, the ethical issues involved in human research with IVF. Risks of the research to the embryo top the list. Risks to the woman—referred to as "the oocyte donor"—is number eight on a list of twelve.

Risks are not even the only threat IVF poses to a woman's well-being. The innumerable manipulations of her body, and the suffering they cause her, also threaten her well-being. Yet this issue is absent from the ethical and medical literature on IVF. It is an issue about which writer Julie Melrose has thought a great deal, though not specifically in the context of in vitro fertilization.

Through her own experiences as a medical and surgical patient, Melrose came to focus on studying medical ethics issues, particularly in women's health care. In an interview, Melrose stated:

> There is a discrepancy between the way the doctor defines a surgical procedure and the way the person experiences it. Doctors have a tendency to look at surgical procedures in a technical and mechanical way. If they see a way that they can manipulate the body to accomplish what they want without posing an extremely high risk, they define that procedure as a piece of cake. From their position as mechanics, it *is* a piece of cake, that is, an easy procedure for them to perform.
>
> My feeling is that the human body has an integrity of its own and that it cannot be violated, even in a way that the doctor may see as minor, without there being physical and emotional consequences for the person on whom the surgery is performed.
>
> Women often believe doctors when they say something is a piece of cake and believe that they shouldn't make a big deal about it but then, during and after the procedure, they often feel that it *was* a big deal and it did not feel like a piece of cake to *them*. Their immediate, and often lingering, response to the procedure in fact has depth and has strong emotions connected with it and may have changed them in significant ways.

What chance do the women who endure all the procedures involved in IVF have of becoming pregnant? As of 1981, the probability of getting a live birth once a woman had been selected for egg recovery was about 0.029 using Steptoe and Edwards' current techniques, IVF expert Dr. John Biggers of Harvard calculated in a *New England Journal of Medicine* article. If an egg were actually recovered, the probability would shoot up to 0.044. The chances of achieving a pregnancy then, even with repeated operations, "are extremely small," he wrote. But suppose techniques for egg collection and embryo transfer were completely perfected? Even then, if a single embryo were produced and transferred, the procedures might have to be repeated about four times for pregnancy to occur in 50 percent of the patients, and eight times for success in 70 percent, Biggers calculated (Biggers, 1981).

Wood states that in the successful IVF clinics in Australia, the United States and England, the success rate in terms of pregnancy per laparoscopy varies from 15 to 25 percent. (The many unsuccessful clinics, of course, have much lower rates.) Biggers accepts this figure. But he observes that one question one must ask when such a figure is quoted is: Is that the success rate in *early* pregnancy? If so, the figure does not take into account loss of the embryo or fetus later in pregnancy. In other words, while 15 to 25 percent of women may become pregnant, they may not all give birth.

When the Norfolk team removed the spontaneous abortions and miscarriages from its figures, it came up with a success rate of about 13 percent (Jones et al., 1983). So the most experienced IVF team in the United States has an 87 percent failure rate.

"It's taken the Norfolk group since 1978 to do *that* well," Dr. John Buster, the ovum transfer pioneer, commented in 1983. "And they're the best. They're terrific. Other groups have a much lower success rate right now. So it's difficult to get it [IVF] to work."

Buster temporarily suspended his own IVF program in Torrance, California, after performing twenty-five to thirty embryo transfers. "We got three positive pregnancy tests but none went on," he said. "This is the experience of many people who've done this. My God, it's been just terrible!"[7]

Of the thousands of women hoping to get a baby through the 200-odd IVF programs across the globe, the vast majority have been disappointed. The cycle of hopes raised (she's accepted into the program) and dashed (doctor could not get an egg), raised (got an egg) and dashed (egg was abnormal), raised (got a normal egg) and dashed (embryo did not implant), raised (embryo implanted) and dashed (miscarried) harms women in ways pharmacrats have not acknowledged.

Every fresh failure generates the same grief symptoms experienced by a couple that loses a baby through sudden infant death or stillbirth, cautions Valerie Edge, R.N., project coordinator of the IVF program at Baylor College of Medicine, Houston (COG, 1984).

Nancy was one of the "lucky" women who had a successful embryo transfer after her first laparoscopy in an Australian program. She was pregnant. Part of her cheered, while another part cautioned that the chances of success were small. "It was this incredible turmoil that I was in," she explained. After about a month, she lost the pregnancy.

"I wasn't really surprised when I lost it. Some other people who I've talked to in the program feel devastated. I didn't. I just felt real sad. I felt grief-ridden for a while, but I didn't think about giving up."

After her second laparoscopy, while she, still sore, was recovering from surgery, the doctor told her the eggs they had just harvested had been abnormal. "When I went in [that] second time and my egg didn't even fertilize, that was harder than the first time because I thought, 'Well, I've lost a pregnancy, but next time they're going to get it.'"

There were six more "next times"—seven operations in all— and they still had not "gotten it" by the time Nancy was interviewed in 1981.

When eggs are retrieved, when pregnancies take and hold, doctors consider those pregnancies high risk. They monitor them through a variety of invasive means including ultrasound and amniocentesis. Ultrasound allows the doctor to visualize the baby in the uterus. (One reporter, describing this, wrote that IVF mother Anthea Polson had "a womb with a view.") Risks of amniocentesis include hemorrhage, perforation of viscera and infection. In one study, about 20 percent of women undergoing the procedure reported cramps and discomfort lasting from a few hours to a few days (Golbus, 1974).

According to her husband John, Lesley Brown was nervous about the amniocentesis. After a first unsuccessful attempt to do it, she telephoned John. She was sobbing: "Mr. Steptoe tried to do the amniocentesis today, but he couldn't manage it," she said. "I was too worked up. Now I'm getting pains in my tummy. I'm sure I'm going to lose the baby." Lesley knew there was a slight risk that the amniocentesis might cause a miscarriage and this upset her (Brown, 1979, pp. 118–119). (In fact in 1980, one woman in an Australian IVF program did miscarry her test-tube baby at 20 weeks following amniocentesis [DM, 4/30/80].)

In a final manipulation of a woman's body in the IVF programs, doctors delivering test-tube babies often do so by cesarean section, subjecting the woman to the risks of major abdominal surgery. Steptoe performed a cesarean on Lesley Brown because she developed toxemia, a life-threatening condition characterized by swelling of hands and face, excess weight gain, protein in urine and elevated blood pressure. Brown developed toxemia three weeks before the operation and she spent those and several preceding weeks in the hospital. While ob/gyns generally maintain that the cause of the condition is unknown, evidence from a number of demonstration projects targeted at preventing toxemia indicates that it may be a disease of malnutrition.[8] If it is, Brown's toxemia could have been hospital-induced, for she had been eating hospital fare.

In his book, Steptoe describes the various needles, tubes and knives introduced into Lesley Brown's body and the manipulations performed on her organs during the cesarean: shot of atropine injected to dry up excess respiratory secretions; rubber tube passed into trachea; heart monitoring equipment applied to chest; separating bladder and womb; pushing Lesley's stomach until the baby's shoulders appeared in the wound in her abdomen, etc. After delivering the baby, Steptoe lifted the womb out of the body to demonstrate to the cameras that Lesley had no oviducts and so could not have conceived naturally. The baby was examined, weighed and handed to Steptoe. He recalls:

"A jubilant Bob and Jean joined me, and I passed Louise, as she was to be named, to Bob. It was his brain, skill and perseverance and Jean's hard-working devotion which had led to this wonderful moment of achievement. We stood briefly together for the cameras to preserve the moment and then returned Louise to her cot and her guardian nurse" (Edwards and Steptoe, 1980, p. 165).

During their triumph, Lesley lay unconscious on the table.

She later recorded her memory of the birth: " 'Lesley, Lesley,' someone was shaking me awake. 'Do you want to see your baby?' The anesthetic had hardly started to wear off. My eyelids felt like lead as I tried to open them. Through a haze, I saw the outline of a little baby being held in front of me. 'It's a little girl,' a voice said. Then I must have fallen straight back to sleep again" (Brown, 1979, p. 172).

Many test-tube babies have been born prematurely and have had the health problems associated with prematurity. Sharna, born in 1981 in Australia, was twelve weeks premature and weighed just over two pounds. She was put on a ventilator in the neonatal intensive care unit and was fed intravenously (McLean, 1980).

One child, a twin born after physicians implanted two fertilized eggs in his mother's uterus, underwent corrective heart surgery soon after birth. Within a few days, doctors operated on him again to remove part of his severely inflamed bowel. They announced they would perform major heart surgery on the boy when he was six months old.

Australian newspapers focused less on the boy's precarious health than on Australia's "feat" in producing the world's first test-tube twins. So did the IVF team. Professor Carl Wood stated of the twin births: "This is a great step forward in test-tube technology." Dr. Alan Trounson was commended by the head of his team for his work in "developing" the two embryos that became the twins.

The second twin had a slight case of jaundice due to premature birth. Referring to a resort area, the pediatrician said the child's jaundice looked like "a good Surfers Paradise suntan."

The twins' father kissed his wife after the cesarean section (surgery Wood described as "a perfectly normal cesarean") and said: "Well done, darling. You've made me a very proud man."

The twins' mother? According to the *West Australian*, she "had vowed never to go through it again."[9]

After the ordeals infertile women endure, are those who do finally bear a baby happy? Not always. Consider the woman who wrote to the newsletter of Resolve, an organization that counsels the infertile: "Since I had longed for a baby so desperately, I felt as though I could neither permit myself any negative feelings nor be less than the perfect mother." But the baby was colicky "for three horrid months, a period of time during which I never slept more than three hours or so at a time." One day a neighbor, having heard of her infertility history, said to her, "You must be so-o-o happy!" The new mother burst into tears and sobbed: "I hate the little bitch and the whole damn motherhood scene." The startled neighbor confided that she had hated her colicky baby too.

The mother continued: "In truth, I was a victim of my successful pursuit of fertility. As I have finally discovered, at one time or another most mothers dislike their kids and wish for something besides motherhood. . . . I am finally getting to the point where I can enjoy the baby for what she is, not for the hoped-for fulfillment of all the fantasies that infertile people are prey to" (*Resolve Newsletter,* Dec. 1977; April, 1979).

Neither of these formerly infertile women were in IVF programs. Lesley Brown, of course, was. "It really shocked me once when I shouted at the baby because she kept crying," she wrote of Louise. "It wasn't a question of not loving her. It just seemed as if I didn't deserve her if I behaved like that. There were so many childless women who would have made better mothers, if they'd been given the same chance" (Brown, 1979, p. 187).

Notes

1. For example, the Health Systems Agency report recommending approval of the Norfolk IVF clinic stated: "Thus, inasmuch as this program does not exist elsewhere in this country, disapproval of the project may constitute denial of a fundamental right to individuals desiring the procedure, and may, thus be legally indefensible." Why does the patriarchy give serious attention to this "right" of women—the right to submit to experimentation in an attempt to reproduce—and not to other rights such as those of equal protection under the law and equal pay for equal work? Why is its interest in women's rights so selective?

2. Anthea Polson of Australia, like other women in test-tube baby programs, was told that external fertilization was her only hope of bearing a child. After ten unsuccessful operations to repair her damaged tubes, she consulted a new physician. He asked her if she would like to go and see Professor Carl Wood who was launching an in vitro fertilization program in Melbourne. Polson recalled: "He said he thought Prof. Wood was my only hope" ("Test-tube baby made dream come true," *Sunday Times,* Australia, 7/6/81).

3. The information on Yvonne Simpson comes from a newspaper article headed "Blind Mother Refused." The article was sent to me from Australia without the name of the newspaper or date. The information on Anne-Marie Sykes appears in "Doctor 'Is Not Playing God,'" (Sydney) *Sun,* 5/18/78. The information on Rosa Dowling appears in the *New York Times,* March 18, 1979.

4. It is not easy to separate out the forces that shape a woman's desire to bear a child. See the discussion by Barbara Menning (1977, pp. 96–106) of these motivations for parenthood: parenthood as a way to conform to societal pressures; as a reliving of one's own childhood; as a desire to compete with one's own parents; as role fulfillment; as a "rite of passage" to adulthood ("Infertile people frequently relate stories of feeling like perpetual adolescents until they finally achieve parenthood by some means. This attitude seems particularly focused on the woman. . . . The man may show his credentials in other ways, most specifically in his education and his work."); and finally, parenthood for its own sake, loving children and wanting them in one's life.

If we want to be mothers and cannot, that may cause us great pain. But pain and suffering can sometimes have a positive value. As Hannah Arendt observed: "The human condition is such that pain and effort are not just symptoms which can be removed without changing life itself; they are rather modes in which life itself . . . makes itself felt. For mortals, the easy life of the gods would be a lifeless life" (quoted in DeCrow and Seidenberg, 1983, p. 130). Actively dealing with our pain (rather than handing it over to the pharmacracy for a technological "fix") can spur our growth. Our pain can impel us to look for more varied ways of living our lives fully.

Dr. Janice Raymond argues that surgical treatment for people labeled "transsexuals" results in their becoming much less than they could be as human beings and I think that IVF could have the same result for infertile women. For an important discussion on this point, see chapters on "Therapy As a Way of Life," and "Toward a Development of an Ethic of Integrity" in Raymond, 1979.

5. Read between the lines in the following papers to see what kind of manipulation and suffering women endured in infertility work-ups and treatments: Steptoe and Edwards, 1976, pp. 880–882, and Steptoe and Edwards, 1970, pp. 683–689.

6. Dr. Alexander Lopata of Melbourne speaking before the American Fertility Society, March 1981 in Atlanta.

7. Buster closed down the IVF program to devote all his resources to embryo transfer but plans to reopen later after hiring more personnel.

In 1983, Dr. Martin Quigley, head of the IVF team at the University of Health Sciences Center at Houston, estimated conservatively that 100 to 200 centers were then doing IVF or talking of doing it in the next twelve to eighteen months

(Kolata, 1983). Because it takes a large experienced team of twelve to twenty people to run a successful IVF program, established IVF team leaders like Quigley are concerned that novices may not achieve anywhere near their success rates. But will novices take pains to make sure women understand that? One woman who entered a newly opened IVF program in 1983 told me she had about a 20 percent chance of getting pregnant. In fact, her chances were much lower. If the experience of established IVF groups is any guide, the team working with her would most likely have no pregnancies at all in its first year of operation. Even the established groups have what Quigley calls "batting slumps"—periods when, for unknown reasons, none of the patients get pregnant. So even had she gone to the country's most experienced IVF group, Norfolk, she would not have been assured of having so high as a 13 percent chance of actually bearing a child.

8. Dr. Tom Brewer, an obstetrician who directed a prenatal nutrition program among the poor in Costra County, California, for twelve years, and Gail Brewer, author and childbirth educator, present the evidence for toxemia as a disease of malnutrition in their book, *What Every Pregnant Woman Should Know.* They explain: When a pregnant woman's diet is deficient, the liver, lacking vital nutrients, begins to malfunction. It cuts down on the synthesis of albumin, a protein critical for maintaining blood volume. When albumin synthesis drops, the water which should be in the blood circulation leaks into the tissue, causing swelling. With the mother's blood volume so low, the placenta fails to get enough blood and the nutrients the blood carries. Malnourished, it malfunctions. The fetus does not gain the necessary weight. Placental insufficiency, the Brewers maintain, is caused by the reduction in blood volume. If too little blood reaches it, the placenta may deteriorate, breaking off from the uterine wall in a catastrophe called placenta abruptio.

9. Sources for the section on the test-tube twins were: "Test-tube twins are doing well," *West Australian,* June 9, 1981; "Test-tube twins 'A big step forward'," *Sun Herald,* June 7, 1981; "Test-tube twin improves," *West Australian,* June 9, 1981; "World's first—they're twins," *Weekend News,* June 6, 1981.

Part Four

RELATED TECHNOLOGIES

10

Sex Determination:
A Question of Gynicide

In 1955, four research groups working independently in Copenhagen, Jerusalem, New York and Minneapolis developed amniocentesis, a procedure involving the insertion of a long, hollow needle through a pregnant woman's abdomen and into her uterus. Through the needle, physicians withdraw some of the amniotic fluid, which surrounds the fetus and contains embryonic cells. Technicians can distinguish between XX (female) and XY (male) cells in this fluid. So amniocentesis can be and is used as a prenatal sex detection test.

Sociologists studying the record of two hospitals in a large city in western India for a twelve-month period in 1976 and 1977 found disturbing evidence of the consequences of this use. In the first hospital, all ninety-two women who sought amniocentesis for sex detection wanted to abort the fetus if it were female; all wanted to retain the fetus if it were male. In the second hospital, 700 predominantly middle-class women underwent amniocentesis for sex detection. Of these, 450 were told they would have a daughter and almost all (430) aborted the female fetuses. The remaining 250 mothers were told they were carrying male fetuses and every single one of them elected to carry the babies to term, even those who were advised of a possible genetic defect in the child.

The sociologists conclude: "The pattern we have documented of inducing abortion when the foetus is female continues the traditional practice of female infanticide" (Ramanamma and Bambawali, 1980).

Clearly, the technology of sex control can translate sexual prejudice (a "preference" for male children) into a sexist reality. The number of women relative to men could well be reduced. This is

188

what one medical ethicist terms "previctimization"—women being destroyed and sacrificed before they are even born (Raymond, 1980).[1] This can be accomplished today by *sex determination* (evaluation of fetal sex through such a technique as amniocentesis followed by abortion of female fetuses) and may someday be accomplished through *sex predetermination* (techniques, such as sperm separation, to ensure that a male embryo is formed in the first place).

Sociologists rarely see the previctimization of females as a problem. In studying sex preference, they seldom question its morality. "Rather," according to sociologist Jalna Hanmer of England's Bradford University, "one can detect a tendency to cope with possible criticisms by implying or stating that all is not as bad as it might be." The researchers, for example, tell us that when sex predetermination methods are available, the anticipated increase in males over females will decline after a few years (an assertion others have effectively challenged)[2] or that only a minority will use these techniques.

Despite the widespread misperception that reliable sex predetermination techniques are already available, no such methods have had their effectiveness convincingly demonstrated. But if such techniques do become available, are we so sure that males will be valued over females? Yes. Folk customs expressing male preference, the sex preference studies, and social and economic structures that select on the basis of sex, all indicate this.

First, folk customs. The notion that boys are better is implicit in ancient beliefs on the prediction or determination of a child's sex. An age-old belief that the right side of the body is the more valuable side and that right-handedness is associated with strength and justice coincided with innumerable theories that boys emanated from the right. Sons were produced by the right testicle, under one theory, and by the right ovary under a later one. Left-handedness was associated with weakness and evil. Girls came from the left. It was popularly believed in antiquity that men copulating with the left testicle tied up would produce a boy.

Certain ways of predicting fetal sex revealed the presumption that sons were superior to daughters. For example, according to Arabian, Indian and Jewish traditions, if the woman was particularly happy and untroubled, the fetus was male (Cederqvist and Fuch).

P. J. McElrath argued in his 1911 book, *The Key to Sex Control*, that boys were made of superior stuff. Fresh, vibrant sperm and newly released eggs produced sons. Aged, weak sperm and stale eggs produced daughters (Whelan, 1977).

From the scripture of Father–God religions, from the folk sayings and practices of peoples around the world, I could present an endless list showing that sons are more highly treasured than daughters. A sample:

—A German adage goes: "A house full of daughters is like a cellar full of sour beer."

—A Chinese proverb: "Eighteen goddesslike daughters are not equal to one son with a hump."

—The Talmud states: "When a girl is born, the walls are crying."

—In India shortly after a Hindu marriage, the husband performs the ceremony *Garbhadhana,* in which he and his wife pray for the conception of a son. Three months after the conception, they perform another of the sacred domestic ceremonies, the *Pumsavana,* for obtaining a son. Mantras prescribed in a Hindu sacred text can also be chanted in an attempt to transform a female fetus into a male (Ramanamma and Bambawali, 1980).

—In the past in Korea, rituals designed to produce sons were common. They were called "son praying." A drastic form involved burning the woman's navel through cautery. Blue salts and musk powder mixed with wheat dough were placed over the woman's navel and cauterized with salt moxa. This was generally done two hundred to three hundred times on a sonless woman. According to researchers Chung, Cha and Lee (as cited in Williamson, 1976), this "seeding of sons" through cautery was practiced widely into the 1920s or 1930s. They write: "Sometimes cautery was carried to an extreme by zealous husbands who believed that the more salt burned, so much the better. Instead of burning mox on the navel, the husband brought a red-hot iron rod against the navel of his wife and held it there while the wife screamed in unbearable pain."

Studies confirm what the folk customs tell us. Sociologist Dr. Nancy E. Williamson has reviewed the sex preference research around the world and conducted her own studies. The evidence that parents in many countries would rather have a predominance of boys over girls is "overwhelming," she writes. Daughter preference is so rare she refers to it as "this deviant preference."

An example: In a 1954 study of American college students, 92 percent of males and 66 percent of females surveyed wanted a son for an only child, while 4 percent of males and 6 percent of females wanted a daughter. Twenty years later, other researchers replicated the study with similar results (as cited in Williamson, 1976, p. 31).

Son preference prevails in the United States and in developing countries but the degree differs vastly. In developing countries, son preference is "much, much stronger," Williamson said in an interview. "It borders on obsession." Studies show that couples in the United States often want a balanced family—one child of each sex. But there is a decided son preference here as well, expressed as much in birth order as in numbers. Studies have consistently found that people want the first-born to be a son and, if they want an uneven number of children, more sons than daughters (Westoff and Rindfuss, 1974). Men desire sons much more strongly than women do, the studies reveal. Women, however, still want a first-born son and, if the number of children is not even, more boys than girls.

Professor Gerald Markle, a sociologist from Western Michigan University, examined sex preference studies, conducted his own and concluded: "There is a consensus among most scientists that the adoption of sex-choosing by the general population would lead to an excess of male infants" (Markle and Nam, 1971).[3]

On a worldwide basis, girl preference is rare. In fact one study of factory workers from six nations found that the alternative to boy preference was not girl preference but was, rather, a desire for "either." Those wanting a girl did not exceed 5 percent among any of the six groups of workers (Williamson, 1978, p. 9).

Women would also choose sons over daughters, though their son preference is weaker than men's.[4] But is it really a "choice" they would be making? Choice, one commentator has noted, is intrinsically connected with the *power* to choose, a power systematically undermined by patriarchal values. "The fact that women 'choose' male children in a culture where women are programmed not to value themselves can hardly be termed choice," she wrote (Connors, 1981, p. 206).

A woman's son preference may not be a "preference" at all, but rather something that is maintained by force and ideology. Within the traditional patriarchal family, women are rewarded for bearing sons and punished for failing to do so. Women may "prefer" a son because they prefer not to live as outcasts, poor and despised.[5]

A wife's status increases when she produces sons who will carry on her husband's name and inherit his wealth (Williamson, 1976, p. 19). A married woman in Taiwan, according to a 1968 sex preference study, gets her first bit of security in her husband's family when she bears a son and the quality of her life will largely depend on the ties she develops with that son. "Until a woman bears a male child," the researcher observed, "she is only a provisional member of her husband's household, merely a daughter-in-law; with the birth of a son, she becomes the mother of one of its descendants, a position of prestige and respect" (quoted in Williamson, 1976, p. 143).

Women in many cultures who failed to produce a man-child have been subjected to pity, contempt, social disapproval and social displacement. They have suffered a lack of personal security. Some have been physically beaten, some divorced, deserted, some even killed. The severity of the punishment varied with the time and culture:

—In traditional Korea, a man would desert his wife if she bore no son (Williamson, 1976, p. 96).

—Henry VIII annulled his marriage to the aging Catherine of Aragon because he wanted a male heir. Another wife, Anne, disappointed him by bearing a daughter, Elizabeth, and then bringing forth a stillborn son. He had her beheaded.

—In 1982, the controlled Chinese press began publicizing the abuse of wives who gave birth to daughters, noting that the offending husbands and in-laws had been punished for their actions. In one case, a teacher from northeastern China, Gao Lihua, married a soldier, Chen Xudong, and subsequently bore a daughter. Her in-laws advised their son to divorce her. Chen came home on furlough and beat his wife, leaving her with a brain concussion and facial injuries (Wren, 1982).

—In the United States, pressure—though in a different form—can also be exerted on women to produce sons. The husband's "disappointment" at the birth of a series of daughters can place a "strain" on the marriage, arousing fear in the wife that she might not be able to hold onto her man (see Rorvik and Shettles, 1971, pp. xvii–xxiii).

In addition to folk customs and sex preference studies, the presence of social and economic structures that select on the basis of sex also indicate that males will be valued over females once sex control techniques are fully developed.

Boy preference is not simply a personal preference but something embodied in institutions, in customs and in laws. For example, in rural areas in many countries, parents have often felt the need for a son who will take over the family farm and provide for them in their old age, society being so structured that a daughter could not do that for them.

Sons and daughters have different access to goods, services, status and power because they live within a sexual caste system. Sex selection technology, then, cannot be seen as an isolated phenomenon. "Sex selection takes place every day in this society without a specific biomedical technology," Dr. Janice Raymond notes. "These procedures merely carry out, on a technological level, what happens on other levels" (Raymond, 1980, p. 209). We see the results of sex selection every time we read the list of male names on the masthead of *The New York Times* or look at the composition of the Soviet Politburo, OPEC, the American Medical Association or the Pittsburgh Pirates.

There is yet another reason why sons are valued, especially, by men. The sons, through whom men pass on their name and property, assure men a form of immortality. The father transmits his name to his son as a way of signifying that his life has been transmitted to the child; surnames have become male "life lines" (Stannard, 1977, p. 302). A daughter cannot build a father's immortality; she will go off and help another man build his by bearing children who will carry his surname.[6]

In view of the importance of sons and the pressures that can be exerted on women to bear them, I want to examine a statement a medical ethicist made in justifying the abortion of "wrong sex" fetuses. Dr. Karen Lebacqz of the Pacific School of Religion argues that aborting a fetus because of its sex rather than because of a genetic defect like Down's syndrome is only a difference of degree. Parents, she adds, have a right to abort a child for a serious reason, including a threat to the integrity and unity of the family. "And I can see instances in which to abort a child because it's the unwanted sex is done because that child would be a threat to the integrity of the family unit," she said (Chedd, 1981).

Lebacqz fails to ask Background questions before arriving at her analysis: Why might the "unity" and "integrity" of the family be threatened by the birth of, say, a female: Is it threatened because the husband is intent on a male heir to carry on his name and bring him immortality and perhaps, through a relative's will, an inheritance? Is family unity and integrity threatened because the wife fears that if she does not bear a son, a "strain" will be placed on the marriage and her husband might divorce her, leaving her and her daughters to fend for themselves in a society where child support payments are meager and, after the first two years, seldom paid and where women earn 59 cents to every dollar a man earns? Is it that the parents have a set of gender stereotypes they want to impose on the child born to them and if the "wrong sex" is born, they will have to switch and impose a less desired stereotype? What does Lebacqz mean by "unity" and "integrity" anyway? Are these words here anything but platitudes obscuring the power difference between men and women in the family?

If we need further evidence that patriarchal cultures value males over females, it presents itself in the history of infanticide. Sociologist Jalna Hanmer came to examine infanticide from what at first seems a roundabout way. Something puzzled her when she considered polyandry, the system under which a woman is married to several men at the same time: If certain women have numerous husbands, what happens to all the women who must be left without any husbands at all? She learned that those women do not exist. They were destroyed at birth. As one encyclopedia informs us: "Polyandry ... seems to be associated with scarcity of women owing to the practice of infanticide of females."[7]

Infanticide, which usually involves the murder of girl children, is, Hanmer believes, more properly called femicide or gynicide. Since "gynicide" is not in the dictionary, my definition of it is adapted from Webster's for "genocide": The use of deliberate systematic measures (as killing, bodily or mental injury, unlivable conditions, prevention of births) calculated to bring about the extermination of women or to destroy the culture of women.

Societies that practiced infant gynicide include: the Greeks, Romans, Chinese, Tibetans, Eskimos, Arabs, Japanese, Indians and the Maori of New Zealand.[8]

From antiquity into the Middle Ages there was a statistical imbalance of males over females. One method of limiting population is the destruction of females, the "breeders," reported classical scholar Sarah B. Pomeroy, "and the most likely reason for sexual imbalance in a population is female infanticide" (Pomeroy, 1975, p. 46).

It was the father, in many places, who decided to keep or to kill the infant. During the "lifting up" ceremony of many patriarchal primitive tribes, the father either lifted up the infant, acknowledging it as his own, or did not, leaving the child to be killed or to live as an outcast. Similarly, according to an ancient Roman custom, a newborn was placed on the ground and was allowed to live only if the father raised it. This is the origin of the expression "to raise a child" (Stannard, 1977, p. 299).

Collier's Encyclopedia informs us that infanticide "cannot be classed as callous brutality." No? This is how girl children were killed: thrown in ditches; suffocated; skulls smashed against a hard surface; exposed on a mountaintop; abandoned on the bark basin onto which they were born; drowned; buried alive. In the Hellenistic period in Greece, exposure of infants was widely practiced. Sometimes people would collect the exposed infants who, in most cases, would automatically have slave status. Some slave dealers took these girl babies and sold them as prostitutes (Pomeroy, 1975, pp. 140–141).

Another form of sex selection did not involve outright destruction of females. Systematic neglect of female infants—underfeeding them and denying them needed medical care—sometimes co-existed with the practice of infant gynicide. When infanticide was illegal, neglect alone could lead to the desired result without any law violation.

Neglect could be responsible for suspiciously low rates of survival among female infants in ancient Greece and Rome and in some countries today. Studies cited by Williamson report evidence of female neglect in modern times in Pakistan, India, Ceylon (Sri Lanka) and Bangladesh.[9] Additionally, in northern Algeria, where strong son preference prevails, female infanticide or female neglect are reputedly practiced today.

There are two methods of eliminating the female before birth. First, let us consider *sex determination* (as opposed to sex predetermination).

In 1982, Britain's *Guardian* reported that physicians in India were setting up businesses that provided the service of detecting female fetuses through amniocentesis and aborting them. A husband-and-wife team in Amritsar, Punjab, pioneered the new service. Physicians in Delhi, Bombay and Calcutta followed suit. A doctor from the All India Institute of Medical Science in Delhi said he knew of at least fifty physicians who were busily aborting female fetuses for large fees. Only female fetuses were being aborted, even in cases where the parents had three sons and no daughters, he had found.

In July, women's groups, along with some leading doctors, began a campaign to ban amniocentesis for sex determination.[10]

Amniocentesis is the technique most frequently used to detect sex but there are problems with it. The test can only be done late in pregnancy and the abortion performed in the second trimester around 18 to 20 weeks. The risk of a woman's death in abortion is six times greater in the second than in the first trimester. So a search for simpler, earlier methods of sex detection is underway.

A more effective technique than amniocentesis would be the analysis of fetal cells sloughed into the cervical canal. This, unlike amniocentesis, can be done in the first trimester when abortion is safest. In China, researchers inserted suction tubes into the cervices of women and aspirated fetal cells. They correctly detected the gender in 93 percent of cases, they reported. Their "Anshan aspiration" technique appears to be so safe, simple and accurate that it could be widely used. This would have ominous implications for women. In the Chinese study, after 100 experimental sex predictions, thirty planned abortions of "wrong sex" fetuses occurred. One aborted fetus was male; twenty-nine were female (Teitung, 1975).

Since 1975, nothing more has been heard from China about this test and it is likely that the government is not encouraging its use. In July 1982, the state's *Health News* reported disapprovingly that some women were having fetal tests in hospitals to determine the sex of their unborn child and then undergoing abortions if a daughter were detected. (The tests were unspecified and could have been amniocentesis or the Anshan technique.) This technologically advanced form of gynicide was occurring concurrently with a few cases of the old infanticide. The previous month, a peasant near Shenyang fished a sack out of a river and found a dead female infant tied to a stone. This was the ancient Chinese method of killing unwanted daughters. A report several years earlier had mentioned eight baby girls found suffocated in a sack left at a Communist Party office (Wren, 1982).

American researchers experimented with a technique similar to Anshan aspiration that could theoretically detect sex as early as the ninth week of pregnancy. But the accuracy of this test proved to be lower than that of amniocentesis—only 86 percent. In five out of thirty-six cases, males were born after females had been predicted (Rhine, 1975).

Several new methods for determining the sex of fetuses were tried in the 1970s and 1980s after technical improvements made identification of male cells easier. Researchers found that the male sex-chromatin could be stained. This allowed a more accurate discrimination between the cells of the mother and fetus. Researchers have attempted to detect fetal sex by examining the pregnant woman's saliva (Rosenzweig and Adelman, 1976), cervical mucus (Goldstein, Luckesh and Ketchum, 1973; Manuel, Park and Jones, 1974), and blood. In one study involving removal of blood from pregnant women attending a prenatal clinic between the fourteenth and eighteenth weeks of pregnancy, the probability of correct prediction for a boy was reported to be 82 percent, and for a girl, 91 percent (Grosset, Barrelet, Odartchenko, 1974).

Other researchers attempted to use a machine, the fluorescence-activated cell sorter (FACS), to isolate fetal cells from the mother's circulation and then examine the fetal cells for sex determination. The method, they found, was not useful for determining fetal sex (Schroder and Herzenberg, 1980). Still other researchers tried using ultrasound over the mother's abdomen to see if they could detect fetal penises, scrotums and labia majoras (Schotten and Giese, 1980; Weldner, 1981).

Rather than detecting the sex of fetuses and selectively aborting them, a leading embryologist and pioneers in IVF have suggested moving back a step. Scientists might detect the sex of the embryo (rather than the fetus) and implant in wombs only those embryos of the desired sex.

As we saw in Chapter 5, a cow embryo can now be sexed by removing some of its cells but many embryos are damaged in the process (Foote, 1979, p. 19). In the 1960s, IVF pioneer Dr. Robert Edwards and a colleague accomplished this in rabbits as well. They cut off small bits of early embryos (blastocysts), examined cell nuclei in order to detect the sex and then transferred the embryos into females. They found, upon the birth of the offspring, that they had correctly predicted the sex. (The birth of the offspring coincided with the death of the mothers. For unspecified reasons, the researchers killed the pregnant rabbits and delivered the offspring surgically. Then they killed the offspring too, determining their sex by examining their reproductive tracts.)

One of the offspring had no head. They speculated that they might have cut too deeply into the embryo or part of the embryo might have protruded through the slit they made in the cell wall, causing the loss of head-forming tissue (Gardner and Edwards, 1968).

The two researchers suggest that in attempting to control the sex of offspring of farm animals and human beings, enough embryos might be obtained by maturing ovarian eggs in the laboratory.

Two years later, Edwards and geneticist Dr. Ruth Fowler wrote: "Eggs fertilized in the laboratory and cultivated to the blastocyst stage could be transferred back to the mother. . . . Since there would be several [human] blastocysts from one couple, a degree of selection could be exercised in deciding which one to return to the mother.

For example, the sex of the baby could be predetermined" (Edwards and Fowler, 1970).

Both embryologist Dr. Clifford Grobstein and Dr. Laurence E. Karp, director of an IVF program at Swedish Hospital Medical Center in Seattle, have also suggested sexing embryos and discarding those of the unwanted sex (Grobstein, 1981, p. 122; Karp, 1978).

It may be possible to step back even earlier in the female's existence to eliminate her. Earlier than the fetal stage. Earlier even than the embryo stage. Perhaps the type of sperm that engenders females might be isolated and discarded. Here, we move into *sex predetermination*. Edwards, who suggested that one of the earliest future applications of research on human IVF may be sex predetermination, admitted that sexing sperm would be ethically preferable to sexing embryos. However, he thought sperm sexing was then infeasible (Walters, 1979, p. 49).

Not everyone agreed. Researchers believe sperm can be "sexed" because there are two types of sperm—one producing males, the other, females. It will help at this point to look at the way in which a child's sex is determined: Egg and sperm cells have twenty-three chromosomes, rod-shaped bodies that contain the genes or hereditary factors. One of these, the sex chromosome, determines sex. All eggs contain an X sex chromosome. Half of a man's sperm contains an X chromosome and are called gynogenic (female-engendering). The other half contains a Y chromosome. These are androgenic (male-engendering). If an egg is fertilized by a gynogenic sperm, the child will be female (XX). If it is fertilized by androgenic sperm, the child will be male (XY).

It was only in 1923—relatively recently—that the existence of gynogenic and androgenic sperm was discovered. This discovery made techniques to separate the male and female sperm seem possible. Little time was lost. By the 1930s, researchers were experimenting with sex selection methods. In 1969 and 1970, two discoveries making it possible to count the X and Y sperm gave a major impetus to the study of sex predetermination.[11]

Most attempts to predetermine sex are based on the assumption that there *must* be differences between "male" (androgenic) and "female" (gynogenic) sperm, just as there *must* be substantial enough differences between male and female human beings to justify a different status for each. Researchers assume that these differences would be significant enough to enable them to separate and selectively use the sperm. As Dr. Robert H. Glass of the University of California at San Francisco has noted, many attempts to separate "male" and "female" sperm presuppose that "the Y chromosome confers on the sperm a unique physical property that allows differentiation from the X sperm." The theories go that "male" sperm must swim faster or stronger than the "female," or have a distinctively shaped head, or emit a different electrical charge.

In fact, it is not clear that such differences exist. Sex selection based on techniques that separate the male and female sperm may be impossible because these two types of sperm are too similar in size, shape, weight and motility to allow them to be differentiated. It is reasonable that these sperm types would be similar, for they come from the same original cell.[12]

Methods of sex predetermination "ranging from the ingenious to the incredible" (Short, 1979) fall into four categories. To date, none has met with marked success.

1. *Separation techniques* to segregate androgenic and gynogenic sperm, followed by artificial insemination with the "right" sex sperm. These techniques include centrifugation and sedimentation (spinning sperm at high speeds so the heavier sperm will settle out); electrophorosis (using alleged differences in electrical charges of the two sperm types to separate them); racing (placing sperm in a test tube full of viscous liquid and letting the two sperm types "race" each other to the bottom); and ultrasound (snapping off the heads of "wrong" sex sperm with sound waves.)

2. *Discrimination against either X- or Y-bearing sperm inside the woman's body after intercourse.* It has been proposed that one type of sperm might be filtered out with a special condom or diaphragm but no studies have been published on this.

From the early 1930s to 1942, researchers in sex predetermination focused on the acid–alkali method using baking soda douches to discriminate against "female" sperm and produce a boy and vinegar douches to produce a girl. (Actually, Dr. Felix Unterberger, the German obstetrician who developed the method, and other researchers explained that while they had experimented with alkaline douches, they had never tried vinegar douching for a girl because they had never had a patient who felt strongly enough about having a daughter to try it [Gordon, 1978, p. 765].) When repeated trials failed to confirm early positive results, researchers largely abandoned the method.

"One of the few things you can say with certainty in this field is that acidity and alkalinity do not have differential effects on X and Y sperm. That method has been thoroughly discredited," said Glass, who tested this theory (Diasio and Glass, 1971).

3. *Timing of intercourse* to provide the best circumstances for fertilizing the egg with the "right" sperm, either androgenic or gynogenic. In 1961, Dr. Landrum Shettles introduced a timing-of-intercourse method which in more than twenty years has not been demonstrated to be effective.[13] Dr. Rodrigo Guerrero developed another technique that is exactly the opposite of Shettles'. While Shettles advised intercourse two or three days before ovulation for a girl, Guerrero advised the same procedure for a boy. Shettles suggested intercourse at ovulation for a boy; Guerrero suggested that that procedure would yield a girl. Guerrero's method, like Shettles', remains unproven.[14]

4. *Antigen–antibody reactions between sperm and egg.* In the 1970s, work was conducted on the antigen–antibody reactions between sperm and egg. The possibility that this immunologic sperm treatment will have practical application is remote. The method is based on evidence that the Y chromosome carries an antigen that causes the female to make antibodies against it. Theoretically, antibodies produced against either androgenic or gynogenic sperm could be injected into the female, rendering those sperm inactive. If, for example, antibodies against the X sperm were injected, only Y sperm could fertilize the egg. One man has a patent on such an immunologic technique (Netwig, 1980). But the alterations in sex ratio are slight with this method (Rinehart, 1975).

Those are the basic methods of sex predetermination. Year after year, men work in their laboratories spinning sperm, building elaborate machines to separate the sperm, constructing obstacle courses for the sperm to run, shooting electrical current through the sperm to separate "male" from "female," dreaming of a way to snap off sperm heads with sound waves. They search hard for some slight difference between male and female sperm—sperm that arose from the same original cell—and some method of amplifying that difference.

In addition to these basic methods of sex predetermination, three of the other new reproductive technologies could also be used to predetermine the child's sex.

1. *Embryo transfer.* Before being implanted in a woman's womb, cells from the embryo might be snipped off and examined under a

microscope to detect its sex. If the embryo were the wrong sex, it could be discarded.

2. In vitro fertilization. As we saw in Chapter 7, Steptoe and Edwards have proposed freezing human embryos for later implantation and Wood's IVF team in Australia is already doing this. This procedure would provide enough time before implantation to determine the embryo's sex.

3. Cloning. Cloning, or asexual reproduction, has not yet been achieved in humans. It involves taking a single cell from a person and inducing it to begin dividing so that it produces an organism genetically identical to the parent. The sex of the child would be the sex of the person who donated the body cell. Rockefeller University president Dr. Joshua Lederberg, who received a Nobel Prize in 1958 for his research in the genetics of microbes, has written: "Nuclear transplantation [cloning] is one method now verified to assure sex control, and this might be sufficient motive to assure its trial."

Proponents of sex predetermination have offered several rationales for its use, including population control. In 1973, John Postgate proposed, as the solution to the world's alleged population problem, the distribution of a pill assuring the birth of boys. This "man-child" pill, made freely available to all, could be used mostly in Third World countries where the desire to breed male children "amounts to an obsession," according to Postgate. The resulting deficiency of females (breeders) would limit the number of babies who could be born in the following generation, thereby reducing population growth. Further, couples would stop producing child after child in an attempt to get the desired number of sons.

Postgate describes how women would live in a world in which many of their kind had been eliminated. "All sorts of taboos would be expected and it is probable that a form of purdah would become necessary. Women's right to work, even to travel alone freely, would probably be forgotten transiently. Polyandry might well become accepted in some societies; some might treat their women as queen ants, others as rewards for the most outstanding (or most determined) males."[15]

Dr. Ho Guan Lim, permanent secretary and director of medical services of the Singapore Ministry of Health, apparently shares the conviction of Postgate and others that sex predetermination would help solve the population problem. In 1975 he set up a clinic at the Kandang Kerbau Hospital, hoping that if couples could have the son they desired, they would limit their families to two children in conformity with the government's policy.

The clinic, experimenting with what proved to be an inefficient method of gender control, closed in 1977. But it left an ominous record. Of the thirty-one women who had definite gender preferences and attempted to use the method, every single one wanted a boy. A glance at a chart accompanying a report on this clinic (Williamson, 1978) provides women with chilling information:

Boys preferred	31
Girls preferred	0
Boys born ("Successes")	14
Girls born ("Failures")	17

Another rationale for sex control is therapeutic. The practice will help eliminate sex-linked genetic diseases, proponents argue. In 1980, Steptoe and Edwards announced that they would pioneer experiments to help couples determine the sex of the child with a method involving timing of intercourse. Edwards explained that the aim was to combat the genetic disorders that produce hemophilia and some forms of muscular dystrophy. This therapeutic rationale is intrinsic to many of the new reproductive technologies, ethicist Dr. Raymond noted, adding: "For it focuses the discussion off the social and feminist dimensions of the issue onto the more personal, curative, and supposedly benevolent aspects of the technology."

Sex control will be a boon to mental, as well as physical, health some argue. "The direct psychological effects of being able to control the sex of child in line with preferences would seem to be considerable, and almost wholly positive," researcher Edward Pohlman concluded. "The conception of children of an undesired sex is often undesirable from a mental health standpoint." Many psychotherapists, he explained, believe that the birth of a "wrong sex" child may lead to sex role confusion, which may lead to homosexuality or to psychological problems.

The difficulty with his explanation goes beyond the fact that, as he admits, there is no adequate research to support the psychotherapist's belief, and beyond the erroneous assumption that homosexuality is in itself problematic. The difficulty is this: "Sex role confusion" is a political term masked as a psychological one. Members of a sexual caste, like those of a racial caste, are expected to keep to their place. If women reject various subservient roles, then they are "confused" about their sex role. If Blacks in John Dollard's 1936 study, *Caste and Class in a Southern Town*, had gone to the front, rather than the back door of white homes, and failed to display other signs of subservience before whites, they would have been exhibiting "race role confusion."

Sex predetermination, besides contributing to mental health, is also alleged to provide an expansion of options and increased freedom. Researchers Saul Rosenzweig and Stuart Adelman, noting that "fetal sex determination in the first trimester in pregnancy with selective abortion may soon be widely practiced," refer to sex predetermination as "this new step in human sexual autonomy." They further observe: "Parents may soon be able to engage in total family planning, i.e., control of family size, spacing between children, sex of offspring, and male–female sequence."

Social scientists do not stand alone in defending sex predetermination. Dr. Clifford Grobstein, embryologist, justifies it in terms of increased individual freedom and control over reproduction. "In general terms, the rationale is to utilize expanding options and capability to make beneficial choices in terms of purpose rather than of accident or chance," he writes.[16]

Dr. Ronald Ericsson, who has developed one method for obtaining male offspring, also has benevolent reasons for his work. He "says his intention is not to promote boy babies but to prevent the tragedy of unwanted children" (Minden, 1981).

We have masses of people in the studies saying that they do not care for one type of human being (female), that they "prefer" another type (male), and this is being treated as perfectly acceptable. We must question the use of the word "preference" in this context. We are not talking about preferences for vacation sites—the seashore rather than the mountains. We are talking about human beings and whether ones with certain biological features will be allowed to come into existence.

Several commentators have speculated on what might happen in a society in which sex predetermination techniques were available. The society they envision is a horrifying one for women. One social scientist makes a revealing comparison between research on sex predetermination and on nuclear weapons: both are unstoppable. "Nuclear weapons were perfected despite a keen awareness among many researchers of the frightening implications of their work," he wrote. "Scientific curiosity, competition between scientists, and the like, will probably drive researchers on towards means of controlling sex of offspring, whatever the consequences" (Pohlman, 1966).

What are those consequences? The sex preference studies indicate that, globally, sons will be sought more often than daughters and the proportion of men to women (the sex ratio) will likely rise. How life is structured in future, female-scarce societies would vary with the cultures. Commentators speculate that in such societies, several men might share one wife in a polyandrous marriage, and rises might occur in homosexuality and prostitution. The scarce women might be secluded and pressured into marrying and reproducing, further reducing the control women have over their bodies. During a militaristic buildup, males might be regarded as cannon fodder and their conception planned with that purpose in mind. The government might legislate the circumstances under which people could use sex predetermination technology and occasional scandals in the administration of the laws might surface. Black markets in "boy-pills" and "girl-pills" could arise (Postgate, 1973; Luce, 1978; Etzioni, 1968; Hanmer, 1981; Pohlman, 1967). Since women read more books, see more plays and visit more museums than men, less culture would be "consumed," as one sociologist phrased it (Etzioni, 1968). Criminality, he noted, would increase because males are a disproportionate percentage of criminals.

The sex preference studies also indicate that with the availability of sex predetermination techniques, we would have a nation of older brothers and younger sisters (Westoff and Rindfuss, 1974). Whatever characteristics are associated with being firstborn would be concentrated among men. Those characteristics are ambition and success. Studies in sociology and psychology indicate that firstborns have advantages over those children born later. William Altus, who, as professor of psychology at the University of California at Santa Barbara, conducted some of these studies and reviewed others, summarized: "The dice are loaded in favor of the first-born."

The firstborns are more likely to achieve socially, educationally, and economically and to have higher IQ scores than later children. Several studies have shown that firstborns are overrepresented among college students.

With sex predetermination, then, women could be permanently deprived of the advantages of being firstborn. "A nation of younger sisters does not bode well for women as a group" (Hanmer, 1981).

Altus believes the preeminence of firstborns is largely due to the fact that parents treat them differently. They tend to be stricter with the first child and have higher expectations of achievement from him. Furthermore, the firstborn is the only child who, for a time, does not have to share his parents with other siblings. Firstborns may receive a disproportionately high share of emotional attention and economic support from the parents.

And secondborns? One study on secondborn women indicates that a woman from a two-child family tends to disparage herself more and suffer from lower self-esteem if she has an older brother than if she has an older sister (Altus, 1966).

"What are the implications of being second-born and knowing at some early age that you were planned-to-be second?" Dr. Roberta Steinbacher, chair of the Urban Studies Department at Cleveland State University, asks (Steinbacher, 1981).

Suppose mistakes occur, as they inevitably will, and a couple planning on a son have a daughter instead. How will that daughter be treated? Even now, being the "wrong sex" is a common experience, especially for girls. What does it do to children to know they are not what their parents wanted?

Other potential consequences of the use of sex determination are the radical reduction of the number of women in the Third World and increased poverty among women in developed countries. Postgate, as noted, has advocated a policy that would lead to the first consequence. As for the second, if selective abortion were the primary means of sex determination, poor people would have less access to that means. The availability of abortion for poor women is already severely restricted, Steinbacher points out. So more firstborn males would be born among the privileged while the number among the poor would remain the same. This, Steinbacher noted, would ensure that throughout the world "increasing numbers of women in the future are locked into poverty while men continue to grow in numbers, in positions of control and influence. Whatever selection method is utilized, the end result will carry with it the lasting opportunity for institutionalizing sexism in birth order."

Finally, the burden of the technology itself falls on the woman. It is women who must take their temperatures daily, chart their menstrual cycles and douche before intercourse. It is women who must bear the physiological effects of amniocentesis. It is women who face the risks of abortion for sex selection in the second trimester when the procedure is six times as life-threatening as in the first trimester. It is women who must endure repeated, and occasionally painful, courses of artificial insemination.

Commentators on sex predetermination assume that only those who want the technology will use it. But we cannot assume it will not be used coercively, perhaps on an unknowing people. Theologian Emily Culpepper has pointed out that DES (diethylstilbestrol) was given to some pregnant women who were told they were receiving vitamins. The drug has since been associated with serious abnormalities in the children of such women. (To convey that the decision on use of the technology may be made by someone other than the mother, sociologist Hanmer and colleague Hilary Rose use the term "sex predetermination" rather than the liberal terms "sex choice" or "sex selection."[17])

Dr. R. G. Edwards, co-progenitor of the world's first test-tube baby, has given some indication of how he views the coercive use of sex predetermination technology. As we saw earlier, he correctly determined the sex of rabbit embryos by analyzing the outer cells. He described the technique's potential use in humans and commented: "Imbalance of the sexes could probably be prevented by recording the sex of newborn children, and *adjusting the choice open to parents*" (my emphasis) (Edwards, 1974).

In discussing sex predetermination, most scientists focus on foreground issues (the expansion of options; disease prevention; population control) and ignore the Background question: Gynicide. If many women in the Third World are eliminated through sex predetermination, if fewer firstborn females exist throughout the world, if the percentages of poor women and richer men rise in the overdeveloped nations, then it is indeed gynicide we are discussing.

Hanmer observes: "A new offensive against women may be opening up in the sex war, one that social scientists seem determined to ignore in the pursuit of choice for happy families" (Hanmer, 1981).

Notes

1. Previctimization, she explains, is analogous to philosopher Mary Daly's notion of the *prepossession* of women. Before a women can be possessed, she must first *be,* but the possession takes place before her movement in be-ing can break through to consciousness. Prepossession, Daly writes, "involves depths of destruction that the term *possession* cannot adequately name" (quoted in Raymond, 1980).

2. I asked sociologist Jalna Hanmer, who has studied the sex preference literature, on what evidence these advocates based their reassurance that the sex ratio will eventually balance itself. "None whatsoever," Hanmer replied. "That is what's so astounding: None."

Nor does sociologist Dr. Nancy E. Williamson believe that the sex ratio (proportion of males to females) will naturally balance itself. Such a view, she writes, "implies an 'invisible hand' guiding people to adjust their private interests and behavior to the societal good." She thinks there is little reason to suppose such an adjustment would naturally occur. If couples thought it was to their advantage to have another boy or to have a firstborn boy, they might well do that even if their actions were harmful to the society as a whole, or for women as a group (Williamson, 1976, p. 861).

3. A few do not agree. Dr. Saul Rosenzweig and Dr. Stuart Adelman of the departments of psychology and psychiatry, Washington University in St. Louis dispute with Markle that widespread adoption of sex-choosing will lead to an excess of male infants. They argue that when they analyze data from recent studies, they find it indicates a preference for a balanced number of sons and daughters in a given family (Rosenzweig and Adelman, 1976; 1978).

But the contentions that sex-choosing would lead to an excess of males and that most people want a balanced number of sons and daughters can both be true, as Markle points out. The norm would be for people to want two children, one of each sex with the boy arriving first. A minority would want only one or three children and these would choose either one boy or two boys and one girl. That minority could throw the sex ratio, which is usually 105 (males):100 (females) out of balance.

"So it's not that everyone will choose a lot more boys," Markle said in an interview. "It's that a 'small' excess of boys raising the sex ratio from, say, 105:100 to 115:100 would be highly significant."

Another point is that due to flaws in their design, many sex preference studies may have underestimated the degree of the son preference they found. The studies can leave quite different impressions depending upon the questions they posed to people, and the questions posed vary from study to study. For example, if one asks for preferences for a two-child family, people overwhelmingly vote for one of each sex. If one asks for a choice based on the assumption that only one child is possible, the proportions of boys desired soars dramatically. To get more meaningful responses, a demographer and two mathematical psychologists developed a sex preference measurement technique, the Coombs scale, which Williamson regards highly. This scale does not rely on the respondent's first choice about number and sex of children. Instead, Williamson notes, it asks a series of questions to get at the person's underlying preference structure.

"This approach has found more evidence of boy preference in the U.S. than the simple first-choice measures," Williamson writes.

The National Center for Health Statistics, which periodically conducts the National Survey of Family Growth, used a short version of the Coombs scale in 1973. Its results indicated that son preference is still "quite pervasive in the American culture . . . all the recent emphasis on sexual equality notwithstanding." (A national sample survey conducted two years later obtained similar results.) About half the married women aged 14 to 44 interviewed revealed an underlying preference for sons while about one third preferred daughters. Only one fifth clearly preferred an equal number of sons and daughters.

This evidence from a national sample is somewhat at variance with other data that have been interpreted as indicating preference for balance, data based on more superficial sex preference measurement techniques. Demographer Lolagene Coombs comments: "When choices beyond the first are taken into account, the IS [sex preference] scale values show much more underlying boy preference" (quoted in Williamson, 1978, p. 8).

Williamson notes, furthermore, that most large U.S. studies with information on sex preference have interviewed only wives. This is a major failing of the studies. Most studies have ignored the fact that the wife's wishes alone will not determine what sex child is chosen. Wives are subordinate to husbands in the family as women are subordinate to men in society, and it is likely that that fact affects whose "choice" will prevail. Evidence suggests that the husband's influence would be in the direction of increasing male births (Westoff and Rindfuss, 1974).

Researchers Rosenzweig and Adelman observe: "Since most major decisions usually reflect the wishes of the dominant spouse, it is obvious that the possibility of sex choice will open up a new area of potential marital conflict." They suggest that future family planning programs may have to incorporate some form of "sex-choice counselling" (1976; 1978).

4. Psychoanalysts have often maintained, in a belief that at first appears to be consistent with evidence from sex preference studies, that women usually prefer giving birth to a son. This opinion was probably based on Sigmund Freud's discredited theory that bearing sons would solve women's so-called "masculinity complex" and symbolically compensate them for not being men. The birth of a daughter has even been considered a contributory cause in psychiatric disturbances following the birth.

Yet the findings of European researchers refute the supposition that women pregnant for the first time want to bear a son and that the arrival of a son is more satisfying to the women (Uddenberg et al., 1971). They found that women who have daughters are less likely to suffer from mental disturbances after birth than women who have sons.

Irrespective of the sex they had wished for, women giving birth to boys were more often disturbed after the delivery than women bearing girls. Paradoxically, those who suffered the most from mental disturbances were the women who wished for a son and then bore a son. The researchers explained that finding in this way: Some of the women stating a preference for a son were not expressing their true wish but were instead bowing to convention and to their belief that their husbands wanted sons. Three studies, in fact, have found evidence that women want sons in order to please their husbands (Williamson, 1976, p. 61).

One explanation why women may, on whatever unspoken level, be more pleased with the birth of a daughter, is that most pregnant women identify themselves with the expected child and therefore want a child of their own sex. Two studies that found that children generally prefer their own sex support this explanation, the researchers note. Boys prefer sons and girls prefer daughters (Kohlberg, 1967, cited in Uddenberg et al., 1971; Hartley, Hardesty and Gorfein, 1962). As boys grow older, they retain their preference for sons. But girls change. As adults, they suddenly "prefer" sons too. The Uddenberg study suggests that, on a deeper level, women, like little girls, want to have daughters but some force intervened as they grew to make them say they would choose sons.

5. See Emecheta (1979) for a vivid portrayal of how failure to produce a son can affect a woman's life.

6. See the powerful Nigerian novel *The Joys of Motherhood,* which expresses the importance of sons to men (Emecheta, 1979, p. 166).

7. Encyclopedia Britannica, 1980. Another, Collier's (1979), tells us: "In some primitive communities . . . the disposal of girl babies has led to polyandry resulting from a shortage of marriageable women at a later date."

8. A few details. *Greece:* Studies show a preponderance of male children in

classical Athens, providing evidence of infant gynicide (which we know was practiced). In one study of wealthy and influential families, the ratio is five males to every female. (However, women were so devalued that they may not have been consistently counted. For example, Herodotus reported that Cleomenes died childless, leaving only a daughter.) Nonetheless, there is other evidence that males did in fact greatly outnumber females. Priam had fifty sons but only twelve daughters, Homer states, relating a Bronze Age or, less probably, a Dark Age tradition. Andromache, the sole girl-child in her family, had seven brothers (Pomeroy, 1975). *Japan:* During the Tokugawa period (1600–1868 A.D.), some districts reportedly registered nine male births for every female birth. The implication is that seven or eight out of every nine girl babies were destroyed (Rinehart, 1975). *India:* During the early days of the British occupation, the Radschucmors of India killed nearly 10,000 baby girls every year (Rorvik and Shettles, 1971).

9. In Hellenistic Greece, women's lives were shorter than men's by five to ten years and Pomeroy, the classical scholar, has theorized that that may be partly due to their diet, which was inferior to that of boys. Xenophon praised the Spartans for nourishing their girls as well as their boys for it was unusual among the Greeks to do that. Even a male infant at his mother's breast may have been nourished better than a female infant, for the "mother's ration" given to Ionian women in 489 B.C. in Persepolis was twice as much for women who had borne boys as those who had borne girls (Pomeroy, 1975, pp. 228 and 85).

In Rome, too, there was a sexual imbalance—fewer females than males among upper-class Romans. One cause of the imbalance, which may have been more important than either female infanticide or woman's shortened life span, was the preferential treatment of boys (Pomeroy, 1975, p. 165).

10. Malhotra, 1982. Following the public stir, authorities in Amritsar served notice on the pioneering husband-and-wife team that their practice was contrary to law and medical ethics, and they were subject to prosecution. The couple said it would contest the order on the grounds that it contravenes the fundamental right of every citizen to carry out his vocation.

The Good Parents Group of Nutley, New Jersey, supports the practice of aborting the female fetuses of the poor in India (it calls this "Therabort") and has offered to help finance a model therapeutic termination clinic. Women found to be carrying male fetuses would not be permitted abortions at the clinics unless the fetus were defective. "With therapeutic-termination the submerged one-third of humanity can have mostly sons," its brochure stated (Good Parents Group, 1978).

Now in his seventies, William I. Battin, Jr., incorporated the Good Parents Group, a charity, in 1955, with his wife Helen who serves as secretary. He runs the nonmembership group from his small brick house on a tree-lined street in Nutley. Battin, a graduate of Swarthmore College, worked for a gas and electric company and studied population problems in graduate school at night in New York in the 1940s. He came to believe that if the poor had all sons, and if future mothers all came from the upper classes, poverty would be reduced. The upper-class women could provide good homes for the babies. They could afford food for themselves and therefore their babies would not have birth defects associated with maternal malnutrition.

In 1972, Battin began publishing yearly editions of Son-by-Choice, a booklet expounding his philosophy and giving instructions on sex selection by a method of unproven efficacy. He has the booklet distributed free in India.

His group, which encourages large families among "leading citizens," offers to pay the poor in India to have all sons, an offer none have taken up. The group also offers to provide a "pronatalist service" for women seeking abortion. It would pay the women to undergo an amniocentesis and, if the fetus is found to be male, pay them more to bear the baby.

11. L. Zech, a Swedish researcher, found a way to stain chromosomes in 1969. She discovered that one portion of the chromosome showed up brightly when put under a fluorescent microscope. The next year two British researchers, Dr. Peter Barlow and Dr. C. G. Vosa, stained sperm with quinacrine and found that in the heads of about half the sperm they could see a fluorescent spot (called the F or Y body) which appears to indicate the presence of the Y chromosome. So they have provided a chemical test to identify X and Y sperm.

This discovery gave those working in sex selection the opportunity to identify human androsperm without having to do a timely and costly fertility test. Before these discoveries, they would experiment with their sperm separation methods, take the separated sperm, inseminate lab animals or cattle with it, and then see what sex offspring they got. After these discoveries, anyone with an idea for sex selection could take the sperm he had attempted to separate, stain them, place them under a microscope, count the number of Y chromosomes and see if they had changed the sperm ratio from 50:50.

12. To understand how gynogenic and androgenic sperm originate from the same cell, we need to look at the way sperm is produced. During this process, four spermatozoa—two carrying the Y chromosome and two carrying the X—will be produced from the very same primitive sperm cell, the spermatogonium. In the first step of production, the spermatogonium divides in half to create identical cells. Each of the new cells (or primary spermatocytes) carries a full complement of chromosomes, that part of the cell where the DNA or hereditary material is kept. In the next phase of sperm production, the primary spermatocytes split into two cells, one carrying a Y chromosome and the other an X. These secondary spermatocytes each have half the number of chromosomes. These two "half cells" are identical (they sprang, remember, from the same primitive cell) except that one has a Y chromosome and the other an X. Finally, these half cells split again, forming spermatids, which eventually mature and become sperm.

13. Williamson, 1978. For favoring the conception of a girl, Shettles advised that the woman should douche before intercourse with diluted white vinegar, thus increasing the acidity of the reproductive tract. She should have intercourse flat on her back two or three days before ovulation when the acid environment prevails. Penetration should be shallow at the time the man ejaculates. She should not come to orgasm, as that is alleged to increase alkalinity. (However, despite Shettles' belief, there is no evidence that the woman's orgasm causes any chemical change in the vagina.)

To favor the conception of a boy, Shettles advised, the woman should douche with an alkaline baking soda solution. She should have intercourse at or close to the time of ovulation when her secretions are the most alkaline. The man should penetrate her deeply from the rear to help ensure that the sperm will be deposited at the cervix. She should come to orgasm. To increase the sperm count, the man should have abstained from ejaculation from the start of the woman's cycle until the time of ovulation.

14. Glass, 1977, p. 124. Those wanting a boy, according to Guerrero's method, would have intercourse on the sixth, fifth, and fourth days before the expected day of ovulation, as indicated by a rise in the basal body temperature, and would avoid intercourse until three days after the temperature rise. Those wanting a girl would avoid intercourse until two or three days before ovulation was expected (Whelan, 1977, p. 117).

15. Let's look more closely at the rationale Postgate cites for gynicide: curbing the population explosion. Postgate wrote that the population explosion has caused a world protein shortage, serious shortages of raw materials and a global pollution problem. Author Clare Boothe Luce, who also advocates a "man-child" pill, cites the same population menace. She traces all international problems, including a potential nuclear war, to the root cause: "uncontrolled fertility of the female of the species." Domestic problems, she writes, "are the omnipresent, inescapable side effects of the pressures on the planet's limited resources generated by the unlimited fertility of women."

Numerous books and articles have refuted the notion that overpopulation is the root cause of hunger and depletion of the world's resources. (See Frances Moore Lappé and Joseph Collins, 1977, *Food First: Beyond the Myth of Scarcity*, Houghton Mifflin Co., Boston; Susan George, 1977, *How the Other Half Dies: The Real Reasons for World Hunger*, Allanheld, Osmun and Co., Montclair, N.J.; Peter Adamson, June 1977, "Population Control," *New Internationalist*, 52; Latin American Working Group, Toronto, Fall 1974, "Population control," unpublished; Anuradha Vittachi, June 1980, "The aspiration bomb," *The Internationalist*, 88.) They demonstrate that the problem is not too many people or too little food but antihuman decisions about what crops to grow and where to distribute them. Several note that during the 1973–1974 famine in the Sahel, the export of cash crops from some parts of the Sahel actually increased. Adamson observes: "Fertile land in Latin America grows Del Monte fruit and pink carnations for North America while children are malnourished only a few fields away."

Commentators also note that the problem is less a population explosion in the underdeveloped world than a consumption explosion in the overdeveloped world. Vittachi points out that the poor world has 75 percent of the world's people, but consumes only 15 percent of the world's energy sources and 30 percent of the world's food grains. A person born in the rich world, then, will consume about thirty times as much as a person born in the poor world. Consequently, the 16 million babies born each year in overdeveloped lands have about four times as much impact on world resources as the 109 million babies born each year in underdeveloped nations.

Further, critics such as the Latin American Working Group point out the close links between earlier eugenicists and today's population controllers or neo-Malthusians. "The main fear gripping the entrails of the eugenicists and today's neo-Malthusians is the swelling tide of inferior humanity rising to overtake the material resources and wealth of the world, thus threatening the hegemony of white western civilization."

Despite difficulties in demonstrating that a "population explosion" is truly what threatens life on the planet, professionals continue to bring up gynicide as a possible solution to the population problem. For example, two researchers write that in populations where boys are an asset to parents and girls a burden: "Interruption of pregnancies with female fetuses would probably be acceptable" (Cederqvist and Fuchs). Such a proposal for population control perhaps "deserves some consideration," they conclude.

Other professionals also mention, without condemnation, proposals to reduce the proportion of the world's women relative to men in order to lower population growth (Rosenzweig and Adelman, 1976; Revelle, 1974).

16. Grobstein, 1981, pp. 121–122. A bioethicist for the National Institutes of Health, Dr. John C. Fletcher, has also advocated support for safe, effective sex predetermination methods that increase the parents' ability to choose the timing of pregnancy and sex of their children (Thorne, 1982).

17. When cattlemen attempt to use sex predetermination to enlarge their dairy or beef herds, it is obviously ridiculous to speak of the cows themselves "selecting" the sex of their offspring, Hanmer and Rose note. But it can be argued that when the technology arrives, women may freely choose the sex of their children. "How free is choice in a society where some people are more powerful than others," they ask, "and where societal forces including the mass media create 'need'?"

11

Surrogate Motherhood:
Happy Breeder Woman

Tom, a Moslem from Lebanon, married Jane, an infertile American woman. Jane wanted to adopt a child but Tom did not. He wanted to father his own. While the Vietnam war raged, he got an idea. Maybe he could find a woman who would agree to be inseminated with his sperm, bear the baby and turn it over to him and Jane. He knew many men were dying in Vietnam, leaving widows with children, and thought one of those widows, needing money for her children, might do it. "The Lord intended women to have children and I thought maybe one would want to do what came naturally and maybe help somebody else out while helping herself and her family," Tom recalled (Keane, 1981, pp. 20–30).

In September 1976, Tom and Jane contacted attorney Noel Keane in Dearborn, Michigan, to discuss Tom's idea. After that meeting, they read a newspaper account of a man who had hired a blond office worker to bear a child for him. The last of his family line, the California man wanted a child to carry on his name. So he had placed an ad for a woman in *The San Francisco Chronicle* ("Childless husband with infertile wife wants test-tube baby. English or Northwestern European background. Indicate fee and age.") The office worker had just borne him a daughter for a fee of $7,000.*

Keane now knew what to do for his clients. He ran ads for a surrogate mother in several Michigan college newspapers. Seeing the ad, a reporter called, interviewed Tom and Jane and wrote a story. In response to the ad and the newspaper story, two hundred people

---

* The man stated that he still wanted a son. "I can't afford it right now," he said, "but I may try again."

wrote to Keane. (One was a man volunteering the use of his 27-year-old girlfriend. "She smokes cigarettes but she doesn't drink or take drugs," he wrote.)

Keane eventually found a surrogate (breeder) for Tom and Jane. Moreover, he had queries from new clients who wanted breeders and, soon, an invitation to appear on *Donahue,* the national television show. After that appearance, his business accelerated as viewers who wanted to use a breeder or to be one called him. He made many more appearances on *Donahue* as well as on other programs, continuing to do so long after the thrill of television celebrity had worn off. "I now went on shows like *Donahue* for a simple reason," he wrote. "Other than placing classified ads, the only effective way of finding surrogate mothers was through television and news articles" (Keane and Breo, 1981, p. 173).

Keane began to refer to the sale of breeder women as a "movement," a "cause," and to himself as a "pioneer" and a "champion" of breeders, whom he called "surrogate mothers."

In the next few years, others quickly jumped into the act, setting up some sixteen surrogate mother, or breeder, businesses across the country. Many were launched by physician-attorney teams, others by those who spoke of their backgrounds vaguely. One had previously worked for "a major insurance company." Another told me that he had made motion pictures, designed buildings and served as a consulting engineer on missile programs.

The firms opened up in: Louisville, Kentucky, 1979; Philadelphia, Pennsylvania, Hollywood, Los Angeles, and Malibu, California, 1981; Chevy Chase, Maryland, Denver, Colorado, and Tulsa, Oklahoma, 1982; and Columbus, Ohio, Tempe, Arizona, Springfield, Massachusetts, New York, New York, Lincoln, Nebraska, Norfolk, Virginia, Northridge and Costa Mesa, California, 1983. By May 1983, an estimated seventy-five to one hundred babies had been born to breeder women nationwide.

John Stehura, president of The Bionetics Foundation, Inc., which helps arrange surrogate pregnancies, fears that hiring surrogates is too financially burdensome for middle-class American couples. But this burden may be lifted. He thinks the price paid to women for reproductive services will come down once surrogate motherhood is more commonplace. The industry can then go to poverty-stricken parts of the country where half the current $10,000 fee may be acceptable, he told me in an interview.

The development of embryo transfer technology may bring the price down still further. Today's surrogate mother contributes half the baby's genes through her egg. Consequently, those hiring a breeder want her screened carefully for physical, intellectual and racial traits. But once it is possible to have what Stehura calls an "authentic" surrogate—a woman into whom an embryo is transferred and who herself contributes none of the child's genes—clients will find the breeder's IQ and skin color immaterial.

The genetic makeup of the woman is "much more important right now because she contributes 50 percent to the child, but in the future, it's going to be zero percent," Stehura said. He is monitoring the progress of embryo transfer technology so that once a dozen or so babies have been created, he will be ready to step in with his service.

Another surrogate firm run by attorney William Handel in North Hollywood is also planning to arrange the transfer of embryos into surrogate mothers. Noting that he keeps in contact with practitioners in the reproduction field, Handel told me in 1982 he was certain experimental work in this area was currently going on at IVF clinics connected with hospitals.

As we saw in Chapter 7, the Monash University IVF program in Australia has already established one viable pregnancy by transferring an embryo conceived with a donor egg. This is one procedure that could be used with surrogate mothers.

Once embryo transfer technology is developed, the surrogate industry could look for breeders—not only in poverty-stricken parts of the United States, but in the Third World as well. There, perhaps one tenth the current fee could be paid women, Stehura speculated. Asked what countries he had in mind, Stehura replied: "Central America would be fine." It is "inevitable" that the United States go to other parts of the world and "rely on their support" in providing surrogates, Stehura thinks. Comparing the United States to the city and Central America to the country, he pointed out that "the cities are always supported by the country."

An "authentic" surrogate from the Third World won't even need to be very healthy. "The mother could have a health problem which could be quite serious," he said. "However if her diet is good and other aspects of her life are O.K., she could become a viable mother for a genuine embryo transfer."

Using Third World women as surrogates, Stehura maintained, would benefit them because the women would earn money with which to raise their other children.

Media helped create the phenomenon of surrogate mothering (often termed surrogate "parenting," a word choice that obscures the fact that we are talking here only of *female* breeders). "The true fathers of the surrogate-mother story, perhaps, are the *Phil Donahue Show* and *People* magazine," Keane wrote.[1]

The pattern set early on has continued through the present. Those who, like Keane, have an economic motive for promoting surrogate motherhood are generating the news about it. They go on television and explain why trafficking in breeder women is noble. What sociologist John Dollard wrote of defensive beliefs used to justify oppressive practices applies as well to the rationale these proponents offer for their businesses. This rationale stresses a partial and inadequate element in the situation (the suffering of infertile couples) and obscures a clear vision of the actual social forces. Certain facts about surrogate motherhood are highlighted in media discussions while others are buried.

Although entrepreneurs in the surrogate industry emphasize the unhappiness of infertile couples in justifying their practices, in fact not all are confining their advocacy of surrogate motherhood to the infertile. Sometimes the "empty arms" the firms are attempting to fill belong—not to barren women, but to single men, or fertile women, or couples with adopted children. Some proponents of surrogate motherhood are making a conscious political decision not to highlight these other potential employers of surrogates at a time when they need public approval of the procedure in order to get laws passed legalizing it.

Keane annoys some of his colleagues by being quite open about the other employers of breeders. He wrote: "Single men are increasingly seeking surrogate mothers as a solution to having children without romantic entanglements." For men who want a child but not a wife, surrogate motherhood offers a "dramatic option," Keane believes. Now a man can go out and have a child any time he wants. "And if he prefers to have a boy, there's a 75 to 85 percent probability we can arrange it by separating the sperm before insemination," Keane claimed (Krucoff, 1980). (That probability has not been demonstrated, as we saw in the previous chapter.)

Keane says he works with single men now. At least two breeders have already birthed children for separated or divorced men (Parker, 1982; Donahue, #02033). Single women are also seeking breeders, Keane maintains.

He sees nothing wrong with using breeders for women who are perfectly fertile and he may do so in the future. If a fertile woman chooses to have children by a breeder, Keane is willing to represent her if he already has enough surrogate mothers for the infertile.

Alan A. Rassaby, research fellow in the Centre for Human Bioethics at Monash University in Melbourne, also defends the use of surrogates for career-related reasons, stating that a busy female executive's or model's need for a surrogate may be just as great as that of an infertile woman. Unfortunately, he added, one can expect the career woman to be discriminated against in times of "scarce resources" (the "resources" being women's bodies).

Unlike Keane, other surrogate entrepreneurs frown on the use of surrogates for fertile women and require proof that clients are married and that the wife cannot bear babies. Because they are more selective than Keane and exercise greater control over surrogates and clients, some of Keane's competitors imply that their businesses are more reputable than his. They are critical of the fact that he is willing to accept a wide variety of clients—single men,[2] transsexuals (one, to date), and, in the future, fertile women. They are not criticizing Keane's ethics, but rather his poor political strategy for winning public acceptance of, and favorable legislation regarding, surrogate motherhood.

As I write, there are no laws in the country on surrogate motherhood. But there are statutes against baby-selling and these statutes could cause surrogate firms trouble. Until laws are passed legalizing surrogate motherhood, any public indignation aroused over the practice could threaten the emergence of this "whole new sector of the economy," as The New York Times referred to it (November 1980). Adoption agencies, the Catholic Church and Concerned United Birthparents (a group of women who, years earlier, had given up their babies for adoption and suffered greatly from it) have opposed surrogate motherhood at public hearings.

"Keane will take anybody who walks in the door," William Handel, of Surrogate Parent Foundation, told me. He disapproved: "It's kind of a hard thing to say morally, because these are not necessarily my morals, but considering his position, I think that simply for political and P.R. reasons, you've got to play it very conservatively and very safe. It's difficult to take potshots at someone who's doing this for a married couple who cannot have children. But it's easy to criticize someone who's doing it for a gay single male, which he takes on all the time." (In fact, Keane says he has never dealt with homosexuals but "would consider them on a case-by-case basis" [Miller, 1983].)

Handel said he was not morally opposed to using surrogates for gay men. Two such men, physicians with high incomes in a stable relationship, asked him to arrange a birth for them. He declined. He is trying to get some favorable legislation on surrogate motherhood passed, he explained, and so he runs his business conservatively.

"I told them it was a *political* choice I was making not to take them on. Chances are that the two of them would have made phenomenal parents."[3]

In Michigan, state legislator Richard Fitzpatrick, who introduced the second legislation in the country on breeder women, made "a conscious decision for political purposes" to apply his legislation only to married couples and not to single men seeking breeders. He did this, he stated, because "it is a highly sensitive and controversial issue enough as it is without getting into other aspects. Even those who strongly support it understand that the most important thing right now is to get the concept of surrogate parenting into the law" (Gaynes, 1981).

In addition to the fact that infertile couples are not the only ones purchasing the services of surrogate mothers, there is another fact media discussions of surrogate motherhood bury: Adoption agencies do have children that infertile couples could adopt. Those who defend the use of breeder women mention, in passing, that these children are not the "right kind," and therefore couples have little alternative but to hire (white) breeders.

"While there are plenty of babies to adopt, they are not, quote, 'desirable' babies, if that's the right word to use," Dr. Michael Birnbaum of Surrogate Mothering, Ltd., in Philadelphia told me. "There are plenty of babies of mixed racial background. There are plenty of babies with handicaps, but most couples want a perfect baby if they're going to adopt it, and those kind of babies are hard to come by."

Harriet Blankfield of the National Center for Surrogate Parenting in Chevy Chase, Maryland, told me that most of the infertile couples she personally knew were not interested in adopting an older child or a handicapped child. She added: "When it came to wanting a child—no matter how desperately they wanted a child—they didn't want to take what they would consider second-best.... That may not be a good term but that, verbally, is how they felt emotionally."

I raise this issue not to argue that these couples should adopt special-needs children (feeling as they do, it is likely that both they and the children would be harmed by such an arrangement), but rather to point out that the desire to nurture a child for its own sake is not their prime motivation. They want only a child that meets certain specifications.

The child here is viewed as a commodity. Dr. Richard Levin of Surrogate Parenting Association in Louisville has referred, perhaps jokingly, of the baby as a "product" and Keane refers to the child as an "investment." (Keane wrote: "How can the husband be sure he is indeed the father of his 'investment' short of isolating the surrogate from other male contacts?" [Keane, 1981, p. 265]. Levin said that surrogates in his program must agree to paternity testing to ensure that the baby was fathered by his client and not the surrogate's husband. "We only take the real product," he said [Donahue #04150].)[4]

A main function of the genetic, medical and psychological screening of surrogates is to ensure quality control over the product the breeders will produce. "Do you get to choose blue eyes, brown eyes?" television host Phil Donahue asked Keane. "As a matter of fact, they [the couple] do," Keane replied. "They take portfolios that are available on each surrogate and it lists the characteristics." Keane adds that they can and do find out the surrogate's IQ.

The view of baby-as-commodity came into sharp focus in the Stiver–Mallahoff case. In January 1983, a surrogate mother delivered a defective product—a baby with a small head, probably indicating mental retardation—and all parties involved initially rejected the baby and announced it would be put up for adoption. The baby had a strep infection and the man who contracted for the child's birth— Alexander Mallahoff of Queens, New York—instructed the hospital to "take no steps or measures to treat the strep infection or otherwise care" for the child, according to an affidavit filed by Lansing General Hospital in a successful effort to secure a court order allowing it to treat the child.

On the *Donahue* television show, Ray Stiver of Lansing, Michigan, husband of the surrogate, Judy, charged that Mallahoff "asked the hospital to put this baby to sleep, and then he asked my wife to start over and make a new one for him. It's just like buying a defective piece of merchandise." Mallahoff denied that he had done this.

Mallahoff contended that he was not the child's father and blood tests proved him right. Under intense and degrading questioning on national television as to exactly when she had had intercourse with her husband following the artificial inseminations, Judy Stiver said she had abstained for at least thirty days after, but had not been told it was necessary to abstain before, when the pregnancy might have occurred. The Stivers, after learning on camera that Ray was the child's father (the blood test results were called in to the television show), said they would take the baby. Mallahoff had said that if the child proved to be his, he might put him up for adoption but that if it had been normal, he would have taken the baby.

In those cases in which a married couple is involved, why would an infertile wife agree to her husband's artificial impregnation of another woman? There are several explanations. First, this woman would be subject to all the pressures on infertile women discussed in Chapter 9.

Moreover, for many women, the alternatives to childrearing look dismal. One woman who obtained a child through a surrogate explained: "All I ever wanted from life was to get married and have children." Then she had a hysterectomy at 25 (Keane, 1981, p. 58). She had worked in banks but could not imagine doing that for the rest of her life. "There's got to be more," she said, believing that "more" was a child. (Similarly, Lesley Brown, mother of the first test-tube baby, had worked in a factory wrapping cheese and could not bear the prospect of spending the rest of her days in the factory.)

Sociologist Hanmer believes there is another motive: It is socially structured so that, for many women, the only way she can get affection is to have children. "Children love you," she observes. "It's actually possible for women to have love relationships with children. It's extremely difficult to have them with men."

Fear of abandonment can be another motive for a woman agreeing to the insemination of a surrogate. Consider Tom and Jane, the pseudonymous clients of Noel Keane seeking a surrogate. Jane explained that she had wanted children ever since she was a little girl who played with dolls. Her husband came from a Lebanese culture where children were prized as a symbol of manhood and her unsuccessful attempts to conceive a child had shaken her marriage "to its foundation" (Keane, 1981, p. 13). When a woman like Jane "chooses" to hire a surrogate mother, then we must ask what happens to her if she does *not* choose this. It may mean that her husband will leave her.

Fear of social ostracism and emotional and economic abandonment does seem to have motivated the West Indian woman who traveled by bus from New York to Detroit in an unsuccessful attempt to hire a surrogate through Keane. Married to a Nigerian, she would soon be moving to his country. She feared that, under pressure from his relatives, her husband would divorce her for her failure to bear him a child (Fleming, 1978).

We watch a series of women appear on television to explain that they *want* to be surrogate mothers, that they are giving the gift of life and helping infertile couples, and that we, the public, need to be educated as to the nobility of the transaction between couple and surrogate. We like these women. They are kind and intelligent. Lawyers, psychiatrists and physicians appear on television with the women and present what they call a discussion of the issues raised by surrogate motherhood:

Should the breeder be married or single? Should she have had other children or none? Should the couple meet the breeder? What kind of counseling should be done with the couple? The surrogates? What records should be kept? What if the breeder refuses to give up the baby? Can the surrogate be forced to have an abortion if the fetus is found to have Down's syndrome? Can the natural father require the breeder to undergo an amniocentesis? Can the breeder sue the father for damages arising from the pregnancy? If the couple divorces before the baby is born, who is responsible for the baby? Is the child illegitimate? Can the sperm donor deny the breeder an abortion? What if the couple dies before the child is born? If a breeder is being paid for bearing a baby, does control over the child revert to her in the wake of missed payments?[5]

These questions keep our eyes focused on the foreground. But, as with all these technologies, there is something more going on than an attempt, motivated by compassion, to fill the empty arms of childless couples with babies. That "more" is in the Background.

In surrogate motherhood, the woman is again seen as the vessel for a man's seed, just as she was under Aristotelian/Thomistic biology. According to Aristotle, woman merely supplied matter which the active male principle formed and molded into a human being. Men played the major role in reproduction while woman served as the passive incubator of his seed. That Aristotelian biology was back became clear to me when, in 1980, it was revealed that Joseph Orbie, a single, 30-year-old man, was looking for a surrogate mother who would bear him a son. He planned to hire a sex predetermination researcher who would attempt to remove the X sperm from his semen and inseminate the breeder with the remaining Y sperm (Donahue, #07290).

As we saw in Chapter 10, producing sons for men has been a prime function of woman. Now, through technology, men may someday be able to employ her for this purpose with minimal human involvement. Like the surrogate who would lay on the examining table at a sex predetermination clinic to be inseminated with Orbie's processed, supposedly male-engendering sperm, women can serve as mere vessels for the incubation of men's sons. Though they supply the eggs (at this point, still) and nurture their babies within their bodies, their connection to the child is not acknowledged. They are to disappear after the child's birth, leaving the man as the parent. In fact, under proposed legislation in Michigan, the child of a surrogate mother would be considered not *her* child, but the offspring of both the man who provided the sperm and that man's wife.

That the surrogate mother is viewed as a vessel for the man's seed is evident from the language consistently used to describe her. The women are referred to as inanimate objects—incubators, receptacles, "a kind of hatchery" (Schroeder, 1974), rented property, plumbing—and they have come to speak of themselves in this way.

Though the babies born to surrogate mothers to date have all been their own children, conceived with their own eggs, the women often maintain that they are not. Some of the surrogate applicants Dr. Parker interviewed asserted that their babies belonged to the adoptive couples and they denied the possibility that they might feel any loss when they gave up their infants. Among the reasons the women gave for not expecting any emotional involvement with their babies, Parker reported, were "I'm only an incubator," and "I'd just be nest-watching" (Parker, 1983). A psychotherapist who worked with Handel in California said the attitude of many surrogates she interviewed amounted to: "I'm not the mother. I'm the plumbing providing the opportunity for her to be the mother" (Krier, 1981).

One surrogate mother told me: "I never looked at the baby as *my* baby. It was *their* baby. I just felt like I was doing like my chickens do. I was just hatching it and all the other chickens would take care of it."

References to the woman's body as property are common. For example, Sanford Katz, professor at Boston College Law School and chair of the American Bar Association's Family Law section, commented: "I wouldn't consider this [surrogate motherhood] buying a baby. I'd consider this buying a receptacle" (NYT, 1980, May). A *Western Journal of Medicine* article referred to the surrogate as "the woman attached to the rented womb" and to her child as "her tenant" (Karp and Donahue, 1976).[6]

Advocates of surrogate motherhood often bring up the biblical story of Abraham, Sarah and Hagar like a trump card, implying that the practice is ancient, God-endorsed and, therefore, moral.

> Now Sarai Abram's wife bare him no children; and she had an handmaid, an Egyptian, whose name was Hagar. And Sarai said unto Abram, Behold now, the Lord hath restrained me from bearing: I pray thee, go in unto my maid; it may be that I may obtain children by her. (*Genesis* 16:1–2)

Sarah allowed Abraham to take concubines for his sperm to be reproduced in the world, Raymond explains. Today the Judeo–Christian tradition that a woman was valued insomuch as her ability to reproduce, has become medicalized so that it is incarnate in technology. This enhances the ethic that if a woman cannot reproduce naturally, Raymond adds, she must do it in some other way. Now the woman might take the egg of another woman into her body or—with surrogate mothering—not even bear the child.

"It is almost like allowing your husband to take a concubine so that his issue may be reproduced in the world," Raymond said. "That is, to me, the overriding ethic: that his issue may be reproduced. It's the same old story, only this time it's made much more possible by biomedicine."[7]

It is often asserted that the person benefiting from the surrogate mother's "gift" is the infertile wife, not the husband. For example, Alan Rassaby asserts that satisfying the desires and needs "of a number of women" would be the primary benefit of surrogacy (Walters, 1982, p. 104).[8] Despite this reversal, the statements of Keane, Levin and their clients make it clear that Raymond is right: The overriding ethic is that the man's issue may be reproduced in the world.

Take the case of surrogate Elizabeth Kane (a pseudonym). She told a television audience that she was willing to accept any health risks involved in the pregnancy. "I felt that strongly about giving a baby to another woman that needed one. It was a gift that I had to give at any cost." Earlier she explained: "I had wanted to have another baby for a woman for ten or twelve years because I had always felt . . . an empathy for women with empty arms" (Donahue #12170).

But the woman who received Kane's baby did not have "empty arms." She and her husband had a three-year-old adopted son. The husband explained that they sought a surrogate because another adoption would have been difficult and because "we wanted, if possible, to have a child that was biologically related to me." He thanked his wife for "suggesting and initiating and supporting *me* [my emphasis] in doing this thing." Asked how she thought Kane could give up the baby, the wife, in her reply, indicated that the child was really for her husband: "I think she was just doing it as a gift of love, you know, for mankind. You know, she had some feelings as to how a person, like, in my situation would feel not being able to have a child and knowing how my husband wanted one so deeply."

Alice Baker (pseudonym) will also be bearing a child for a

couple who is *not* childless. Baker, a 30-year-old woman in Alexandria, Indiana, with four children of her own, was attempting, at the time of our interview in December 1982, to become pregnant for a couple who already had an adopted girl. (She had earlier borne a baby for a couple who adopted a child during her surrogate pregnancy.)

Levin's statements too reveal that the surrogate "gift" is more to the husband than the wife. Conceding that childless couples could adopt an older or handicapped child or a child of another race, he adds: "But these people want a child related to them, who will carry on their [i.e., the husband's] bloodline. The women often say, 'I want my husband's baby even if someone else carries it'" (Krucoff, 1980).

Keane, too, revealed that the underlying ethic is that a man's issue might be reproduced. When his policy of screening the surrogate mother but not the father was criticized, he observed: "Well, I'll say every man has a right to reproduce himself" (Donahue #02033).

The clients of breeder firms also make it clear that Raymond's analysis is on target. For example, Mrs. Wallace, a woman whose fertility had been destroyed by an IUD-induced infection, said that a surrogate mother was her only hope for her "to have my husband's child" (Donahue #04150).[9]

Sometimes the wife already has children by a previous marriage but, because of a subsequent loss of fertility, cannot provide her second husband with children of his own. One woman, after bearing two children, had a hysterectomy and later remarried. She and her husband sought a surrogate. After meeting the surrogate, the wife said: "I felt so bad that I couldn't give my husband a child—but now I can" (Krucoff, 1980).

Keane's clients included couples in similar situations. Keane relates the story of a male client who was obsessed with having a child while his wife, who had diabetes and kidney problems, seemed unenthusiastic. It was a full-time job for her to care for herself. Despite that, the husband insisted that he wanted to hire a surrogate mother. About two weeks after the couple contacted Keane, the wife left her husband. Keane reported: "She left a note saying that she could not stand the pressure being put on her to have a child" (Keane, 1981, p. 138).[10]

Since no laws exist on surrogate motherhood, it is uncertain whether courts will hold the contract between a man and breeder woman valid. Perhaps they will not; statutes against baby-selling seem to prohibit paying women to bear babies.[11]

When Surrogate Parenting Inc. opened in 1979 in Louisville, it stated that Kentucky law allows the payment of a fee to a surrogate mother, an interpretation of the law that state attorney general Steven Beshear challenged. "The Commonwealth of Kentucky does not condone the purchase and sale of children," he stated in January 1981. Beshear brought a civil action to enjoin Richard Levin's corporation from engaging in its business but has not pressed the suit since then. Surrogate Parenting Inc. has continued operating and even expanded into the international field, matching American breeders to couples in France, Canada, Mexico and Australia.

Those running surrogate businesses want laws passed explicitly legalizing their practices. Some are working closely with legislators to write those laws. "We're actively involved with Assemblyman Mike Roos in developing a surrogate parent law," attorney William Handel of Surrogate Parent Foundation in North Hollywood, California, told me. He added later: "We helped write the legislation so it's got everything we want in it."

The first legislation on surrogate motherhood was introduced to the Alaska house of representatives in April 1981. Nine states are now considering such legislation.[12] To date, none has passed any. A number of proposed laws constitute a massive move against women's civil rights. They would establish unprecedented medical and state control over the woman's body, would attempt to make the contract between man and woman binding, and would give the sperm donor a greater right to the child than the mother. For example, proposed legislation in Michigan would give the sperm donor and his wife full rights to the child immediately upon birth.

The "binding contract" provision is one for which Keane and other proponents of surrogate motherhood have argued. Keane believes that women who sign a surrogate mother contract ought to be legally bound to give up their babies.

Under one draft of proposed legislation in Michigan, if a woman changes her mind, the judge of probate courts holds a hearing. While the question is being decided, the rights to the child remain with the sperm donor. Unless the woman could demonstrate "by clear and convincing evidence" that her child's best interests would not be served by terminating her parental rights, the judge would enforce the contract and order the baby given to the sperm donor and his spouse. (In keeping with the notion that the baby belongs to the man who furnished the sperm, the mother would be legally prohibited from attempting to form a mother–child relationship with her baby.)

Such provisions in draft legislation worry Jalna Hanmer: "When they can legally force a woman to give up the child, then the way opens up to horrible abuse." Annette Baran, author of *The Adoption Triangle,* has a similar concern. A woman cannot know in advance how she will feel as she progresses through the pregnancy and the child's birth, Baran points out, so she must retain the right to change her mind. "You cannot indenture her and her unborn child before the fact," she said in an interview. Some surrogate mothers and applicants have never birthed a child and may be surprised by the feelings pregnancy arouses in them.[13]

One version of Michigan legislation is based on the notion that sperm donors and surrogate mothers are fulfilling comparable functions and ought to be treated comparably under the law. Under this legislation, the natural father (who furnished the sperm) and his spouse would be considered the legal biologic parents just as under the Michigan artificial insemination statute, the natural mother and her husband would be considered the child's parents.[14] Explaining the rationale behind this draft of his bill, Representative Richard Fitzpatrick told me: "We believe that philosophically if a man has the right to sell the use of his reproductive organs as we currently have in the law at this time—that a man can be compensated for the donation of his sperm—certainly a woman should be able to be compensated for the donation or utilization of her reproductive organs. So we go into the law and snuggle up as close as possible to all the regulations on artificial insemination in relationship to parentage, inheritance, and all that." Allowing men to sell sperm but forbidding women to sell their eggs and wombs would constitute sex discrimination against women, Fitzpatrick and others argue.

I asked feminist leader Andrea Dworkin to comment on the argument that sperm donors and "womb donors" were comparable and that forbidding women to sell their bodies constituted sex discrimination.

"I suppose if one swallows a seriousness pill and tries to take the argument on its own terms, you'd have to point out the difference between an ejaculate of the body and the body itself which seems to me something that an ancient Greek philosopher might have pointed out—so ancient is that mode of logic," she said. "It's the difference, for instance, between tears and the eye. You could collect tears in a glass but that's different from taking someone's eyes."

She continued: "There *is* no analogy between the sperm of a man and the womb of a woman. There is none. They are not analogous in any way. To underscore it: Not physiologically, not ethically, not reproductively, not morally, and by no means are they analogous in terms of their meaning to the integrity of the person. What this argument underscores is that men have not yet grasped that women are not baby-making machines, and that women's bodies are not commodities best suitable to be sold. There seems to be no notion of personhood and integrity that applies a priori to women in men's minds. Otherwise it [surrogate motherhood] would be unthinkable."

When a woman volunteers to be a breeder, advocates of surrogate motherhood assert that the woman's act is an expression of her individual will. She wants to do it; she is a free person; what right has the state to interfere with her will?

"No one is forcing a woman to enter into this contract," a spokeswoman for Assemblyman Mike Roos said in response to the objection that surrogate motherhood was reproductive prostitution. (See Chapter 14.) "She enters into it of her own free will for whatever reasons she wants. It's anything but prostitution. This is a woman's free choice to use her body any way she wants to. And that's what freedom is all about."

Feminists like Andrea Dworkin do not agree that that's what freedom is "all about." They argue, rather, that legislators and those in the human breeding business are developing a specious notion of what freedom and equality are and are applying it in their proposed legislation.

Dworkin notes "the bitter fact that the only time that equality is considered a value in this society is in a situation like this where some extremely degrading transaction is being rationalized. And the only time that freedom is considered important to women as such is when we're talking about the freedom to prostitute oneself in one way or another."

She observes that the "freedom for women" argument is conspicuously absent in the speeches of establishment people when they are talking about other aspects of a woman's life. "You never hear the freedom to choose to be a surgeon held forth with any conviction as a choice that women should have, a choice related to freedom," Dworkin said. "Feminists make that argument and it is, in the common parlance, not a 'sexy' argument. Nobody pays any attention to it. And the only time you hear institutional people—people who represent and are part of the establishment—discuss woman's equality or woman's freedom is in the context of equal rights to prostitution, equal right to some form of selling of the body, selling of the self, something that is unconscionable in any circumstance, something for which there usually *is* no analogy with men but a specious analogy is being made."

In response to the assertion that some women *want* to be breeders, Dworkin argues that the social and economic construction of the woman's will is what is at issue. This will is created outside the individual. In both prostitution and surrogate motherhood, Dworkin writes, the state has constructed the social, economic and political situation in which the sale of some sexual or reproductive capacity is necessary to the survival of the woman. It fixes her social place so that her sex and her reproductive capacity are commodities.[15]

Proponents of surrogate motherhood insist that the woman's will is interior, somehow independent of, and unaffected by the culture in which she lives. When a woman sells the use of her vagina (as a prostitute) or her womb and ovaries (as a surrogate mother), they assert that these are acts of individual will.

"This individual woman is a fiction—as is her will—since individuality is precisely what women are denied when they are defined and used as a sex class," writes Dworkin. "As long as the issues of female sexual and reproductive destiny are posed as if they are resolved by individuals as individuals, there is no way to confront the actual conditions that perpetuate the sexual exploitation of women. Women by definition are condemned to a predetermined status, role, and function" (Dworkin, 1983).

One of the actual conditions that perpetuates the exploitation of woman is her economic status. In the United States, women earn 59 cents for every dollar men earn, a proportion that remains constant regardless of the woman's employment or educational level. Most women are confined to the female job ghetto—that handful of jobs in which the pay is low and there is little or no mobility. Working women, typically, are: secretaries, typists, file clerks, receptionists, waitresses, nurses, bank tellers, telephone operators, factory workers, sales clerks in department stores or cashiers in supermarkets, elementary school teachers, beauticians or cleaning women (MacKinnon, 1979). Those women who manage to avoid job ghettos encounter sex discrimination in salaries, promotions, benefits and/or sex harassment (Pearce and McAdoo, 1981).

Within such an economic world, it is hardly surprising that money motivates women to become breeders. Remember that Tom, the man who sought a breeder, was looking for a Vietnam war widow in need of money to raise her children. One man searching for a surrogate mother described the ideal surrogate as a woman who had lost her husband. "Maybe she's struggling to make ends meet and could use the money," the unidentified man told the *Detroit Free Press* (2/4/77). In fact, when the call went out in 1980 for Australia's first surrogate mother to deliver a child for $10,000, one applicant was an 18-year-old widow left penniless after her husband was killed in an accident. Another was a 23-year-old whose husband was terminally ill and who said she urgently needed the $10,000 to provide some security for her child. More than half the ninety applicants were divorced or single. They ranged in age from single 17-year-olds to a widow of 44, and included a former prostitute (*ST*, 12/14/80).

Dr. Howard Adelman, a psychologist who screens breeder candidates for Surrogate Mothering Ltd. in Philadelphia, told *Ob/Gyn News:* "I believe candidates with an element of financial need are the safest. If a woman is on unemployment and has children to care for, she is not likely to change her mind and want to keep the baby she is being paid to have for somebody else" (Miller, 1983).

Dr. Philip Parker indeed found that slightly more than 40 percent of the surrogate applicants in his study were unemployed or receiving financial assistance.[16]

Rich women, Keane wrote, "are not likely to become surrogate mothers" (Keane, 1981, p. 236). When Keane placed ads for surrogate mothers in newspapers, he received responses from Pocatello, Idaho, to Jacksonville, Florida, and most of the women said they needed the money (*Chicago Tribune,* 12/4/77). There were plenty of women willing to reproduce for payment. At that time, Keane was under the impression that his clients could pay a fee to the surrogate. But when, after receiving a judge's opinion in March 1977, he realized that they could not, the number of volunteers dropped to almost zero (*Detroit News,* 5/4/78).

Keane could not get enough breeders if he could not pay them. He brought a lawsuit to have the payment of a fee to a surrogate mother declared legal. He lost the first round of his suit in 1980 when Wayne County (Michigan) Circuit Judge Roman S. Gribbs sided with the prosecuting attorney. That attorney had argued: "the fact remains that the primary purpose of this money is to encourage women to volunteer to be 'surrogate mothers.' Plaintiffs have initiated this lawsuit because few women would be willing to volunteer the use of their bodies for nine months if the only thing they gained was the joy of making someone else happy by letting that couple adopt and raise her child. Thus, contrary to plaintiffs' exhortations, in all but the rarest situations, the money plaintiffs seek to pay the 'surrogate mother' is intended as an inducement for her to conceive a child she would not normally want to conceive, carry for nine months a child she would normally not want to carry, give birth to a child she would not normally want to give birth to, and, then, because of this monetary reward, relinquish her parental rights to a child whom she bore."[17]

Some entrepreneurs in the surrogate mother business are sensitive to the criticism that poor women, having few opportunities to earn money, would have no choice but to become breeders. Handel, for example, says that this criticism is unfounded for he does not accept indigent women into his program. The women must have good incomes before he will accept them. However, he also noted that his company is getting middle-class and working women who, with their husbands, are using the money to set up a fund to send their children to college or to make a down payment on a house.

One surrogate mother I interviewed told me she and her husband had used the money she had earned through child-bearing to keep their small trucking business going during hard times. "We own semis [tractor trailers] and right now is a bad time with Reagan," she told me. "So we used the money to help keep the trucking company going."

Judy Stiver of Lansing, Michigan, who became a surrogate for Alexander Mallahoff of Queens, New York, is an inventory clerk earning less than $5 per hour and her husband is a part-time bus driver. Stiver said she became a surrogate in order to pay off her family's bills and, possibly, take a vacation.

Who knows what pressures are being exerted and will be exerted on even middle-income women to contribute to the family income in hard times by breeding? The pressures might range from extremely subtle and nonverbal to violent. Women may themselves suggest, even enthusiastically, that they help out the family by breeding for payment, but this does not mean that in a society that defines women by their reproductive function and consistently underpays them for their labor, that the women are acting of their own "free will."

Furthermore, that indigent women are not being accepted into many surrogate programs now, as asserted, does not mean they will not be accepted in the future. As we have seen, some of the entrepreneurs are being cautious about how they run their businesses in the early years when public opposition to it could prevent them from getting laws passed legalizing it. Once the laws are on the books, it will no longer be necessary to labor under self-imposed restrictions as to who can be accepted into the program. Stehura already sees it as "inevitable" that entrepreneurs will come to use poor women as surrogates and pay them as little as one tenth the current low breeder wage.

So a woman's economic status helps construct her "will" to sell her womb. So does her emotional structure. It has been engrained in women that one of the most important roles we play is tending to all others, fostering their growth and happiness. Their needs and difficulties should be our major concern and dealing with them should take precedence over other claims, including any "selfish" needs of our own. Of course nurturing is a highly valuable activity. What is wrong here is that only women—not all human beings— are supposed to engage in it and engage in it to the exclusion of other valuable activities. This is what social worker Margaret Adams terms "The Compassion Trap" (Adams, 1971). Under the social pressure to be nurturing, one single element of woman's psyche has hypertrophied while other qualities have withered.

Pharmacrats searching for surrogate mothers or egg donors exploit woman's emotional structure. They appeal on the media for compassionate women to come forward and "give the gift of life" to a sorrowing couple. They call these women "special" and praise them as selfless, loving, sensitive and big-hearted. (Even though they may, in the very next breath, call them "rented wombs" or "receptacles.") When women are called upon to relieve the suffering of others by sacrificing—even prostituting—some part of themselves, many leap at the chance out of what Adams calls the "overriding need to feel useful and wanted in a social system that in other respects does not accord women much, if any, value or opportunity for really significant participation."*

The social manipulation of women's psychological resources, Adams argues, has much in common with the exploitative view of women as purely sexual objects. "What I am talking about is an exactly similar process in which not physical sexual attributes, but psychological ones, are subject to similar prostitution and misuse."

The manipulation of women's psyche is an exploitation difficult to resist because it is so hard to change our emotional structure.

"The worst thing you can do to someone is mess with the core of her in some way and I think *that* is what is going on in the appeal to surrogate mothers," a friend told me. "You violate or exploit a person's sense of herself. I think it's the most horrendous crime against another person. Murder is a crime against the physical

* I am applying Adams's insights to surrogate motherhood. She does not write about this phenomenon in her article.

self but there is also a long list of crimes committed against the selfhood of women and this is one of them."

Besides a woman's economic status and her emotional structure, another condition that perpetuates her exploitation and shapes her "will" is her social status. No matter what her individual talents or her unique character might enable her to do, this social system fixes her reproductive function as primary. As bioethicist Alan Rassaby observed in a different context, society places a greater premium on a woman's childbearing role than it does on her employment prospects. Given that childbearing is the prime function for which women are valued, it is not surprising that some women only feel special when they are pregnant and assert that they love reproducing. This enables some men to use what I call the "Happy Breeder" argument in explaining why women are willing to be surrogate mothers. It is comparable to the "Happy Hooker" justification for prostitution.

In a study of Keane's surrogate applicants, Parker found that some women who had already borne babies saw surrogate motherhood as a chance to earn money while enjoying a pregnancy. Parker reported that the applicants "described a feeling regarding their [previous] pregnancy that varied from a tolerable experience to the best time of their life such that they wanted to be pregnant the rest of their lives. This latter group felt more content, complete, special, adequate, and often felt an inner glow; some felt more feminine and attractive and enjoyed the extra attention afforded them" (Parker, 1983). (Since, in his study, he does not give the number, I asked Parker *exactly* how many of the 124 applicants had said they felt this way. He said he did not have the specific numbers and that if I were going to quote him, I could use "the term 'some.'" He added later that "a few" women said, "I feel better when I'm pregnant than when I'm not pregnant.")

In defending surrogate motherhood, other men such as Laurence E. Karp, M.D., and Roger P. Donahue, Ph.D., have asserted that some women just love to be pregnant. Much has been made of the possibility of exploiting poor women through surrogate motherhood arrangements involving embryo transfer, Karp and Donahue write. They, on the other hand, worry about denying women a livelihood through surrogate motherhood. A few women have called their offices to volunteer their services if such embryo transfer schemes should ever be carried out.

"They state that they love being pregnant and would arrange to always be in this condition if it were not for the matter of having to keep the babies," Karp and Donahue write. "They think that hiring out their uteri would be a fine way to make a living. On reflection it seems inconsistent to categorically deny such women this kind of livelihood, while we permit and even encourage people to earn money by such dangerous means as coal mining, or racing little cars around a track at 200 miles per hour" (Karp and Donahue, 1976).

Rassaby has a similar concern. Without denying that some surrogate mothers may be the victims of an unfair social order, he asserts that some women may prefer exploitation to poverty. He believes it would be "counterproductive" to deny them the "option" of exploitation (Rassaby, 1982, p. 103).

"If men generate the ethic—which I firmly believe they are doing in this case—that women are really happy when they are pregnant, that's nothing new," ethicist Dr. Janice Raymond commented in an interview. "They've said that for ages. Now they are just saying it in a different context and are zeroing in to apply it to a specific population of women—in this case, surrogate mothers."

Raymond makes a crucial point about the social construction of a woman's will: Men are controlling not only what choices are open to women, but what choices women learn to want to make. Women may have a will to be pregnant, she added, but we have the potential to want other things as well. This potential is kept largely unfulfilled.

"Not only do women not go into certain things, but they don't even have the motivation to *want* to because the choices have been so limited," she said. "That is what I see as most drastic: Not the fact that our choices are being controlled, but that our *motivation* to choose differently is also being controlled."

While men like Karp and Donahue assert that some women really love to be pregnant, this becomes a self-fulfilling prophecy that closes off all the other choices a woman might make. Pointing to the social forces in the Background generating a woman's desire to be pregnant-all-the-time, Raymond asked: "Why aren't men—all these reproductive biologists—saying in the same breath, 'Women love to be doing science,' or 'Women love to be doing philosophy'? You never hear that. They keep beeping out those messages, 'Women love to be pregnant,' and limiting the choices for women. And women will fulfill those choices.'"*

---

* Of course many women do, have and always will resist their conditioning in a male-supremacist society. Nonetheless, it is nearly impossible to overestimate the effect this conditioning has on restricting, in a thousand different ways, the lives of women.

Because the social control over a woman begins at an earlier stage than that of the woman's actual decision-making, because it begins by controlling her motivation to choose, people can argue that women freely decide to be surrogate mothers. When television host Phil Donahue raised the question of women being used as baby factories, Janet Porter, a surrogate volunteer, replied: "But a woman still has to choose to be a surrogate mother, you know. She's not gonna be hogtied and have it done to her, you know." Donahue responded: "Yes, that's true."

Both ignore the sophisticated level of control the dominant class exerts over women.

Dworkin has a final comment on this issue of "free choice." The notion that the selling of the body is the highest expression of what freedom means in a capitalist society, she said, is a grotesque application of laissez-faire principles of capitalism. The argument that a woman has an absolute right to sell her body as a commodity and that that is a cherished freedom, is also grotesque.

She added: "These are very bizarre ideas of freedom. If you read in philosophy and in history and in all of these very important male disciplines, nothing is more important than the question: What is freedom? There is never a very simple answer to it. So how come the answer is so simple when the question is asked about women? And how come it's so functional? You have all these philosophers writing tomes about what freedom is, and I think any student of philosophy will agree that no one definitively answered the question. How come with women it amounts to some answer that has to do with buying and selling?"

Parker is conducting a long-term study of breeder women. Since a researcher's values can affect the way he designs and interprets a study, Parker's values, about which he is explicit in his writings, bear scrutiny. He defends financial gain as a legitimate motive for bearing a child. There is no evidence that breeding for the purpose of earning money has any adverse consequences—psychologically, medically or legally, he asserts. Financial reward from "a grateful husband" may even be motivating some wives to bear children now, he speculates. Parker implies that both situations—wives and breeders bearing babies for money—are appropriate. Some feel that money as a motivation for producing a child degrades the whole process of procreation, he observes, and comments: "I can see no reasonable justification to force this moral tenet on the rest of society." His basic position is stated succinctly: "I believe that a married couple's use of a surrogate mother to bear the husband's biologic child falls into the category of a fundamental right." (He does not name the belief system under which one has a fundamental right to use a woman's body and spirit for one's own purposes, but I can accurately describe it as patriarchal.)

Parker defends the surrogate motherhood business by invoking his studies: "Also, I have so far found no evidence to support the notion that surrogate motherhood with or without a fee, leads to serious adverse psychological consequences and therefore (as some people feel) should be prohibited" (Parker, 1982).

I suspect Parker sees no "evidence" of harm for a reason similar to that which Thomas Aquinas cited in maintaining that it is appropriate for men to kill and eat animals. Aquinas argued: "There is no sin in using a thing for the purpose for which it is" (Singer, 1975). And animals (imperfect beings) supposedly exist for men (more perfect beings) to use. Parker, with his patriarchal values, may see no harm in using a woman for the purpose for which she supposedly is intended: reproduction. (Remember what Tom, the surrogate seeker, said: "The Lord intended women to have children and I thought maybe one would want to do what came naturally.") It does not seem to Parker to injure the integrity of a woman when she sells her body, her self, as a commodity.[18]

Besides studying the surrogate mothers, Parker counsels them. Generally, in each surrogate firm, a psychologist or psychiatrist like Parker is involved, as well as a lawyer and a physician. (The lawyer draws up the contract. The physician examines the breeders to determine their health and fertility, inseminates those chosen, and frequently sees them for monthly check-ups until the obstetrician takes over.) The psychologist screens the breeder candidate for mental suitability and sees the pregnant breeder for counseling roughly on a monthly basis. Handel's program is slightly different. "We're the only group in the country that insists on group therapy for the surrogates," he said. (Dworkin commented: "It's like they're not going to take a chance that a woman might have an independent thought.")

Parker believes that the pregnant surrogate should be offered special prenatal classes specifically tailored for surrogates and that support groups should be organized for pregnant and postpartum surrogates. Noting that women in one support group formed a closely knit community, he added: "This feeling of camaraderie and sharing complemented and tended to support the empathetic feelings toward the parental couple." This does suggest that the benign view of breeding-for-pay is reinforced in these groups.

Annette Baran, co-author of *The Adoption Triangle,* appeared on a television program with one professional operating a surrogate business. "His attitude is that he's got them in therapy during the whole period," Baran commented. "They recite in chorus, 'We're doing something great for somebody else. We're carrying somebody else's baby.' It's really a brainwashing affair. He plays violin strings and talks about these poor [infertile] people with their *only* alternative today."

Those in the surrogate industry assert that the women are "giving the gift of life" and placing a baby in the "empty arms" of a childless woman. Surrogates appearing on television say the same thing. Janet Porter, for example, explained her willingness to be a surrogate in terms of her "need to give." She was happy with her own child and wanted to give to others the joy she had. (While sperm vendors rarely assert that they are selling their sperm because they want to help the infertile, surrogate mothers often say that compassion motivates them. However, about 90 percent of surrogate applicants Parker interviewed required a fee to bear a baby [Parker, 1983]. A "need to give" was not enough motivation.)

Again and again in interviews, the surrogate mothers repeat the same statements: "I'm filling the empty arms of a childless woman. I'm giving a gift of love, the highest gift anyone can give. It's their child, not mine. I'm just a chicken hatching eggs."

"It's incredible," Dworkin marvels. "It's like—the gift of love, the highest gift a chicken can give?"

There may well be isolated occasions in which one woman, seeing the suffering of a friend, does truly make a gift of a child to her. That is very different from a situation in which lawyers, psychiatrists and gynecologists are forming companies for the purpose of selling women's reproductive capacities to strangers—some of whom already have children or are unwilling to nurture "second-best" children—and are appearing on the media to solicit women and create a need for this new "service." They pretend that the first, rather noble, situation is the same as their own exploitative practice and use the same vocabulary to describe both: "the gift of love."

Is it true what the surrogates predict—that they will feel only a slight sadness at giving up their babies?

Elizabeth Kane, who had referred to herself as an incubator during her pregnancy, proved to have the complicated emotions of the actual human being she is: "The first time I saw the adoptive mother hold the baby, it was thrilling," she said. "But I also went through depression—for example, on the third day in the hospital when my milk came in and the other woman was feeding the baby. And when I said good-bye to the baby, it broke my heart. I cried for weeks every Sunday because he was born on a Sunday" (Blair, 1982).

Parker interviewed twelve surrogates who had delivered babies. He found that the women expressed "transient grief symptoms" that were highly variable. "One stated that she had almost no consciously experienced feeling of loss," he wrote. "Another described one episode of deep crying, while still another related repetitive symptoms such as crying daily at the time of delivery and sleeplessness, both lasting about one month."

In writing the above section, I recalled an interview I had had with Joe, the midwestern farmer who allowed me to watch embryo transfers in cows. He told me that on his farm, they took a calf away from its mother at seven months in order to dry the mother up so she could rest and prepare to produce the next calf. The farm expected a calf a year from each cow; it was in the business of selling these calves, which would eventually be slaughtered for beef. A portion of our interview:

JOE: We take the calf away from her. We call it weaning. They bawl for four or five days and before you know it, why they're out in the pasture eating and they sort of have given up on their calves. Within two weeks they've just about forgotten their calves.

ME: The cows actually cry?

JOE: Yes, sure they cry. They bawl terribly. Not with tears. It's more of a yelling kind of thing. No, they don't have tears to show emotions but they certainly are very vocal about it.

ME: So the cows have real emotions, then?

JOE: Not emotions like humans have. They've been seven months with this calf. They know it's their calf and this is their main job, raising their calf. They don't want to give it up. But it's not exactly the same as with humans. I suppose it is very similar. Where humans show tears and depression, with a cow it's just excitement, bawling and this type of thing.

How deep *is* the woman's grief when her child is taken from her? Will that grief be viewed any more seriously by men who regard the woman as a rented receptacle than the cow's grief was viewed by men who see a cow as a machine for producing marketable products, calves? Like the cow's grief, could the woman's be misread as "just excitement"? Could a woman's crying be interpreted not as an expression of sorrow, but "more of a yelling kind of thing," or, as Parker medicalized it, a "symptom"?

How sensitive is Parker to women as complex human beings when he writes that the twelve women who delivered a baby and received a $10,000 fee did not seem to have any adverse psychological consequences merely because they received a fee, and adds, as if providing evidence that paying for women's bodies can actually have a *positive* psychological consequence: "As a matter of fact, one surrogate expressed that spending some of the money on items for the house helped her to deal with feelings of loss" (Parker, 1982).

One feminist with whom I discussed the loss experienced by surrogate mothers commented: "It is drilled into us in every conceivable way that we women have this maternal instinct, maternal love. We are told that if we have an abortion, we'll suffer a great psychological trauma and sense of loss. Now they're saying: 'Well, as long as you know it's not yours, you can give it up. No problem.' They're conditioning women to say: 'It's not my baby. It's your baby because you paid for it.' How fast they change! They switch propaganda on us as it suits their needs."*

Now, if you are a breeder woman, giving up your baby can even be therapeutic. In one study (1983), Parker found that 35 percent of the women volunteering to be surrogates had lost at least one fetus or child through abortions (26 percent) or surrender of the baby for adoption (9 percent). The experience of relinquishing the baby appeared to help the surrogate deal with prior voluntary losses of a fetus or child, he maintained.

"A few consciously felt that they were participating in order to deal with unresolved feelings associated with the prior losses. The only applicant who was herself adopted had been 'forced' to relinquish her baby at age 14 and wanted to repeat the experience of relinquishment and master it."**

Asked if the 35 percent rate of abortion and adoption surrender differed from the rate found in a similar nonsurrogate population of

---

* Another example: When justifying embryo transfer, Dr. John Buster, a pioneer in the technology, asserted that the real mother of the child was "the woman who nurtures and shapes a child for nine months. If that isn't being a mother, what is?" (Donahue, #08223). Yet when justifying surrogate motherhood, surrogate entrepreneurs often assert that the woman who "nurtures and shapes a child for nine months" is *not* the real mother; she's just a living incubator. This makes the practice of taking the woman's child from her seem more palatable.

** Parker's use of quotation marks around "forced" seems to indicate disbelief in the woman's account of her own experience.

women, Parker replied: "We don't know." That data is not kept, he maintained. If the percentage is similar, Parker's theory is of questionable validity.

I asked Parker *how many* women actually said they wanted to be surrogates in order to atone for a previous abortion or to master feelings associated with the previous loss of a child. Parker did not give me numbers. He did tell me that not all the women who had had abortions said they wanted to be surrogates as a result of those abortions. In fact he added: "Some of them totally denied that there was any causal connection." He said he thought there generally *was* a causal connection "even if they [the women] are not aware of it," and he would count those denying the connection among the surrogates atoning for a previous abortion. So Parker dismisses the women's own felt experience when it contradicts his theory.

I do not know the depth of grief surrogate mothers are experiencing. I do not know whether women are eagerly signing up as breeders in an attempt to benefit from the therapy allegedly anticipated in giving up their children. Maybe it is true that some women can surrender their children without great pain and loss. But I do not think we are going to find out from Parker, the man who believes that use of a woman for paid breeding is a "fundamental right" of the user.

Besides justifying surrogate motherhood as "therapeutic," Parker serves another useful function for the surrogate industry: He explains away some of the opposition to surrogate motherhood with his insights into the irrational psychology of the opponents. The strong opponents have unconscious fantasies of adultery and incest that are triggered by the concept of surrogate motherhood, he maintains. And/or, the opponents' unacceptable anger and hostility toward children may be stirred up and expressed by condemning the surrogate who will give up the child she bears. Keane wrote: "Such irrational opposition, he [Parker] says, should be identified and discredited" (Keane, 1982, p. 254).

Parker told me that whenever you separate reproduction from sex from marriage, you tend to encourage in people the onset of fantasies that make people uncomfortable, particularly fantasies about incest. Knowing that Parker emphasizes the need for studies in evaluating surrogate motherhood and that he discredits opponents of the procedure by pointing out that they have no data on which to base their criticisms, I asked him for the scientific basis for his assertion.

"That's based upon my talking with some people," he replied.

"It's not a controlled study at this point, no. That's based upon my own clinical impression, talking with some people informally—some of them even during interviews ... and some of it is my own speculation."

Surrogates are being paid to perform one of woman's biological functions. This is not the first such arrangement. For centuries, women were paid to nurse the babies of others. Embryologist Dr. Clifford Grobstein sees the connection between the two roles: "If a favorable ethical and social consensus develops, the role of wet nurse (which is accepted in many cultures) could probably be expanded fairly rapidly to include surrogate childbearing."*

Under medical control, as physician reports reveal, wetnurses were screened, inspected, controlled, devalued and viewed as cows. We will see a comparable control exercised over surrogate mothers.

First, consider the way physicians controlled wetnurses. Dr. Isaac A. Abt, who supervised wetnurses at the Sarah Morris Hospital in Chicago, reported on his experience in 1917. Maternity hospitals and foundling asylums referred women to Dr. Abt. He would inspect them for milk production, squeezing the women's breasts to see if the milk shot out or only dribbled. He did not accept dribblers.

Once hired, the women moved into the hospital. They got room, board and $8 per week. They were required to do light work. Their rooms were inspected for cleanliness. Dr. Abt wrote: "The personal hygiene of the wetnurses is carefully supervised. It is insisted that they shall bathe regularly and that they shall be attired at all times in clean clothes."

The wetnurse was compelled to retire at 9 P.M. and rise at 8 A.M. During the night, she was not permitted to nurse her own baby. In the afternoon, between milking periods, she was allowed some leisure time: "During this time she may exercise or rest.... If she goes out for a walk, she takes her baby with her; this precaution helps to keep her out of mischief. She is not allowed to leave the institution after dark, and is required to be in her room by 8 P.M." (Abt, 1917).

The women did not put the foster babies directly to the breast. Instead, apparently for "sanitary" reasons, they expressed their milk into sterile bottles.[19] Dr. Abt reported: "All the wetnurses milk at the same hour under the supervision of a head nurse and assistants.

---

* Wetnursing was made obsolete around 1925 with the development of an artificial breast—the baby bottle—and a substitute for mother's milk. The development of an artificial womb and placenta would make surrogate mothering obsolete.

Thus the operation is pretty well controlled.... It is necessary to exercise watchfulness in supervising the operation, because it has been our experience in times past that wetnurses have practiced deceit, either by diluting the milk or by substituting cow's milk for their own product."

Dr. Owen H. Wilson of Nashville also emphasized that the wetnurses must be watched. They have sometimes carried milk bottles in their bosoms and emptied them into the receptacles, he warned. (What must the lives of those women have been like that they were desperate enough for money to do that?)

Just as physicians controlled wetnurses, so too are controls exerted over today's breeders (see Ince, 1984). The contracts women sign with the various surrogate mothering firms are similar. Generally the woman agrees to abstain from intercourse during the insemination period to assure the man employing her that he is the father of her child. She agrees not to smoke or drink during the pregnancy and not to use any drugs, including aspirin, without the doctor's written permission. She agrees to be present for psychological counseling during the course of the pregnancy. She is contractually bound to obey all medical instructions of the inseminating physician and her obstetrician. Although routine obstetrical practices have been subjected to devastating critiques in government hearings and reports and numerous books, if the physician wants to use those practices on her, she must submit.[20] She agrees not to engage in any activities that would be against her doctor's advice and that—he felt—would endanger the birth.[21] (The physician who inseminates and/or conducts prenatal exams on a surrogate mother may see himself as serving the interests of the couple or lawyer who hired the surrogate mother rather than the woman herself, just as a veterinarian sometimes sees himself as serving the interests of the cow's owner rather than the cow. For example, take the case of a surrogate mother who changed her mind and refused to give up her child to Keane's clients. The surrogate, her physician wrote to Keane, had been bothered during her pregnancy by severe nausea and vomiting and had at one point considered an abortion. "We firmly discouraged the abortion, as the patient's *agreement and responsibility* [my emphasis] were thoroughly reviewed." The physician's letter, Keane wrote, "indicates he is working for the success of the arrangement.") The breeder must adhere to a strict prenatal schedule. Keane requires no fewer than one visit to the obstetrician per month during the first seven months of pregnancy and two visits—at two-week intervals—during the ninth month. Fitzpatrick, who worked with Keane on the draft, added a similar provision to his law regulating surrogate motherhood. The Michigan draft law, House Bill No. 5184, would legally bind the breeder to obey all medical instructions of the inseminating physician and the obstetrician.

"That's got to be a denial of every civil right, even under this [Reagan] government," Dworkin commented. "When you're in prison, you have more rights than that over your own body."

Also under the draft law (since superseded by another version), the surrogate would have to sign a contract agreeing not to abort the fetus unless her doctor thought that was necessary for her physical health.*

Handel requires that the surrogate keep his firm informed of her whereabouts at all times. Asked why, he replied: "Because she's carrying my client's child. It's nice to know where she is at all times. If she moves, we have to know. If she changes employers or insurance, we have to know. If anything traumatic happens in her family such as a death or a job loss—anything that could materially affect the contract in any way whatsoever—we have to know. If anything comes up, we deal with it. She breaches the contract if she does not tell us."

Besides being controlled, wetnurses and surrogates are devalued. Physicians and lawyers set the value of the women's services and assess it as minimal. In 1917, Dr. Arthur D. Holmes, director of a Bureau of Wetnurses in Detroit, noted: "We placed notices in the local papers and with the members of the profession, asking women who had had stillbirths or lost their babies to register at our bureau, guaranteeing them $7 a week, board, room and necessary laundry.... We soon had quite a number" (Hoobler, 1917). Dr. Apt of Chicago observed: "We pay wetnurses $8 a week. We do not like to have any one pay them more, for it is the middle and lower class people, of no great means, who need them most."

Surrogate professionals are also setting a low wage for a surrogate mother's labor. Dr. Richard Levin figures that, counting the inseminations, the nine months of carrying the child and six weeks of recovery, the woman is giving up to a year and a half of her time. (He does not mention her labor in giving birth.) "So the fee we set—$10,000—comes out to be less than minimum wage," he states. "Less than I feel comfortable with" (Keane, 1981, p. 220). But

---

* However, the Supreme Court held in 1973 that the right to privacy, as protected by the Ninth Amendment, encompasses a woman's right to end her pregnancy. Whether a woman's right to have an abortion can be waived by signing a contract is not clear. Contracts between private individuals that impose unconstitutional conditions may be held invalid (Young, 1982).

they have a sliding scale because Levin, like Dr. Isaac Apt before him, is concerned that middle and lower classes not be priced out of surrogate services. "If a couple says they have only $3,000," Levin explains, "I ask a mother to lower her price or try to find one who is willing to do it for that amount."

Currently a surrogate receives $10,000 or less for the following: repeated artificial inseminations; time taken off from work for doctor's visits, psychological counseling and for the birth; pregnancy-induced fatigue, nausea, weight gain, discomfort, skin stretching, loss of sleep; altered or suspended sexual activity; possible miscarriage (several surrogates have suffered from them already); painful labor ("I thought I was going to die from the pain," Keane quotes one surrogate mother as having said.) Additionally, she runs a one in five chance of undergoing cesarean section, major surgery with a significant complication rate. (Several breeders have already been subjected to this surgery.) Many women contract infections following the surgery. The recovery period can be even longer than six weeks.[22] The agreement Keane has the surrogate and sperm donor sign states: "The Surrogate and her Husband, if married, understand and agree to assume all risks including the *risk of death* [my emphasis] which are incidental to conception, pregnancy, childbirth and postpartum complications" (Keane, 1981, p. 293).

The surrogate may also suffer from postpartum depression, a common experience among birthing women in this culture, and from any additional anguish involved in giving up a child which is in every way *her* child, conceived with *her* egg, carried in *her* womb, and birthed through *her* labor.

"The miscarriage was absolutely horrible," one surrogate mother recalled. "I was surprised at how powerful my feelings were. I mean, I had been saying to myself all along, 'It's their baby. It's Judy's baby. I am only carrying it for them.' But when I lost the baby, I was depressed for weeks. That was the beginning of the end for me and the dentist and his wife" (Keane, 1981, p. 177).

How did Handel arrive at the $10,000 figure for all this? "It's an arbitrary figure we came up with that we thought was reasonable."

Others find these conditions "reasonable":

—Under one piece of proposed legislation, if the surrogate miscarries prior to the fifth month of pregnancy, no compensation other than medical expenses will be paid. However, if she miscarries after this time, 10 percent of the fee plus medical expenses would be awarded (Gaynes, 1981).

—One surrogate mother from Joppatowne, Maryland, received $3,000 when she became pregnant for a couple from Colorado. She received another $10,000 after the baby was born on March 24, 1983. Her contract stipulated that the $10,000 would not have been paid had the baby been delivered stillborn (SPN, 1983, May).

There is a sense in which wetnurses were, and surrogate mothers are, viewed as cows. In the following racist exchange between Dr. Isaac W. Faison of Charlotte, North Carolina, and Dr. Oliver Hill of Knoxville, Tennessee, in 1917, the men appear to be speaking of cattle. Dr. Faison appealed to other physicians to develop an improved artificial milk for infants. He needed the product, he said, because in his county, few white women were available as wetnurses; few bore illegitimate children. Most available women were "colored," he explained, "a race that cannot be depended on as wetnurses." Dr. Hill rushed to the defense of southern Black women as wetnurses: "They can be cultivated until they are efficient. . . . I really think we have an advantage over you gentlemen in the Northern cities because the negros will come for a small amount of money, if you do not overpay them or pay them in advance. And if you keep them in good physical condition, they give milk of a good quality."

Earlier in the discussion, Dr. Wilson had commented: "If enough cannot be secured from one [woman], herd milk is just as good as individual." Dr. Apt also spoke of a wetnurse as one would speak of a cow: "She produces as high as 56 ounces in twenty-four hours."

In an interview with me, an obstetrician said of surrogate mothers: "They're good mothers. They get pregnant easily. They handle the pregnancy well." When he told me this, it reminded me of Joe the farmer who had essentially said the same of recipient scrub cows into whom embryos were being transferred. They were good mothers with roomy uteri and plenty of milk, he told me.

The arrival of surrogate motherhood has not aroused the "intense emotional response" artificial insemination had evoked for almost two hundred years. Physicians and lawyers had written that AID endangers "marriage, family and society," may create "an anonymous world," is "socially monstrous," and may lead to "radical revolution" in which such concepts as "father" and "family descent," lose their meaning (Rubin, 1965).

There has been no similarly frightened response to surrogate motherhood. AID had weakened men's claim to paternity; surrogate motherhood strengthens it. The practice does not endanger the patriarchal family and is not judged to be "socially monstrous." It will lead to no radical revolution—such as a return to Mother Right—in which the concept of "father" loses its meaning.

The questions prominently raised about surrogate motherhood have been merely questions of logistics: How does one best regulate it so that, for example, women are not refusing to give up their babies, thus thwarting the plans of the men who commissioned for those babies?

In January 1984, several months after our first interview, John Stehura, president of the Bionetics Foundation, informed me that he was moving into the international arena in surrogate motherhood.

"We're bringing girls in from the Orient," he said. "From Korea, Thailand and Malaysia." (He was also exploring the possibility of initiating some pregnancies in those countries and bringing just the babies to the United States, he said.)

According to the first plan, the woman would be paid nothing for her services. The couple adopting the child would provide the surrogate's travel and living expenses. Though such women receive no pay, Stehura said, they benefit from the arrangement because they get to live. "Often they're looking for a survival situation— something to do to pay for the rent and food," he said. They come from underdeveloped countries "where food is a serious issue." These countries do not have an industrial base, but they have a human base, he said. "They know how to take care of children." Since that's missing here, he added, "obviously it's a perfect match."

No women have actually been brought into the United States as of this writing. Stehura said he was negotiating details after having advertised for "girls" in newspapers in the Orient.

The international traffic in women is about to expand.

Notes

1. NBC's *America Alive* was one show that helped promote the practice, staging one of television's cheaper moments. Keane brought a client couple with him onto the show and NBC insisted that, as a precondition of their appearance, a potential surrogate appear with them. It was staged as a dramatic moment, a sort of "This Is Your Life," Keane recalled. The volunteer surrogate, a beautiful blond woman, came on stage to confront the couple who had never seen her before. The impression was given that she would be the husband's breeder. However, some

time later, off-camera, she stated that she had a heart murmur and declined to be impregnated.

2. Harriet Blankfield, head of the National Center for Surrogate Parenting, also accepts single men as clients. She feels she would be open to a discrimination suit if she did not. "Our policy is that we will accept a couple or a single male provided that person or persons pass the screening of the potential parents," she said in an interview, adding that some single men had already been accepted.

3. Dr. Michael Birnbaum of Surrogate Mothering Ltd. thinks that within five to ten years, his firm might change its policy restricting the use of surrogates to married couples. "At this point now," he told me in an interview, "we recognize that we're kind of a trailblazer. This is a new idea and I think that we have a responsibility to those who will come after us to set the right tone in the beginning. To open this up to single couples or to a guy who wants his own kid or whatever—and we've had a couple of requests like that—I just don't think is appropriate. Give us five or ten years to work out the ethics, if that's the right word, and then I think it might be open to anybody who wants to participate. But I think in the beginning, when you've got a new idea in medicine, you've always got to be a little conservative until you do work the bugs out."

4. In view of such language, the questions one attorney poses are relevant: "Is the contract in which the host has agreed to carry the fertilized egg and turn over the child in the nature of an adoption or a kind of predelivery contract for a commodity? Does dealing in embryos in this fashion result in a sort of 'futures' market that should be controlled by a government agency something like the U.S. Securities and Exchange Commission?" (Schroeder, 1974).

5. I compiled this list of foreground questions from television programs concerning surrogate motherhood and from the writings of Keane, George Annas and Barbara Katz.

6. In an editorial on the case of Denise Thrane, a surrogate mother who refused to give up her baby to James and Biorna Noyes, the couple that had contracted with her for it, *The New York Times* commented that Baby Thrane was "residing in a rented womb." It added: "Mr. and Mrs. Noyes may have lost the lease on the womb; their lawyer seems something less than a crack real estate agent; and Mrs. Thrane is claiming her property" (NYT, April 1981). (Thrane kept her baby.)

7. Two points here. 1. According to surveys, many Korean women today would allow their husbands to take a concubine if they were sonless—from 41 to 68 percent of rural women and 25 to 27 percent of Seoul women, depending on the study (Williamson, 1976, p. 95). 2. It might be argued that AID is for women what surrogate motherhood is for men. But when a married woman is artificially inseminated with donor sperm, the overriding ethic is not that *her* issue be reproduced in the world. It is an attempt to produce a child who *appears* to outsiders to be the husband's issue. This is done by matching the sperm donor as closely as possible to the husband.

While there is a centuries-long tradition asserting the centrality of a man's issue there is no comparable tradition concerning a woman's issue. We do not now, and never have had, complex social, legal and economic structures that place the quality of a man's life in serious jeopardy if he fails to impregnate his wife and ensure the reproduction of her issue. For example, we have no history of laws stating that a woman may divorce her husband if he fails to impregnate her but that he has no right to divorce her on grounds of infertility.

When a single or lesbian woman is inseminated, that insemination takes place within a specific social context, one which has never held, through its laws, customs or ideology, that a woman's issue must be reproduced in the world.

There is a vast difference in the context in which AID and surrogate motherhood take place.

8. Rassaby, mentioning the Genesis story, also refers to Sarah who "sought to satisfy her desire for maternity through her maid-servant Agar." As though Sarah were laboring under no imperative to provide Abraham with his issue!

9. Other examples abound in Keane's book. With a tone of amusement, Keane tells the story of Olive May who was 60 years old and obsessed with providing a child for her husband who was 40 (p. 139). Also see the stories of Lorelei and John, p. 167, and Stefan and Nadia, p. 221. Another client (not described in Keane's book) explained: "It may sound selfish, but I want to father a child on my own behalf, leave my legacy. And I want a healthy baby. And there just aren't any available. They're either retarded or they're minorities, black, Hispanic.... That may be fine for some people, but we just don't think we could handle it" (Annas, 1981).

10. For example, see stories of Bridget and Bill, p. 45, and Nancy and Andy, p. 180.

11. Some argue that hiring a breeder is not baby-selling because the father is biologically related to the child and because at the time the contract is signed, the mother is not pregnant and so is under no compulsion to provide for her child. But in 1981, attorney George J. Annas pointed out that the only two legal decisions rendered on this to date rejected this argument. "Both a lower court judge in Michigan and the attorney general in Kentucky view contracts to bear a child as baby selling," Annas reported (Annas, 1981). In 1983, the Oklahoma attorney general said that state law forbids a surrogate from taking money to bear a child for adoption by someone else (SPN, 1983, Oct.). In the only decision to date at all favorable to the surrogate industry, a Kentucky court ruled in October 1983 that payment for surrogates do not violate adoption law because the payment is for termination of parental rights. An appeal has been filed with the Supreme Court of Kentucky (Brozan, 1984).

12. The states are: Michigan, California, South Carolina, Kansas, Minnesota, Oregon, New York. (Representatives in Florida and Pennsylvania are researching the area.)

13. Of 118 surrogate applicants Parker interviewed, 24 percent were single and never married. Of twenty-five women who actually became pregnant, five were single. Thirty to 40 percent of the breeders hired into the North Hollywood program are single or divorced.

14. This is an example of what Dr. Parker calls the "consent-intent" concept of legal parenthood. He explains that, under this concept, the legal parents could be the married couple who voluntarily give informed *consent* to a certain reproductive

procedure with the *intent* of assuming parental responsibility for the child. The "consent-intent" concept of parenthood would include situations involving sperm donors, egg donors and what Parker calls "womb donors," women who bear and deliver the baby (Parker, 1982).

15. For a fuller discussion of this point, see Dworkin's powerful *Right Wing Women.*

16. Additional information from Parker's study of more than fifty surrogate applicants: Almost 60 percent were working or had working spouses. Their incomes (actual 1980 or projected 1981) ranged from $6,000 to $55,000. (We cannot tell from the study if most incomes were closer to the $6,000 or to the $55,000.) The applicants' education ranged from "well below high school" to one woman with a bachelor's degree. Almost 20 percent of the women did not complete high school. About 55 percent either graduated from high school or received a GED. (Here, as elsewhere in his surrogate studies, Parker fails to break the figure down. If 50 percent received a high school equivalency diploma and only 5 percent actually graduated from high school, that would tell us something about the social and economic power of these women.) About 25 percent had some post–high school college courses, business school or nursing school (Parker, 1983).

17. Keane himself had observed: "I am sure that without the money, the response would be very few" (Shepherd, 1981). Parker, who interviewed Keane's surrogate applicants, found that of the first 125 women, about 90 percent said they required a fee to bear babies for clients. "They related a need for the money but the degree of need varied from a feeling that the money would be used to pay bills to a more urgent need for funds" (Parker, 1983).

Keane appealed Judge Roman S. Gribbs' decision. An appellate court in Michigan ruled that the couple, while having a right to use a surrogate, had no right to compensate her. The U.S. Supreme Court refused to hear the case (Brozan, 1984).

18. Women applying as surrogates are required to undergo interviews and counseling with psychiatrists like Parker, and Parker even argues that this requirement should be enforced by law. What kind of counseling are women getting from mental health professionals who hold the common patriarchal view of them as commodities and as baby machines and who see their freedom and equality in terms of their right to sell their bodies? Parker would like to bring many more mental health professionals into the surrogate motherhood industry. Among the numerous occasions he suggests for seeking "psychiatric input" into the process are:

—A need to judge the competency of a surrogate mother who refuses to relinquish her child
—A custody battle between the biologic father and the surrogate mother
—A need to psychiatrically evaluate surrogate mothers who allege that psychiatric damages resulted from the paid-breeding experience, an allegation perhaps made in claiming workman's compensation. (Parker places quotation marks around "resulted," apparently indicating suspicion of any such allegation.)

He recommends that regulatory legislation be passed requiring surrogate applicants to submit to psychiatric interviews which, he states, will help ensure that the women give competent, voluntary, informed consent.

If Parker's recommendations were taken seriously, numerous employment opportunities would be created for psychiatrists practicing an increasingly discredited profession. Among the many books that have critiqued psychiatry and revealed sexist values within it are: Phyllis Chesler's *Women and Madness,* Mary Daly's *Gyn/Ecology,* and Thomas Szasz's *The Myth of Mental Illness* and *The Manufacture of Madness.*

19. There is a persistent suggestion in the medical literature that wetnurses might contaminate the baby. Dr. B. Raymond Hoobler, describing his program in Detroit, declared it was often better to have the nurse live in the hospital rather than in a couple's home: "By bringing only the milk into the nursery, rather than the wetnurse, it seemed to me that the chances of introducing infections were lessened."

20. See Chapter 16, note 3 for a list of books and reports critiquing obstetrical practices.

21. Alan A. Rassaby, research fellow in the Centre for Human Bioethics at Monash University, Melbourne, believes that the activities of the surrogate mother during pregnancy do need to be legally regulated. He leaves the specific nature of these regulations open but raises questions, among them, these two: Should the woman be legally prohibited from engaging in activities, such as skiing, that are potentially but not intrinsically harmful to the fetus? If a baby is born with a disability that can be directly attributed to an activity of the surrogate who was in breach of her agreement or of the law, can she be sued for negligence? (Rassaby, 1982, p. 66).

22. The first surrogate mother hired by a Philadelphia firm was scheduled for a cesarean because she had had a previous cesarean and the physician decided she would have another. There is overwhelming evidence that many women can successfully have a vaginal birth after a previous cesarean (see Nancy Cohen and Lois Estner, *Silent Knife: Cesarean Prevention and Vaginal Birth After Cesarean,* J. F. Bergin Publishers, Inc., South Hadley, Mass, 1983). But if a doctor refuses to consider it and the woman, in a contract upheld by the state, is bound to obey him, then she must submit to this major surgery.

12

The Artificial Womb:
An Escape from the "Dark and Dangerous Place"

It is probable, anthropologist Sheilia Kitzinger writes, that most expectant mothers feel little confidence in their ability to give birth to a live healthy baby without medical help. The fact that women no longer trust their bodies, she explains, is a direct development of male-oriented obstetrics. In the midst of the advanced technology, a woman can feel that she is a mere container for the fetus, "that her body is an inconvenient barrier to easy access and the probing of all those rubber-gloved fingers and the gleaming equipment, and even—ridiculous, but we are talking about *feelings*—that if she were not around, the pregnancy could progress with more efficiency" (Kitzinger, 1980, p. 74).[1]

But such a feeling is not ridiculous at all. Many men are saying just that: that if only we could dispense with the woman's body and put the fetus in a glass and steel "mother machine," babies would be so much better off.

The prospect of developing an artificial womb fills commentators—including obstetricians, ethicists and journalists—with deep enthusiasm.

"The prospect of having an open window on a growing fetus is welcomed by most of those in responsible roles—embryologists, placentologists, fetologists," wrote ethicist Dr. Joseph Fletcher. "Their chance to monitor fetal life in the light, out of the darkness and obscurity of the womb, will add enormously to our knowledge and help us reduce the hazards that face obstetricians and their patients" (Fletcher, 1974, pp. 102–103).

Not just hazards. Actual perils. "Quite simply, the womb has become the most perilous environment in which humans have to live," wrote Gerald Leach in *The Biocrats.*

The womb, commentators agree, is dangerous. This is not a modern idea. Exploring the primordial image of the Great Mother Goddess, in ancient cultures, psychologist Erich Neumann found that the womb is considered both life-giving and death-dealing. It is bloodthirsty, destructive, a mouth full of sharp teeth (the *vagina dentata*). The womb attracts the male and then kills the phallus to achieve fecundation. Like the womb of woman, the earth-womb of the Great Goddess attracts and draws in all living beings for her own satisfaction and fecundation. She is a female who exacts blood. Neumann wrote:

> The womb of the earth becomes the deadly devouring maw of the underworld, and beside the fecundated womb and the protecting cave of earth and mountain gapes the abyss of hell, the dark hole of the depths, the devouring womb of the grave and of death, of darkness without light, of nothingness. For this woman who generates life and all living things on earth is the same who takes them back into herself.... This Terrible Mother is the hungry earth, which devours its own children and fattens on their corpses; it is the tiger and the vulture, the vulture and the coffin, the flesh-eating sarcophagus voraciously licking up the blood seed of men and beasts and, once fecundated and sated, casting it out again in a new birth, hurling it to death, and over and over again to death (Neumann, 1974, p. 149).

Through the ages, belief in the deadly womb persisted. The notion that evil emanated from the womb and ovaries, causing all manner of illness, suffused late nineteenth century American gynecological thought. Physicians were obsessed with woman's womb. Asserting that it was connected with the central nervous system, they often attributed any "nervous disorder"—paralyses, crying fits, insomnia, backaches and headaches—to a disorder of the uterus. "It is almost a pity that a woman has a womb," lamented a University of Chicago professor of gynecology in his 1860s monograph on the uterus (Wood, 1973). Hysteria, a term derived from the Greek word for uterus, was "a very common female trouble ... a complaint intimately allied to the sexual organs of females," according to American gynecologist Dr. Augustus Kinsley Gardner (1821–1876). Treatment of diseases alleged to originate in the womb were often brutal and included surgical removal of the offending organ.

Historian G. J. Barker-Benfield studied Gardner's writings and found the physician comparing the womb to a grave and a prison. He also compared a woman gestating a fetus to a ship bearing a dead man. To Gardner, "the womb's generative power connoted death to men," Barker-Benfield wrote. Obstetricians, he added, soon translated such feelings into the rationale for their control of the deadly dangerous birth process. Gardner wanted to exclude women from midwifery "and even from parturition altogether" (Barker-Benfield, 1976, p. 277; p. 281).

The notion that women's bodies are dangerous, hazardous places which are hostile to the fetus permeates today's obstetrical and reproductive literature. It even came out in a remark made "in a light vein" during U.S. Food and Drug Administration (FDA) hearings on a controversial obstetric procedure. Dr. Theodore King of the FDA panel explained why a study they were discussing found boys more clumsy than girls: "Many of us view that boys, male fetuses, go throughout pregnancy in an alien environment" (Finkel, 1978).

In his book, *Birth Without Violence*, French obstetrician Frederick Leboyer refers to the woman's body as a prison that first keeps the fetus "huddled in submission" and later begins "like some octopus, to hug and crush." The mother's contractions crush, stifle and assault the fetus, pushing it into "this hell," the vagina. The mother is "the enemy" of the fetus, a prison demanding its prisoner's death. "The monster drives the baby lower still," Leboyer writes of the woman, "and not satisfied with crushing, it twists it in a refinement of cruelty."

Such male commentators throw out wildly different explanations to account for the danger posed by the female body:

—The human is the only mammal to walk erect on two limbs and the only one to have trouble bearing offspring. The human skeleton has adapted to the upright walking position in such a way that childbirth has been rendered painful and dangerous. Somehow (and the explanation gets vague here), woman's upright walking position is connected to the puerperal infections that caused the deaths of thousands of women in the seventeenth, eighteenth and nineteenth centuries and to the risks women today run of toxemia and of hemorrhaging to death in childbed. "If man cannot have a normal painless and riskless birth because he continues to walk erect, then perhaps the solution is the artificial womb" (Francoeur, 1970, p. 85). (There is no evidence that the upright walking position causes infection, toxemia or hemorrhage.)

—The fact that many embryos (up to 150 of every 1,000) die in the first month of conception shows that the woman's womb is "an extraordinarily dangerous environment" (Leach, 1970, p. 137). This implies that it is the woman's womb that is killing the defenseless embryos. This is not true. Many defective embryos are conceived and fail to develop. It is not that the womb is killing them. (See Biggers, 1980.)

—Pregnant women live in a world full of cigarette smoke, industrial waste, infectious disease and automobile effluents. Fetuses may someday be safer in an artificial womb than in a woman's body, which does not sufficiently protect them from teratogens—agents that could cause defects (McCorduck, 1981; Grossman, 1971). Moreover, in the womb they are apt to be "victim" to the mother's drug misuse, kidney and heart disease, malnutrition or uterine abnormalities (Lygre, 1979). Birth defects may be reduced for machine-gestated babies for, as one commentator points out, artificial wombs do not smoke, drink alcohol, contract German measles or fall down stairs (Kieffer, 1979).

—Labor is dangerous for babies. Some contractions of the womb can be too hard and long and can actually "batter" the baby (Lerner, quoted in Corea, 1980). Some argue that the artificial womb would eliminate birth trauma (quoted in Walters, 1979, p. 52; Lygre, 1979, p. 27).

The fact that such widely disparate reasons are given to justify the conclusion that the female body is dangerous—a conclusion centuries of men came to long before automobile effluents and industrial wastes entered the world—suggests that there is something more profound going on here than an exercise in rational discourse.

Often commentators feel no need at all to justify the assertion that the womb is dangerous. Fletcher simply states: "We realize that the womb is a dark and dangerous place, a hazardous environment. We should want our potential children to be where they can be watched and protected as much as possible" (Fletcher, 1974, pp. 102–103).

There are other rationales—therapeutic, eugenic, moral, psychological—advanced as well for building artificial wombs and, eventually, practicing ectogenesis—the "machine-based gestation" of a fetus outside a woman's body.

Therapeutic: Within an artificial womb, a fetus could not only be watched and protected, but treated. Its faults could be detected more readily. "Helpful drugs and hormones" could be administered and minor surgery performed with greater ease and control. The fetus could be immunized against childhood diseases (Rosenfield,

1975, p. 139; Kieffer, 1979). If a physician judged a woman "prone to miscarriage," he could flush the embryo out of her and place it in a mother machine (Francoeur, 1970, p. 81).

Eugenic: Artificial wombs would be useful, not only in affording pharmacrats more direct control over fetal development but in practicing a eugenic program, in exercising quality control over the production of children: "it would be even more valuable in enabling us to rear selectively—or even to multiply—those embryos which have received a superior heredity" (Muller, 1935, p. 74). "Sexing" children would be a simple matter (Grossman, 1971; Kieffer, 1979). One commentator has argued that children could more fully realize their genetic potential if gestated in a machine; they would not be subject to oxygen deprivation at birth, which can impair physical and mental ability (Kieffer, 1979). (He seems to assume that the machine will always work, electricity will never fail, technicians will never turn the wrong switch or go off on a coffee break at a critical moment.)

Moral: Artificial wombs might obviate any need for abortion. Unwillingly pregnant women would visit the local Fetal Adoption Center and undergo surgery for removal of the still-living fetus. The fetus would be transferred either to the womb of a surrogate mother or that of an infertile woman or to a mother machine. Abortion clinics would become anachronisms in an era of fetal transplant technology and, presumably, would not be available (Freitas, 1980). Physicians would anesthesize women, locate the fetus in the uterus with a hysteroscope and then pluck the fetus off the uterine wall "like a helicopter rescuing a stranded mountain climber" (Nathanson, 1979).

Psychological: Complete ectogenesis presents this advantage to men: If they fertilize an egg in the lab, grow it and then place it in an artificial womb, they know, beyond any doubt, the paternity of the resulting child. For much of human history, a man could never be certain that he had participated in bringing a particular life onto the earth. Maybe he was the father and maybe he was not. Reproductive technology can alleviate men's anxiety on this score. As Edward Grossman has written: "That part of the population which would use the artificial womb would not have to worry about illegitimacy or doubtful paternity. For the first time it will be possible to prove beyond a shadow of a doubt that a man is the father of his children" (1971).

Benevolent: Most of all, the artificial womb would benefit women. They could skip the morning sickness, heavy steps, kicks from the fetus, labor pains. "And how many women have ever turned down labor-saving devices?" asks one journalist (Rosenfeld, 1975).

If the artificial womb caught on, the "awefulness [sic] associated with pregnancy and childbirth will have nothing to feed on." Motherhood would excite no more awe than fatherhood (Grossman, 1971). By achieving ectogenesis, science could reduce "the delivery of a child to the emptying of a jar" (Rostand, 1959, p. 85).

Women who decide to use artificial wombs might choose to be sterilized (Grossman, 1971). So here too with artificial wombs as with embryo transfer and in vitro fertilization, there is the gentle suggestion that with such a technology available, women might choose—for convenience, for health, for all the most benevolent reasons—to be rendered sterile. Grossman writes as if women have, and will always have, the power to "decide" and "choose," as if most women could not be diagnosed as "prone to miscarriage,"* as if those women who resist the offer of sterilization and try to bear their own babies could not be threatened with a charge of child abuse as a few women who resist hospital birth and cesarean sections already have been.

So men work on artificial wombs and placentas, most often offering a therapeutic rationale—the treatment of newborns with breathing disorders—for their projects. The problems involved in developing such apparatuses are so formidable it is unlikely they will be solved in the near future.

The placenta, a spongy structure, grows on the wall of the uterus during pregnancy. It presents two surfaces: the fetal, to which the umbilical cord is attached, and the maternal. Its main, and highly complex, function is to allow nutrients and oxygen from the mother's blood to diffuse into the fetus's blood, and waste products from the fetus to diffuse back to the mother. It is impossible to overstate the importance of the placenta. It serves as the fetus's stomach, liver,

---

* According to childbirth educator Gail Brewer, president of The Brewer Foundation for Perinatal Education and author of ten childbirth books, the obstetric definition of a "high risk" pregnant woman has been steadily expanding so that today, *most* birthing women fit into the various "high risk" categories.

kidneys and lungs. It also secretes estrogens and progesterone, which help maintain the pregnancy.

Since 1922, researchers have devised various apparatuses in an attempt to study or to perform one or more of the placental or uterine functions. Most involve connecting plastic tubes to the one vein and two arteries of the human umbilical cord, a difficult procedure because of the extreme tininess of these structures. The plastic tubes may also damage the blood cells that pass through them. Sometimes the tubes slip off. The researchers must determine how to transfer the fluid from the fetal to the maternal circulation at just the proper rate and how to prevent an increase of blood volume within the fetus. (Even a slight increase causes the fetus to hemorrhage and die.) They must also figure out how to keep the blood from clotting after they have filled it with oxygen using one of their devices. Researchers have yet to determine exactly what substances the fetus needs—amino acids, trace elements, vitamins, proteins, hormones, enzymes, etc.—in exactly what proportion and at exactly what point in its development. Too much, too little, or none at all of certain substances at critical points could kill the fetus or permanently injure it as it is in the process of forming organs. All these problems suggest the extreme difficulty of replacing a woman's womb with a machine.

Another problem—the psychological effects on a fetus of forming and growing in a stationary machine—are rarely mentioned by those who report on artificial wombs. Embryologist Robert Francoeur is an exception. Within a woman's womb, he points out, the fetus has cycles. Its mother wakes, and it is bounced along with her through her day, her trips to the office or factory, store, friends' homes. It goes up and down stairs, floats in her as she swims at the pool, kicks her resilient uterus, hears her heartbeat. It lies within her while she feels emotions, dreams. What happens to it when all that variety and human contact disappears and it lies still for months in a machine on a shelf?

Some, as we have seen, think the machine will be better for the fetus. Listening to a television news report on the invention of a "baby quieting" device (a record of a pregnant woman's heartbeat and a rhythmic slosh, the sound environment inside a pregnant uterus), a female physician wrote that the male scientists involved were "delighted that no one had to hold a baby to provide these comforts, that they had devised yet another machine to substitute for a mother. I remembered hearing male physicians describe the mechanical-electronic equipment in a newborn intensive care unit in a specialized hospital as 'better than' a uterus" (Demeter, 1977, p. 11).

Let us turn now to men's wombs.

Dr. Robert Goodlin, then of Stanford University School of Medicine, developed an artificial womb that is a high-pressure oxygen chamber. Made of stainless steel with a small round peephole, it is about twice the size of a pressure cooker. Human, spontaneously aborted fetuses of 8, 9 and 10 weeks' gestation were placed inside the chamber, immersed in a salt solution, and put under the very high pressure a sea diver would experience at 450 feet below the sea. At this pressure, the oxygen is forced through the fetuses' skin. Tubes feeding in and out of the womb carry nutrients and oxygen. The problem with Goodlin's womb is that while the fetus can respire, there is no artificial placenta to remove its waste products. Fetuses survived in this chamber for only a few hours; none for more than forty-eight.

Most researchers have concentrated on perfusion experiments.[2] That is, they have connected tubes to the fetus at the umbilical cord, pumped its blood out, removed toxic wastes from that blood, saturated it with nutrients and oxygen, and pumped it back in. (In a variation on this, one research group, working with baby and adult animals rather than fetuses, pumped blood directly into the heart.)

For the perfusion experiments, researchers used adult dogs and newborn puppies, and the fetuses of rabbits, cows, women, ewes and pigs. ("The advantage of the pig as an experimental animal is that its foetuses are of a convenient size and that it breeds at all seasons of the year."[3]) Sometimes they obtained the fetuses by surgically removing them from the mother. Sometimes they got them after spontaneous or induced abortion. (Experimentation on human fetuses obtained from induced abortions has since been forbidden in the United States.) Sometimes slaughter of the mother provided the opportunity to use her fetuses.[4]

Whatever materials or techniques researchers employed—whether they used C-clamps to fix the membranes of the human placenta against the latex rubber basket of an artificial womb or a 2.5 cm-thick Lucite retaining ring; whether they bore 151 holes in the bottom of the artificial uterus for the arterial inlets and venous outlets or fewer holes; whether they simulated the minute arterial branches in the uterus with sections of 18-gauge needles inserted into PE-160 polyethylene tubes or with something else; whether they designed into their apparatuses manometer taps, rubber tubes, stoppers, flowmeters, oxygenators, fluid reservoirs, nylon filters, dialyzers, or magnetic stirrers; whether the pump they attached was a Bluemie-Holter triple chamber B-3 blood pump or a Masterflex No. 7545-15 variable flow pump; whether they kept the artificial womb warm by continuously heating it with a hot-air blower or by immersing it in a vat of hot water—no fetuses attached to these male wombs lived for more than a few days. Most lived only a matter of hours.

But this is not to say that ectogenesis will never become a reality. True, the problems involved are formidable and it may take decades, perhaps very many of them, to solve these problems. But piece by piece, in various laboratories around the world, men are working out the technology for complete ectogenesis. As Robert Edwards, the IVF pioneer pointed out: "A considerable part of the interuterine growth of fetuses can now take place outside the mother." On one end of human life, the first six days of embryonic development can occur in the laboratory, he noted. On the other end, physicians can incubate premature human babies from 24 weeks on. In the middle of gestation, physicians have maintained the lives of abortuses for a few hours or days. "Almost one-half of pregnancy is thus replaceable ex vivo [outside the female body]" (Edwards, 1974). Today, about a decade after Edwards wrote, physicians can begin to sustain fetal life three weeks earlier than he reported—from 21 weeks on. This point is continually going downward. From both ends of human prenatal life and from the middle, then, men are extending the periods during which they can maintain fetal life. It remains to fill in the gaps.

Notes

1. There is a common misperception that after all the exposés of obstetrical practices, the formation of childbirth "consumer" groups, and the establishment of birthing rooms in hospitals, most women can now give birth naturally. This is true for a minority of well-educated women, generally of the upper-middle class. For the vast majority of women, however, intervention in pregnancy and childbirth has escalated dramatically since 1980. "For most women, it's a victory to have a vaginal delivery," childbirth educator Gail Brewer, author of ten books in the field, said in an interview, referring to the increasingly common practice of terminating pregnancy through cesarean section.

2. Among those who have tried perfusion experiments are: R. E. L. Nesbitt, 1970; J. C. Callaghan, E. A. Maynes and H. R. Hug, 1965; L. Lawn and R. A. McCance, 1961; B. Westin, R. Nyberg and G. Enhörning, 1958; A. Astrom and U. Samelius, 1954; C. E. Raiha, 1954; P. Wilkin, 1954; K. E. Kranz, T. C. Panos and J.

Evans, 1962; G. Chamberlain, 1968; W. M. Zapol, T. Kolobow, J. E. Pierce, G. G. Vurex and R. L. Bowman, 1969.

3. References for the experiments: dogs (Callaghan et al., 1962); rabbits (Goodlin, 1963); cows (cited in Chamberlain, 1968); women (Westin et al., 1958; Chamberlain et al., 1968); pigs (Lawn and McCance, 1962); and ewes (Callaghan, 1965; Zapol et al., 1969).

4. In one experiment, researchers inserted tubes down the windpipes of dogs, clamped the tubes, thus cutting off respiration, perfused oxygenated blood into the right side of the heart, and then observed the dogs' physiological condition. "10 minutes after the completion of the period of respiratory obstruction ... sampling was undertaken. All animals that survived the procedure were studied for a period of 3 to 5 days and then were sacrificed for pathologic examination" (Callaghan, 1962).

In another study, fourteen unborn lambs were kept submerged in an artificial amniotic medium for up to nineteen hours (Callaghan, 1962). After exposure to the air, none of these lambs survived for more than a few hours.

Swedish researchers placed human fetuses in a perfusion apparatus they had constructed. ("During the perfusion experiments the fetuses performed movements of the head, body and limbs. These movements were vigorous, even at a temperature of 25 C" [Westin, 1958].) Another researcher from George Washington University also reported movement in one of the human fetuses he placed in a tank with artificial amniotic fluid. The fetus had been removed from a 14-year-old girl by hysterotomy, an operation similar to a cesarean section used on those infrequent occasions when an abortion is performed in advanced pregnancy. (Most abortions are performed at an early stage of pregnancy and do not involve surgery.) "For the whole 5 hours of life, the fetus did not respire. Irregular gasping movements, twice a minute, occurred in the middle of the experiment but there was no proper respiration. Once the perfusion was stopped, however, the gasping respiratory efforts increased to 8 to 10 per minute.... After stopping the circuit, the heart slowed, became irregular, and eventually stopped. The fetus was maintained at 39 to 42 degrees C. in the water bath.... The fetus was quiet, making occasional stretching limb movements very like the ones reported in other human work." The fetus died twenty-one minutes after leaving the perfusion circuit (Chamberlain, 1968).

Other researchers in Maryland found that a fetal lamb they were perfusing rested quietly in the artificial amniotic bath, moving its head or legs about once an hour. "It exhibited a strong sucking reflex as well as a withdrawal reflex when pinched. After 55 hours of perfusion, the fetus abruptly underwent cardiac arrest and stopped extracting oxygen from the umbilical arterial blood" (Zapol, 1969).

In other perfusion experiments not involving animals and designed to study the functions of the isolated placenta, researchers rushed human placentas from the hospital delivery room (sometimes within five minutes of the mother's delivery of her child), to the laboratory where they were quickly attached to the apparatus. There is no mention of whether the mothers consented to, or knew of, the use of their placentas in these experiments (Nesbitt et al., 1970; Krantz et al., 1962).

13

Cloning:
The Patriarchal Urge to Self-Generate

The notion that a man might create a human being by himself, without a woman, is an ancient one embodied in both the legend of the golem of medieval Jewish mysticism (a clay creature that had been given life), and of the homunculus or diminutive man alchemists attempted to create. Boys' urine, blood and sperm were among the ingredients alchemists prescribed for the creation of a little man. One homunculus recipe provided by Paracelsus concludes with: "At the end of this time you shall have a veritable living child, having every member as well-proportioned as any infant born of woman" (Ebon, 1978, p. 113). This is the classic patriarchal myth of single parenthood by the male.

Cloning promises (perhaps falsely) to bring the myth to life.

Here is how: When animals reproduce sexually, an egg and sperm, each containing twenty-three chromosomes, unite. The human fertilized egg has forty-six chromosomes, the number found in every body cell. It can then develop into an embryo. Cloning researchers try to make a cell develop into an embryo without fertilization, that is, asexually. Theoretically, to clone a human they would take a single cell from a person and induce it to begin dividing so that it would produce an adult organism genetically identical to the parent. There are several experimental methods of doing this. One calls for destruction of the egg nucleus, which contains the genetic information. This is termed enucleation and could be done by a laser or ultraviolet beam. The nucleus is then replaced with a cell taken from almost anywhere in the body. Finding itself with the full forty-six chromosomes, the egg is tricked into believing itself fertilized. It begins to divide. At an early embryo stage, it would be transplanted into a woman's uterus, using the technique IVF clinics have developed. Or, in the far future, it might be placed in an artificial womb. The genetic makeup of the resulting fetus is that of the cell donor.

If this method were used, a woman would still have to provide the cytoplasm or "yolk" of the egg and (possibly) the uterus, but, noting this, two commentators maintain: "the child that results can still be the offspring of a man—and of a man alone" (Rorvik and Shettles, 1971, p. 88). (After lengthy discussions of single parenthood by the male, commentators sometimes note in passing, just as I am doing here, that a woman could be the single parent as well if one of *her* body cells were placed in the enucleated egg. But they clearly see this as an aberrant use of the technology.)

In the realm of cloning, as in most reproductive technology, the male is seen as the active principle in reproduction, the female the passive. This was clearly portrayed in the book, *In His Image*, an account of what the author claimed was the first cloning of a human being. Published in 1978, science writer David Rorvik's book caused such a public furor that Congress held hearings to examine cloning. At those hearings, the authenticity of the Rorvik account was thoroughly discredited.

Nonetheless, I take the book seriously as a vision. Consider the plot. Max, an elderly, wealthy businessman, desires a male heir. Before he can die peacefully, he wants "to first remake himself, in effect to be born again." Deciding to spend a million dollars or more, he contacts Rorvik and asks him to find a scientist who can clone him. Rorvik locates "Darwin." Darwin takes his scientific team to a rural area in an unnamed Third World country where Max owns a number of factories and plantations. In this country, rules regarding informed consent are "much more relaxed." At a health clinic Max had established for the people, Darwin begins using female patients as "raw material" for his experiments. He wants their eggs, their wombs. He keeps the women in the dark as to what he is doing to them.

Rorvik asks Darwin if his subjects were being informed of the risks of the experiments, including that of unwanted pregnancy. "He was a bit evasive, which made me think the worst," Rorvik wrote. "At any rate, he said that he was working only with married women, so at least no virgins would suddenly find themselves pregnant after participating in one of his 'studies.'"

Were the women being paid? Rorvik asks. Darwin replies with exasperation that in one hour in his laboratory or operating room, women are paid more than they would be in a month working on one of the local plantations, farms or factories. Rorvik decides the women are benefiting from Darwin's use of them. (Max, of course, owned some of the factories and plantations, and so was setting those low wages.)

Once the cloning technique is worked out, they must find a surrogate mother. Because Max, 67, might want to take the girl as his principal mistress, he insists upon a single, pretty virgin. Max's longtime employee, Roberto, a man given to wearing flashy clothes and ostentatious rings, selects as candidates the prettiest teenagers among the farm and factory workers. Roberto "seemed to be something of a procurer. He would go through the factories and farms and invite various girls to come to the clinic for examination as possible candidates in a 'study.' " (According to a newspaper report, Rorvik had once intended to write "a pornographic science fiction thriller" called *The Clone* [Ebon, 1978, p. 81]. One sees the pornographic elements here.) From dossiers on the "girls," Max selects "Sparrow." Sparrow bears his clone and goes to serve Max and his son in California.

In spinning out a fictional tale of how a man might be cloned, Rorvik is true to the values and obsessions of this culture. The devaluation of the woman, the reduction of her whole being to the two functions men want her to serve (sexual and reproductive), and the racist use of Third World women who are "raw material" for Westerners to exploit as much as is the land on which the women live, all are accurately depicted. So too is the patriarchal urge to give birth to oneself, to be one's own mother, and to live forever.

The promise of immortality is apparently one of the most attractive features of cloning. By creating a being in his own image and with his own genes, a man achieves a genetic continuity he is never sure he has with sexual reproduction. Cloning promises immortality in another form as well. It has been suggested that people could keep copies of themselves as a bank for spare parts. If a liver transplant were needed, one would presumably take it from one's clone with no fear of graft rejection. (How the clone, a human being, would live while waiting to be cannibalized, is not spelled out.) With the constant replacement of worn-out or defective parts, one could live on and on.

In reading literature on any of the reproductive technologies, not just cloning, one sees that desire for immortality expressed time and again. The cycle of birth, growth and death in nature, a cycle venerated in the Goddess religion and epitomized by a woman bearing a child is one against which patriarchal man has long railed.

He does not want to die. He does not want to return to the dark womb of the earth. The inevitability of his death is an affront to him. He dreams of resisting death by cannibalizing clones or transplanting organs or building himself a body out of rustproof steel, or manipulating cells to stop the aging process. He fantasizes about constructing a steel womb—with a glass porthole to let the light in—for the gestation of his clones. His desire to control birth through the reproductive technologies, then, is also a desire to control death.

Cloning seems to promise not just immortality, but a way to control who is born into the world, that is, to practice eugenics. Cloning would remove the chance element from heredity and replace it with conscious selection. Among the rationales commentators Muller (1959), Lederberg (1966) and Fletcher (1974) have given for cloning people have been:

—To predetermine the child's sex. (Its sex would be the same as that of the individual who donated the cell nucleus.)

—To avoid genetic disease by allowing a carrier to clone himself rather than risk producing an overtly diseased offspring through sexual reproduction. (This is also the familiar therapeutic rationale.)

—To clone people with certain qualities that would be useful to society. For example, ethicist Joseph Fletcher wrote that scientists may want to clone people who are impervious to high-decibel sound waves, a quality that would be invaluable for space flights and flights at high altitudes. (Fletcher does not speculate what societies would do if the clones, as adults, did not want to *be* pilots. The notion that these people might have wills seems not to have occurred to him. Such a proposal suggests the creation of a servant or slave class of human beings who, like animals, are bred for specific functions men want them to perform. Just as cows are bred to produce more milk or beef, so human beings would be bred for efficient space flight.)

—To duplicate superior individuals such as Einstein.

"Clonality . . . answers the technical specifications of the eugen-icists in a way that Mendelian breeding does not," wrote geneticist Dr. Joshua Lederberg. "If a superior individual—and presumably, genotype—is identified, why not copy it directly rather than suffer all the risks, including those of sex determination, involved in the disruptions of recombination (i.e., sexual reproduction)."

Besides the promise of immortality and the attraction of eugenics, other rationales offered for cloning are:

—To provide a child for a sterile couple

—To colonize a distant planet using the supply of body cells a biologist could carry through space

—To preserve family likenesses. (Fletcher offers this as one of the "good reasons" for cloning! [Fletcher, 1974, p. 154])

The existence of an artificial womb could accelerate experimentation with clones (as well as with chimeras, which are human–animal hybrids) since it would not be necessary to find human hosts to gestate them. Geneticist Dr. Joshua Lederberg has written that the first attempt to clone a man may be postponed until the perfection of the artificial womb. This "womb," along with prenatal diagnostic tools, would permit researchers to keep the clone-fetus under surveillance and assure its quality.

Assuming that artificial wombs are not available and that the dark and dangerous wombs of women must be used, why would women consent to serve as "hosts" for clones? Dr. James Watson, who won the Nobel Prize in 1962 for his role in the discovery of the structure of DNA, has a theory. He feels that a totalitarian state, which could coerce women into becoming surrogate mothers for clones, need not exist because "the boring meaninglessness of the lives of many women would be sufficient cause for their willingness to participate in such experimentation, be it legal or illegal" (Watson, 1971).

Along with other scientists, Watson, who disapproves of human cloning, has pointed out that in vitro fertilization provides a gateway to this experimentation. Writing seven years before the birth of the first test-tube baby, he warned that soon after that feat's accomplishment, human eggs would become "a readily available commodity," and there would be "a frenetic rush to do experimental manipulation" with them. Hundreds of isolated human eggs would be found in hospitals, he wrote. In the laparoscopy operation, several eggs could be obtained from one woman. While the excess eggs would probably be used for valid experimental purposes, the temptation to try cloning would always be close at hand, he observed.

In the 1960s and 1970s, various scientists predicted that human cloning would be achieved within the lifetime of many of us.[1] Following these speculations, articles reporting on cloning research appeared in the mass media. "Want Your Own Britt Ekland? Make Yourself One," proclaimed a 1969 *Esquire* cover portraying six "clones" of the scantily clad actress. This was a typical presentation of cloning.

At congressional hearings following publication of Rorvik's book, Dr. Robert G. McKinnell, professor of genetics and cell biology at the University of Minnesota, protested that cloning "is not a technique designed for reproductive purposes—rather, it is a method useful in providing new understanding of cell biology." Cloning has been used in the study of differentiation (the processes whereby the fertilized egg gives rise to a diversity of cell types), cancer cell biology and immunology, and promises to be useful to the study of mutagenesis and aging, he pointed out (*Developments*, 1978, p. 14). Another witness agreed, stating that cloning was not an *end*, but an enormously important *means* of studying cell development. "I think people confuse cloning as ends and cloning as means," he said (*Developments*, 1978, p. 90).

It is true that important research uses of cloning—uses that have nothing to do with reproduction—have been de-emphasized in media accounts of cloning. But it was scientists themselves who began speculations on the cloning of human beings. After the public furor caused by the Rorvik book, researchers seem to have closed ranks to downplay the possibility that a person might ever be cloned. Dr. Jonathan Beckwith of Harvard University charged that his colleagues around the country were denying the possible dangers of cloning and underplaying the sophistication of their techniques for fear of public revulsion and legislative reaction (*Developments*, 1978, p. 26).

Cloning has been achieved with limited success in amphibia and, arguably, in mammals. But will it actually become possible to clone a human being? Before dealing with that question, we must briefly look at cloning experimentation in plants and animals.

Every body cell in a plant or animal begins with all the genes necessary for the development of a complete being. As the living organism grows, its cells specialize to form different organs. A cell that becomes part of an eye does not need the genes that could produce a liver. But does it lose those genes?

The assumption on which rests the possibility of human cloning is that it does not, that the nucleus of every cell of every tissue in our bodies contains within it a full blueprint for the development of a complete organism. It is not just the sperm and egg cells that have these vital genes. No matter how cells have differentiated into specialized organs—eye, liver, fingernail—they all contain the latent potential for reproducing a complete adult.

In the early 1960s, Professor F. C. Steward, a cellular physiologist at Cornell University proved that assumption true for plants when he cloned a carrot. The first real success with animals came in the 1950s when two American embryologists, after devising a technique for transferring a nucleus from one cell to another, cloned frogs (Briggs and King, 1952). However, in all their successes, they used not the tissue of an adult frog, but embryonic tissue at a very early stage of development.

In the 1960s, English embryologist J. B. Gurdon followed up on their research, took it a step further, and succeeded in producing adult frog clones using nuclei from fully differentiated intestinal cells taken from feeding tadpoles. Many of the transplants did not develop but a few (1.5 percent) did. They became adult toads (Gurdon, 1962). In producing an adult from a differentiated cell, Gurdon's work in frogs, like Steward's in plants, showed that a mature cell contained complete genetic information and could be induced to express it and form a mature animal.

In England, an Oxford University researcher unsuccessfully attempted to clone a mammal through a new method: fusion. He fused a rabbit egg and body cell together using the biochemical prodding of a virus that he had inactivated with ultraviolet radiation (Bromhall, 1975).[2]

Biologist Peter C. Hoppe of Jackson Laboratory, Bar Harbor, Maine, and microsurgeon Karl Illmensee of the University of Geneva, Switzerland, reportedly succeeded in producing the first true clone of a mammal in 1980 (Illmensee and Hoppe, 1981). They extracted the nucleus from the embryonic cell of a gray or agouti-colored mouse using a tiny glass tube or pipette. Next, they inserted the nucleus into the recently fertilized egg of a black mouse and extracted that egg's original nuclear material. They cultured the egg for four days and then placed it into a white mouse. In this way, they produced three cloned mice, a gray male and female and one agouti female. These clones were not related to the black mice who provided the fertilized eggs or to the white mice who bore them. This experiment, if valid, would show that cloning using nuclei from embryonic mammals is possible.

But questions as to whether the experiment *is* valid arose when members of Dr. Illmensee's staff charged that there were irregularities in his recent research reports. Separate investigative committees of scientists at the University of Geneva and at Jackson Laboratory found no evidence of fraud. Neither did an international review commission. But the commission did find that Illmensee's records contained many errors, corrections and discrepancies that "cast grave doubts" on the legitimacy of the original findings. The commission looked into Illmensee's earlier work with Hoppe, even though the validity of that work had not been contested, and found "no reason to doubt the authenticity of these experiments." But it noted that the results had not been replicated. It urged the team to repeat their experiments (Marx, 1983; Norman, 1984). Scientific research is generally confirmed by other scientists who, using the same methods, repeat the experiments. While the prolonged inability to repeat an experiment tends to cast doubt on the validity of the research, it may be that the original researcher succeeded where his colleagues failed because his skills were superior (Schmeck, 1983, June 4).

In 1983, researchers in Philadelphia reported a significant advance in nuclear transplantation, the procedure employed in one form of cloning. Using a refined technique that causes less damage to the embryos manipulated, they transplanted nuclei from one mouse embryo to the embryo of another mouse of a different breed and color, and then transferred the embryo to the womb of a surrogate mouse mother. Their work resulted in the birth of ten mice genetically unrelated to either the surrogate mothers who bore them or to the females that produced the enucleated egg cells (McGrath and Solter, 1983). The researchers have declined to say whether or not they produced identical mice (clones) although their technique, used with an embryo at a more advanced stage of development, would allow them to do so. (After the embryo has subdivided into numerous cells, they could take several cells from the same embryo, insert them into separate enucleated egg cells and produce clones.) They have successfully used their technique with embryonic cells at a later stage.

Researchers are not waiting for any sort of scientific or tech-nological breakthrough that will enable them to clone a human being. The techniques and tools to clone a man are largely in place now. Working with animal eggs, researchers have developed tech-niques to remove the egg nucleus and insert the donor nucleus from the animal to be cloned. Since these techniques work with mouse eggs, they will work with human eggs that are the same size. The other techniques involved in cloning have all been developed in IVF clinics: acquiring mature human eggs; placing them, once renucleated, in a nutrient medium while they grow to an early embryo stage; transferring the embryos into a woman's uterus.

So rather than waiting for some technological breakthrough, researchers are waiting to learn: Is it biologically possible at all to clone an adult human being? Could it be that a plant and a frog can be cloned while a mammal cannot? (Despite the Illmensee and Hoppe experiments on mice, it has not been conclusively demonstrated that a mammal *can* be cloned. Those experiments remain unreplicated.) Does a differentiated human cell—a skin cell, for example—retain within it, in a latent form, a blueprint for the development of a complete human being? Or, as it becomes specialized, does it permanently lose the necessary genes?

To date, none of the researchers who have successfully cloned have used cells taken from *adult* animals. It may be that cloning will work with some kinds of adult cells (spermatogonia are usually mentioned), but not others.[3] Or it may be biologically impossible to ever clone an adult human. So the fantasy that one could judge which adults are particularly worthy of replication (typically, in the media, such pairs as Albert Einstein and Raquel Welch are envisioned), and then clone them, may never be acted out. Even if it could, it is highly unlikely that a clone would be exactly like its parent.

While its genes would be the same, character and soul do not reside in genes. Furthermore, an environment would act on a clone different than that which had acted upon its parent. This difference begins with the uterine environment. Among pregnant women, there can be significant variations in fetal-maternal circulation and in the way the placenta is formed and attaches to the wall of the uterus. These differences in uterine environment may have subtle effects on mammalian offspring (Edwards and Sharpe, 1971, p. 89; Edwards, 1974; Eisenberg, 1976, p. 324). One of the nightmares evoked by cloning has been that a tyrant like Adolph Hitler could clone thousands of copies of himself to help him dominate the world. But it is conceivable that someone with Hitler's exact genes could look somewhat different and could be a humanitarian.

Though it may never be possible to clone *adult* humans, this does not mean scientists would not be able to clone humans at all. On the contrary, it is likely that they will be able to do so using human *embryonic* tissue as the source of the donor nuclei. They would then know nothing about the accomplishments (or bust size) of the person they were cloning since no accomplishments (or bust size) had ever existed, that person having never lived.

The inability to clone an adult human being would remove for many any motivation to clone humans at all. But there is a motivation for cloning animals. Speaking of domestic animals, cloning expert Dr. Clement Markert of Yale University told a congressional committee: "We can usually improve upon what nature has provided to design breeds of animals more in accord with our own requirements."

One of man's "requirements" is that of cutting up live animals in experiments. Genetically identical animals could be cloned specifically for use in the laboratory.

While we invariably look to see how a technology will affect us, the greatest effect is likely to be felt by animals of other than the human species.

Notes

1. In 1966, Dr. Joshua Lederberg, then professor of genetics and biology at Stanford University and executive head of the genetics department at Stanford's medical school, referred to successful cloning techniques in frogs and wrote: "There is nothing to suggest any particular difficulty about accomplishing this in mammals or man, though it will rightly be admired as a technical tour de force when it is first implemented. (The sentence may be an anachronism before it is published.)" (Lederberg, 1966). Three years later, Dr. Robert Sinsheimer, chairman of the division of biology at California Institute of Technology, estimated that human beings could be cloned within ten to twenty years (Gaylin, 1972). Dr. James Watson's estimate ran a bit longer: twenty to fifty years, perhaps sooner if some nation actively promoted the human cloning venture (Watson, 1971).

2. At Yale, biologist Clement L. Markert worked on yet another method of cloning a mammal. He fertilized a mouse egg in the lab. Then, before the sperm and egg nuclei (called pronuclei) had merged, he removed one of them with microsurgical instruments. This left the egg with half the number of chromosomes it needed in order to develop. (Most of the eggs are destroyed by this process. "Apparently, some irreversible injury occurred, but its nature is so far obscure," Markert, 1977). He immersed the egg in cytochalasin B, a drug that prevents the cell from beginning to subdivide but allows the nucleus to split, producing a double set of chromosomes. Once the DNA has doubled, the drug is washed out. Markert has not succeeded in producing mice by his method, but two other scientists, Hoppe and Illmensee, reported that they had. (Illmensee's work has since been investigated several times although no fraud has been found.) The seven mice they produced had only one parent each but they were not true clones for they did not possess exactly the genes of their parent. Instead, they had half the parent's genes, doubled. However, clones could be produced from these seven mice by repeating the procedure using their body cells. The offspring produced would be genetically identical to their parents. Only females can be produced by this method. Because there is no merging of the nuclei of sex cells—one from the mother and one from the father—in the egg, it is impossible to obtain the XY combination which would be a male. If a Y nucleus doubles, it will be a nonviable YY and will not develop. If an X nucleus doubles, it will develop into a female, XX.

3. The egg cell divides more rapidly than the body cell and this poses a problem in cloning. In order to achieve cloning, the egg and the inserted donor nucleus must be in compatible stages of development. If the rate of division of the nucleus and the cytoplasm are out of synchronization, either the cell will fail to

develop or it will develop into a monstrosity. It is because cells in bodies have great variations in their division rates that cloning might work with some but not with others. Spermatogonia, the precursors of sperm cells, are often mentioned as likely candidates. They have the full forty-six chromosomes, not the twenty-three the sperm cell itself has. If the nucleus of the spermatogonial cell can be transplanted into an enucleated egg, it might provoke normal development and thus generate a clone.

Part Five

THE BIGGER PICTURE

14

Breeding Brothels:
A Caste of Childbearers

During slavery, Black women were considered animals from whom their infant children could be sold away "like calves from cows." One year after the importation of Africans as slaves into the United States was halted, a South Carolina court ruled that female slaves had no legal claims on their children. According to the court ruling, slaveowners could sell children away from their mothers at any age because "the young of slaves ... stand on the same footing as other animals" (Davis, 1981, p. 71).

These women were considered breeders, not mothers. Their bodies could be sold for reproductive purposes just as the bodies of women have been, and are, sold for sexual purposes. It may at first seem unbelievable that women could ever have been viewed as breeders or that, if it were indeed true in an unenlightened earlier century, it could ever happen in our own time and certainly never in the future. But consider:

The Third Reich had a plan to use women as reproductive prostitutes, as breeders. In attempting to "purify" the German race, the Nazis developed a two-part program: extermination and planned reproduction. For this second program, Himmler established the Lebensborn Registered Society on December 12, 1935. Lebensborn ("fountain of life") established homes where "racially valuable" pregnant women could bear children and where those children could be cared for until they were adopted by German families. The term "breeding" first appears in an official document on August 16, 1943, according to journalists Marc Hillel and Clarissa Henry, who have reported on Lebensborn. In that document, Dr. Gregor Ebner, Lebensborn's chief medical superintendent, wrote: "The objective of our breeding must be to bring together people from whom Nordic-minded children are to be expected" (Hillel and Henry, 1976, p. 83).

Lebensborn had several ways of obtaining "Nordic-minded children," only one of which I will discuss here. It involved kidnapping "racially valuable" female children in certain occupied countries—Czechoslovakia, Hungary, Rumania and Poland—for eventual use as breeder women. After bearing several children, the girls were to be exterminated.

No leader of Lebensborn has ever admitted that such a scheme existed and no surviving documents from Nazi Germany mention this plan.[1] A few weeks before Germany's collapse, the SS destroyed the files concerning kidnaped children. But evidence nonetheless exists. Some of the kidnaped girls survived. They are adults now and they have their memories. Hillel and Henry interviewed them, as well as some of the German families to whom they were temporarily entrusted.

One of the kidnaped girls was Alycia Sosinka, born at Lodz, Poland, in 1935 and taken from her mother in September 1942. Lebensborn placed her in a boarding school with other Polish girls. Alycia told Hillel and Henry:

> Life in that barracks was a real nightmare. We were branded on the left hand and the back of the neck [the scars are still visible]. We were very frightened by this branding, but in fact it was not painful. One day we were told: "You will give birth to two or three Germans of good race and then you will disappear." We were also continually given injections. I now believe they were hormonal injections, intended to make us reach the age of puberty more quickly. The other girls, Poles, Czechs, Hungarians and, I think, Rumanians, were subjected to the same treatment (Hillel and Henry, 1976).

Alycia was placed for a few months with a German peasant family. Their daughter told Hillel and Henry that her parents had wanted very much to adopt Alycia but that that had been impossible because the SS had intended to take her back for reproductive purposes when she became 15 or 16 years old.

Nazis are not the only men who conceive of using women quite baldly as breeders. Men in liberal democracies have talked seriously of creating a "caste of childbearers," of using certain women as "professional breeders," of "keeping a stable" of mothers.

As far back as the Depression, when birth rates were declining, American sociologist Kingsley Davis speculated that a policy of paying women who bear babies might lead to the development of professional breeders. Other institutions had taken over many of the functions of the family but not reproduction and child care, Davis wrote. If those functions were to be performed adequately, it would seem that they too must be taken over by agencies other than the family, "agencies which can motivate individuals to perform the given function."

If the government provided financial incentives to women to procreate, it might require women who live by producing children to prove their fitness. "It would thereby produce, gradually and probably unwittingly, a new profession—the profession of child-rearing," Davis wrote. "It would take only one more step to introduce required training for the professional child-rearers, thus elevating both the standards and the social status of this occupational group."

This would be an efficient system in terms of producing both quantity and quality in children: "Suppliers of sperm could be chosen for their biological fitness. Child-bearing women could be chosen for their intellectual and physical qualities." (Davis concluded his article by stating that he was not predicting or advocating a new reproductive institution.)

In 1978, Charles F. Westoff, director of the Office of Population Research at Princeton University, also suggested that some subsidization of reproduction may eventually become necessary. The U.S. population was again low and in about fifty years would begin to decline. If women continued to work outside the home, use contraception and bear fewer babies, how will the next generation be produced? The state may have to provide women with financial incentives for childbearing, he wrote. He refers to Davis' speculations about professional breeders.[2]

Now, with women being bought for breeding service in surrogate motherhood companies, there is increased mention of professional breeders. Lawyers, physicians, legislators and ethicists write of "institutionalizing" surrogate motherhood, of the state regulating the women, of some agency certifying and licensing the mothers.

Professional breeding could become commonplace, attorney Russell Scott writes, if "healthy young host mothers" were offered, not only payment, but social security, educational facilities and other signs of public approval as well.

As social commentator Vance Packard and John Stehura, president of the Bionetics Foundation, have independently suggested, fees paid to "host mothers" would probably vary with the country. Third World women would do it for less. When it becomes possible to transfer embryos routinely, then the way opens up to use these women to gestate babies for wealthier Westerners.

Since, as Andrea Dworkin observes, motherhood is becoming a new branch of female prostitution, it is hardly surprising that the word "stable" crops up in discussions of surrogate mothers. "If they [the doctors] have a number of prospective surrogates on their books, could they be said to be keeping a stable?" asked *The New York Times* in an editorial. Most surrogate firms keep dossiers, complete with photos, on each surrogate so their clients can make their selection from the stable of women. The "girls" themselves do not line up to await the john's selection as they must in brothels; their dossiers line up.

John Stehura's foundation issues a quarterly directory containing photographs of women allegedly willing to serve as breeders (one displays Number 36, "Gabriel," an attractive woman wearing a blouse with a low neckline) and entries describing each available woman. Such a directory of women available for sale makes some in the surrogate industry uneasy. They speak of the need to regulate the industry to prevent such abuses. But the difference between individual portfolios on women shown to clients in the tastefully paneled conference room of a law office and a directory of women published on cheap newsprint and mailed out to anyone who will pay a few dollars for it, is merely one of style, perhaps class, but not one of substance.

Sometimes the reproductive prostitute is or was a sexual prostitute as well. In Britain, a childless couple hired a 19-year-old prostitute for $5,500 to bear a baby for them conceived through artificial insemination with the husband's sperm. The couple entered London's Bow Street Magistrates Court, surveyed the women who paraded to pay their regular fines, and chose one. That woman would not bear them a child but agreed, for a finder's fee of $925, to locate a prostitute who would and did.[3]

Through the centuries, how will social institutions be changed to reflect the fact that men have taken total control of female biological reproductive processes? Of course we do not know exactly. But Andrea Dworkin has described one possible expression of the new reality: the reproductive brothel (Dworkin, 1983). With such technologies as embryo transfer, she wrote, women will be able to sell reproductive capacities the same way old-time prostitutes sold sexual ones. While sexual prostitutes sell vagina, rectum and mouth, reproductive prostitutes would sell other body parts: wombs, ovaries, eggs.

Dworkin's vision is not unthinkable. For centuries it has been

considered acceptable to confine certain women in brothels where
they are controlled, viewed as a collection of body parts infused
with no spirit, no individuality, used as sexual meat. It is acceptable
in a male-dominated society to treat women in this way. Most of us
have learned how to look at the fact of a brothel and not see its
horror. Many a writer has romanticized it.

Setting up stables of surrogate mothers would be establishing a
primitive form of the reproductive brothel. An assembly-line approach
to procreation would be used, but only to a minor degree. ("Some
of the surrogates are pregnant, some are being inseminated, some
are waiting to be selected," an attorney who operates a surrogate
business told me in 1982. "About four or five are waiting to get final
reports in from the physician.") With improvements in technology,
a brothel employing much more sophisticated assembly-line techniques and providing greater control over women becomes possible.

As we have seen in the treatment of farm animals, a model for
such an institution already exists. Many animals in a reproductive
brothel, considered genetically unworthy, serve as breeders for the
embryos of superior animals. This distinction between the genetically
worthy and unworthy is likely to increase. Writing of one scheme
to obtain large-scale genetic improvement in a herd, Dr. Peter Elsden
of the Animal Reproduction Laboratory at Colorado State University
noted that the top 10 to 20 percent of the herd could be superovulated
and used to produce many embryos, while the bottom 90 to 80
percent of the cows could be used as recipients for those embryos.
"Therefore, the lower two-thirds of the herd is being culled in
regard to their own progeny, while the top one-third of the herd is
producing four times as many progeny as normal since the average
number of calves per superovulation treatment is four," he wrote.

As I envision it, most women in a reproductive brothel would
be defined as "nonvaluable" and sterilized and, in this way, their
progeny culled. (Already we have seen use of the new reproductive
technologies in humans linked to sterilization, usually with the
suggestion that sterilization would benefit those operated upon
[Muller, 1961; Fletcher, 1974; Fletcher, 1976; Seed and Seed, 1978;
Djerassi, 1979; *Appendix*, 1979, Edwards].) Certainly women of color
would be labeled "nonvaluable" and used as breeders for the embryos
of "valuable" women. The white women judged genetically superior
and selected as egg donors would be turned into machines for
producing embryos. Through superovulation, "valuable" females as
young as 2 years and some as old as 50 or 60 could be induced to
produce eggs. (Reproductive specialists are now working on expand-

ing the reproductive usefulness of women past menopause. One told me he is treating female infertility patients in their 50s, and added that he found the prospect of enabling older women "scared off maternity because of their age" to have babies much more exciting than work with external fertilization.)

Reproductive engineers would engage in three major activities in the brothel: getting eggs; manipulating them; and transferring embryos.

Getting Eggs

There are a number of ways engineers might get (or, as they put it, "recruit") eggs from women. They could flush them out of women using the technique developed by Richard and Randolph Seed with the medical team at the Harbor–UCLA Medical Center, though this would probably not yield the necessary quantity. They might also try two techniques employed experimentally in animals: placing and keeping tubular instruments inside women in order to continually mine them for eggs; and relocating women's ovaries to make it easier to reach the eggs. They could also keep cultures of oogonia (the precursors of eggs) as a source of genetic material, as they envision doing in animals.

But eggs are far more likely to be obtained from other techniques. In the pages of *Farm Journal* in 1976, Earl Ainsworth, in identifying the factor that prevented farmers from treating sows totally as machines, indicates which ones. "Estrous control will open the doors to factory hog production. Control of female cycles is the missing link to the assembly-line approach" (Mason and Singer, 1980).

The "missing link" to the assembly-line, brothel approach to human reproduction is being forged in IVF clinics around the world where, as we saw in Chapter 7, teams are working intensively to control the cycles of women.

In the brothel, on the appropriate days of their cycles, women would line up for Pergonal shots, which will stimulate their ovaries. Engineers would superovulate only the top 10 to 20 percent of the female population in the brothel. Then, after following the development of the eggs through ultrasound and blood tests, they would operate on the women to extract the eggs. Perhaps they would allow the women to heal from the operation every other month so that women would only be subjected to surgery six times per year.

To obtain eggs, engineers could also do what they now do with certain cows. When the championship cow Sabine 2A died in 1982 during a cesarean section, embryologists from the firm Genetic Engineering Inc. removed her ovaries, obtained thirty-six eggs from them, and froze the eggs. During her lifetime, Sabine's embryos had been fetching $10,000 or more on the embryo transfer market, and when the eggs from the dead Sabine are thawed and fertilized in vitro, they may fetch the same (Brotman, 1983). In the reproductive brothel, as a valuable woman dies, engineers could operate on her, remove her ovaries and salvage eggs from those ovaries, perhaps by using enzymes to eat away the connective tissue and release hundreds of thousands of eggs. They could then freeze the eggs for future in vitro fertilization and transfer into a "nonvaluable" female. A woman could be used for reproduction long after she is dead.

Not only could dead women be used in reproductive brothels. So could women who were never even born. A female embryo could be developed just to the point where an ovary emerges, and then the ovary could be cultured so that engineers could get eggs from it. The full woman would never be allowed to develop. Just her ovary.

Partial ectogenesis—culturing organ rudiments from their earliest appearance to a mature state—is already well established as a technique used in certain biological studies. If various fragmented procedures reported by different scientists could be brought together and, in combination, used in one species, mature organs might soon be produced externally from a fertilized egg, embryologist Dr. Clifford Grobstein has predicted. One of the organs men have extensively investigated is the ovary. By maturing the ovary externally, Grobstein wrote, a supply of eggs for in vitro fertilization could be provided without surgical intervention in a woman's body (Grobstein, 1981, p. 48).[4]

Back in 1923 in his book, *Daedalus, or Science and the Future,* British geneticist J. B. S. Haldane had predicted something similar though his vision, compared to Grobstein's, lacked daring. The *Daedalus* predictions were in the form of a college student's essay written 150 years hence: "We can take an ovary from a woman and keep it growing in a suitable fluid for as long as twenty years, producing a fresh ovum each month, of which 90 per cent can be fertilized, and the embryos grown successfully for nine months, and then brought out into the air" (Reed, 1968, p. 233).

Today in the mass media, keeping ovaries alive and mining them for eggs is presented as a boon to women, as "therapy." In a woman's magazine article, one gynecologist referred to recent experiments at Pennsylvania Hospital and the University of Pennsylvania

School of Medicine in which researchers removed ovaries from rabbits, salvaged eggs from them, fertilized them in vitro and implanted them in surrogate rabbit mothers who delivered healthy offspring. He wrote: "Suppose someday in the future a woman had to have a hysterectomy? She might be able to have her ovaries saved and her eggs fertilized in a laboratory" (Lauersen, 1982). His article was entitled: "New Ways of Making Babies: How Science Can Help!"

Manipulating Eggs

Once the eggs have been "recovered," reproductive engineers along the assembly line could manipulate them in a number of ways:

—Twin the embryos, producing two humans out of one embryo

—Use the eggs of nonvaluable women for clones, destroying the egg nuclei with lasers and injecting the nuclei of valuable men

—Remove the female genetic component from the egg and inject two sperm into the egg, producing a child with two fathers and no mother. (The sperm might be dead or alive. There is some evidence in animals that dead sperm would work [Seidel, 1980].)

—Genetically engineer the embryo for various qualities. If ever partial or total ectogenesis were applied to humans, it would be "no more than a game for the 'manfarming biologist' to change the subject's sex, the colour of its eyes, the general proportions of body and limbs, and perhaps the facial features," wrote biologist Jean Rostand, overconfidently (Rostand, 1959, p. 84). (So little is now known of human genes that such manipulations would be exceedingly difficult.)

—Fertilize them in the laboratory using a culture medium concocted from bits and pieces of women. "We made our culture fluids resemble the female reproductive tract by adding very small pieces of human uterus or Fallopian tube," wrote IVF pioneers Steptoe and Edwards (Edwards and Steptoe, 1980, p. 54). Another reproductive engineer used "minced fragments of fallopian tubal mucosa" (Shettles, 1955).

—Select the sex of the embryo by fertilizing the egg with sperm from either the gynosperm bank or the androsperm bank. Should gynosperm and androsperm not have been separated by then, engineers could sex the fertilized egg by snipping off a few cells to check its gender. Most embryos manufactured would be male. The brothel administration would decide how many female embryos would be needed.

Transferring Embryos

Once the embryo has been manufactured, reproductive engineers would have several options.

They could freeze the embryo in the bank for later use. Or they could immediately transfer the embryo into a woman in the lower 80 to 90 percent of the female population. (These would be the breeders, the women who had been called "surrogate mothers" in the early stage of the reproduction revolution when pharmacrats were conscious of the need for good public relations.)

The transferred embryo might gestate in the breeder for the entire nine-month pregnancy. There will be no "birthing rooms" in the brothel. The assembly-line approach will prevail. The description women gave of their obstetrical experiences in American hospitals in the 1950s are likely to be as apt for the brothel of the future: "They give you drugs, whether you want them or not, strap you down like an animal." "Women are herded like sheep through an obstetrical assembly line, are drugged and strapped on tables while their babies are forceps-delivered." "I felt exactly like a trapped animal" (Shultz, 1958 and 1959).

Alternatively, the engineers could transfer the embryo into a breeder, allow it to gestate for a certain number of months, and then remove the fetus by cesarean section at whatever point at which their incubators could take over. (Today that point is 21 weeks gestation.) In the incubator, they would perform surgery on the fetus, inoculate it or undertake whatever alterations they deemed desirable.

The breeder into whom an embryo is placed need not be alive. This possibility is suggested by several recent cases in which the bodies of brain-dead pregnant women were kept functioning until the fetus had developed enough to be delivered. In one case, a 27-year-old woman suffered a fatal seizure when she was 22 weeks' pregnant. Her husband and other family members wanted the woman's body kept in operation until the fetus became viable. Physicians put her on a life-support system. Their most difficult medical challenges during the nine weeks they maintained the dead woman were keeping control of the woman's many failing body functions and combatting infection, they report. The woman developed diabetes insipidus and Addison's disease and, periodically, a blood infection throughout the whole body. Doctors did blood studies on the dead woman every two hours. They performed a cesarean section on her more than two months after she had been declared dead, extracted a healthy baby and then removed the life-support apparatus. She stopped breathing. Relatives reportedly expressed "a great deal of pleasure" at the birth (*Star–Ledger*, 3/31/83).

"The experience left me with real confidence that this can be done without any great difficulties. . . . In the future, I'll suggest to family members that the option is there," Dr. Russell K. Laros, Jr., of the department of obstetrics, gynecology and reproductive sciences at the University of California, San Francisco, School of Medicine, said (OGN, 6/1/83).

(Immediately over the Newark *Star–Ledger*'s report—"Brain Dead Woman Gives Birth"—appeared a photo of smiling parents holding their infants, the nation's first test-tube twins.)

Perhaps few women, dead or alive, will be required. If pharmacrats have developed an artificial womb, they might place the cultured embryo directly into The Mother Machine. Right now, a fetus produced by artificial insemination, embryo transfer, in vitro fertilization or cloning will need an individual woman to carry it. So reproduction remains a cottage or craft industry. But once pharmacrats develop the artificial womb and placenta, "factory techniques or 'baby farms' could become the mode of production" (Hanmer, 1980).

Within the reproductive brothel, women would be totally reduced to Matter. As we will see in the final two chapters, this would represent the culmination of a centuries-long process.

Notes

1. Everything concerning both aspects of the race purification program—extermination of Jews and planned reproduction—was kept highly secret. Such programs were discussed in code words: "disinfection" for euthanasia; "resettlement" for extermination; "nurse" for breeding woman (Hillel and Henry, 1976).

2. The decline in population is due to a number of factors: the availability of contraception and abortion; later and less permanent marriages; diminishing religious influence over lives; an alleged growing economic independence of women.

3. She found "Miss C." During the pregnancy, "Miss C.," a teenager, realized she could not give up her baby and told her clients. After the birth, they kidnaped the baby. The case came to trial. When the teenager freed herself from prostitution and agreed to supervision, Judge James Conryn awarded her custody of her child. He allowed the father visitation rights for two years (Scott, 1981, p. 217).

4. An attempt to mature an ovary externally could first be made in mice. It would involve these steps: fertilization of an egg in the lab; external development of the embryo to the point where it forms a rudimentary ovary; organ culture of ovary rudiments to produce eggs; finally, use of the eggs for fertilization in the lab to begin the whole cycle again. Improvements in certain techniques would be necessary in order to carry out this procedure but none of the problems involved are insurmountable, Grobstein wrote. If it could work successfully in mice, he added, it would probably be technically possible to apply it to women (Grobstein, 1981, p. 120; also see Rostand, 1959, pp. 20–21).

15

Reproductive Continuity: *Capturing the "Magic" of Maternity*

I want to leave the futuristic vision of reproductive brothels now and go back to the beginning, to the time, centuries ago, when woman was the sole creator of the child. I go back in order to understand how the male's role in procreation—at first perceived to be none at all—affected his consciousness.

In Neolithic society, man knew nothing of his part in procreation and made no connection between sexual intercourse and the birth of a baby nine months later. A woman's body, he saw, ripened with child as a tree ripened with fruit. Clearly a spirit impregnated a woman, perhaps entering her body through the wind, a star, a bird, the rain or the moon.

Humankind revered woman's awe-inspiring power to bring forth life and to nourish that life with the milk of her body. For thousands of years, they worshiped a female deity, the Great Goddess, in the image of this human mother. The Goddess was worshiped for a period five times as long as recorded history, far longer than any other deities (Lederer, 1968, p. 10). (We will return to the Goddess later to record her violent overthrow.)

Man's belief that he played little or no part in procreation affected him deeply as we see in the overwhelming evidence of birth or parturition envy noted by psychiatrists, sociologists, historians, anthropologists and mothers observing small sons.[1] Early man, primitive man and Christian man have all had various methods of trying to make woman's procreative power his own. He has mutilated his genitals in an attempt to render him capable of giving birth. Or simulated labor and delivery (couvade). Or worn women's clothing. Or conducted initiation ceremonies in which the male sponsors of boys give birth to men. Psychiatrist Bruno Bettelheim has written at length about some of these methods.

First, self-mutilation. The Galloi, priests of the goddess Cybele, voluntarily castrated themselves, and ran through the streets holding their genitals in their hands. At a certain point, each priest would throw his genitals into a woman's house and the woman would give him female clothing, a type of clothing he would wear for the rest of his life. This custom, prevalent in Rome from the second century B.C. through the fourth century A.D., shows that men were willing "to become 'female' in order to share woman's superior powers" (Bettelheim, 1968, p. 93).

In less drastic surgery, men often gave women the products of the mutilation—blood or foreskin. Bettelheim suggests that what men expected in return for this offering was "a share in women's great and secret power of procreation, a gift that only women can bestow because only women possess it."

Male expectations in performing subincision appear to be similar. Subincision is an initiation ceremony practiced among many primitive tribes, including the central Aborigine tribes of Australia. The ceremony involves the slitting of the penis in a apparent attempt to make the male genitals into female ones. The subincision hole is called a "vagina" or a "penis womb." The subincision wound, called a "vulva," is repeatedly opened so that it bleeds again, mimicking menstruation. The people themselves compare the blood from the wound to menses. In New Guinea, where the men also practice subincision, a man bleeding from his penis must observe the same taboos a menstruating women must.

One commentator has concluded that "through subincision the young man is supposed to be changed into a woman.... The initiation ceremonies change boys into women, or, rather, man-woman" (Bryk, quoted in Bettelheim, 1968, p. 106).

Couvade, often explained as a custom practiced to distract evil spirits so they do not harm the baby, is another male attempt to take over the function of women. Under the extreme form of this custom, the pregnant woman works until a few hours before the birth, then goes into the forest with some women and bears the child. Within a few hours, she must return to work. Her husband, however, lies on a hammock, sometimes simulating labor and childbirth. While the women nurse and care for him, he fasts or eats a weak gruel. His confinement may last for days or even weeks. The full couvade has been observed on all continents in both ancient and recent time. According to the *Encyclopedia Britannica*, it has been reported as recently as the early twentieth century in the Basque country and in Brazil.

Through this custom, men detract from the woman's importance and pretend to give birth themselves. But, Bettelheim comments, they copy only the insignificant externals of the birth experience, and not the essentials, which they cannot duplicate. "Such an apeing of superficials only emphasizes the more how much the real, essential powers are envied," he wrote.

Transvestism is also an attempt to acquire woman's power. It prevailed in the majority of ancient priesthoods (Walker, 1983, p. 1014). Sometimes, as among the Naven tribe of New Guinea, transvestism plays a part in an initiation ceremony for boys. A boy's male sponsor dresses up in widow's clothing, makes himself look pregnant, is referred to as "mother," and wanders among the people crying out in a high, falsetto voice for his child, the boy initiate.

Initiation ceremonies are rebirth rituals in which the male sponsors of boys give birth to men. Their purpose seems to be to assert that men, too, can bear life. Men frankly act out childbirth in some of the ceremonies. In the Liberian Poro society, the crocodile spirit, a representative of the male group, swallows up the boy initiates, and remains pregnant with them for up to four years. (During this time the boys are living in the bush.) When the boys— now young men—return home, they must pretend to be newborns. Such initiation rituals are sometimes accompanied by the myth that they were stolen from women and sometimes that women were killed to get them (Fisher, 1979, p. 156).

Christian priests rebirth children even today through the power of their God, a phenomenon about which Una Stannard, author of *Mrs. Man*, has written. The early Christians believed one was not truly born until after baptism. Women merely birthed human beings into mortal, fleshly life while men birthed humans into eternal, immortal life through their own amniotic fluid, the baptismal waters. A Catholic rite for the consecration of the baptismal font actually refers to the font as a "stainless womb" (Neumann, 1963, p. 311). In a letter written in 256 A.D., Cyprian wrote: "The birth of Christians is in baptism. He, Christ, generated us from our mother— the [baptismal] water" (Stannard, 1977). As Stannard points out, the Church, embodiment of the Father God, had taken over the pro- creation power of women and become *Mater Ecclesia*. She quotes Tertullian, who said the Church was "the true mother of the living ... the second Adam," and Paul in Galatians in the New Testament who asserted that the Church was "the mother of us all."

Men not only birth; they suckle. It is Christ's word, not woman's milk, which truly nourishes man. Clement, for example, compared seeking Christ to suckling: "For to those babes that suck the Word, the Father's breasts of love supply the milk" (Stannard, 1977, p. 294).

Evidence of a male desire to possess woman's procreative power has been found not only by anthropologists working among primitive peoples and feminists observing Christian practices, but also by psychologists treating adolescent boys. For example, in a paper on the desire of boys to bear children, Edith Jacobson mentioned that among her male patients she had had "occasion to observe . . . an intense and persistent envy of female reproductive ability—an envy which is often disguised by a seemingly normal masculinity" (quoted in Bettelheim, 1968). She protested that pertinent studies on male birth envy had been conspicuously neglected by psychiatrists. Commenting on this protest, psychiatrist Dr. Wolfgang Lederer wrote: "Indeed, of our fear and envy of women, we, the psychoanalytic-papers-writing-men, have managed to maintain a dignified fraternal silence" (Lederer, 1968, p. 153).

That the desire to bear babies is not confined to psychiatric patients is suggested by an acknowledgment in the children's book, The Boy Who Wanted a Baby. Author Wendy Lichtman thanks "the men and boys who were vulnerable and brave in telling me their feelings of longing for that which is not possible" (Lichtman, 1982).

So in the beginning, woman was the sole creator of the child. But at some unknown time, some unknown people discovered paternity, the connection between intercourse and a child's birth. Man then realized that by lying with a woman, he impregnated her and fathered the child she bore. He understood that he was physically linked with the child, that it was flesh of his flesh. He came to see the child as a continuation of himself. In order to understand how the discovery of paternity relates to the new reproductive technologies, we must step back a moment and look at a theory proposed by Mary O'Brien, a sociologist at the Ontario Institute for Studies in Education and a former midwife. In The Politics of Reproduction, O'Brien points out the following: Impressive bodies of philosophical thought have examined certain human biological necessities—the need to eat, to express sexuality and to die—and have shown how these needs have shaped human understanding (or consciousness) and our relationship to the world. Marx transformed our need to eat into a theoretical system in which productive labor remakes our consciousness. The existentialists did the same for death, and Freud, showing how libido shapes our consciousness, for sexuality. But there is another biological necessity that male philosophers have ignored: birth. There is no philosophy of birth comparable to those concerned with labor, sexuality and death.

Yet birth, too, shapes our human understanding. O'Brien notes that the reproductive experience for men and women differs, so men and women have a different reproductive consciousness. For woman, reproduction is a continuous experience. She participates in intercourse. The fertilized egg grows within her body during the nine months of pregnancy. She births the child in an act of labor, sometimes nourishes the child with her milk, and raises the child.

For man, reproduction is a discontinuous experience. He ejaculates his sperm into the woman and then goes about his business. Nine months later, a woman bears a child that is his as well as hers. But he has a hard time imagining that child as his. To make a connection between copulation and the birth of a child much later requires an intellectual act. Paternity, then, is an abstract idea— conceptualizing a cause and effect relationship between copulation and childbirth—while maternity is an experience, O'Brien points out.

Man's sperm is alienated (that is, separated) from him in the sex act and this alienation negates him as a parent. He has no certainty that the child born nine months later is *his* child. Woman's seed, unified with the man's and developed into a baby within her body, is also alienated from her at birth. But she undergoes a process that reconciles her to this separation. Her labor in childbirth confirms for her the certainty that this child is *her* child, and gives her a relationship to the child similar to that which a worker has toward a product. After her labor, she need take no further action to annul her separation from the human race.

When his seed is alienated, man is separated from the continuity of the human species, from a sense of unity with natural process. He does not actually experience a link between generations. While woman has a sense of her connection with the next generation in the labor through which she births that generation, man is isolated within the dimensions of his own lifespan. He has not labored to produce the child, except in the relatively trivial expenditure of energy in sexual intercourse.

Alienation is the separation of a human being from the world and from experience of the world; it is a negation of the self. O'Brien points out, as the philosopher Hegel did before her, that human consciousness resists alienation and negation of the self.

Man's nullity as a parent appears to be unbearable to him. To make that nullity bearable, to neutralize his separation from his seed and from genetic continuity, man had to do something. What he has done is appropriate the child.[2] Defying the uncertainty of paternity, he works in cooperation with other men to assert a proprietorial right to a child, one that nature has not provided for him. His assertion of a right to the child must be supported by ideologies of male supremacy and by a host of social structures. The legal ownership of children and man's need to legitimate on the basis of biological fatherhood can be seen as attempts on the part of the male to reclaim the child, to overcome the discontinuous nature of his reproductive experience. The idea that women contribute only "matter" to babies while men contribute spirit—an idea that, as we will later see, prevailed for centuries—is also an attempt by men to resist the alienation of their seed and reclaim the child.

We see man's appropriation of the child in the laws throughout the world, which, until less than a century ago, gave fathers sole guardianship of children. The father had an absolute right to take the children away from his wife during marriage and, upon his death, could bequeath that guardianship to another male rather than to their mother. Fathers were routinely granted custody of children upon divorce. It was not until 1886 in England that, under certain rare circumstances, a woman could get custody of her children. All but five states in America in the 1890s gave fathers sole legal guardianship of children.[3]

To assure paternity, man had to control the sexual activities of his woman, allowing no other man to impregnate her. Then he could pass his name, power and property down through his sons. In this way (although O'Brien does not state this), he could achieve continuity over time. The creation of the private realm helped men to control their women. Men separated social life into private and public realms in order to ensure themselves exclusive rights to a particular woman, rights buttressed by the woman's physical separation from other men. With marriage and the patriarchal family, two of the institutions men developed to solve the problem of male separation from reproduction, wives who committed "adultery" (a new crime) were severely punished and children born out of wedlock were declared "illegitimate."[4]

It seems to me that whether O'Brien's theory is fully right or not is unimportant. What *is* important is that she has opened up the issue to discussion. She has pointed out how the effect of reproduction on consciousness has been rendered invisible in patriarchal society. She has demonstrated the need for a philosophy of birth, a philosophy that remains to be worked out.[5]

O'Brien has pointed out that because of the discontinuous nature of man's reproductive experience, he lacks a sense of genetic continuity. Reproductive technologies can give him that continuity over time through these means:

—Sperm banks and artificial insemination, which will allow a man to engender children even after he is dead. In fact, the man who originated the concept of frozen sperm banks in 1866, Mantegazza, suggested that a man, while dying on a battlefield, could still beget a legal heir through his frozen sperm at home. More than a century later, Dr. Jerome K. Sherman, American pioneer in techniques for freezing human sperm, observed that by storing his sperm, "man can induce conception in absence of testes, in old age, and long after his death" (Sherman, 1973).

—Sex determination. By ensuring the birth of a son, a man assures himself a form of immortality. He sees himself reborn in his son.

—The creation of an exact replica of a man, his clone. One commentator has noted that "having oneself cloned is yet another effort to assure some form of personal continuity; it is simply more direct than having normal offspring, a child formed by sexual union and incorporating a variety of genetic strains [that is, a mother's as well as a father's]. A human clone would be totally identical to its donor-father, and could step directly into his shoes, as it were, carry on and perfect whatever he had begun, be his heir in the most immediate and literal sense of the term" (Ebon, 1978, pp. 2–3).

Reproductive technologies do more than give males a sense of continuity over time. They are transforming the experience of motherhood and placing it under the control of men. Woman's claim to maternity is being loosened; man's claim to paternity strengthened. Moreover, these techniques are creating for women the same kind of discontinuous reproductive experience men now have. "That is one of the absolutely crucial things about them," comments Jalna Hanmer, a sociologist at England's University of Bradford who has studied the technologies. The woman begins to feel that the baby is not hers, Hanmer observes. The more complex the technologies become, the more a woman must use her intellect to figure out in what way she contributed to the child's birth. Through her egg? Through her womb? Through her labor? As paternity always has been, maternity is becoming an act of intellect— for example, making a causal connection between the extraction of an egg and the birth of a child to another woman nine months later. Meanwhile, those men who extract eggs, culture them, transfer embryos, surgically birth babies, or control the dials on the artificial womb will have a more continuous reproductive experience than men have ever before had.

How will woman's claim to maternity be loosened? As one pioneer in reproductive technology explained to me, in the future there will be three kinds of mothers:

—The genetic mother who "donates" or sells her eggs
—The surrogate or natal mother who carries the baby
—The social mother who raises the child

Under this system of dismembered motherhood, none of these three women will have a compelling claim to her child. Nor does Dr. Joseph Fletcher think she ought to. Fletcher is a medical ethicist associated with the University of Virginia School of Medicine. He believes that a woman whose egg is used to produce a baby should have no claim of any kind on the child born of that egg. Parental relationships need to be "reconceptualized," he writes. "They cannot anymore be based on blood or wombs or even genes. . . . The mere fact of conceiving a child or donating the elements of its conception or gestating it does not establish anybody as a father or mother." Parenthood, he maintains, will have to be understood morally rather than biologically.

As Fletcher notes, with uterine and ovarian transplants, with egg and embryo transfers, "Maternity now is in question too, as paternity used to be."

The modern reproductive technologist championed by men like Fletcher is, in his quest, a brother to the alchemist who looked for one universal medicine, "some powerful substance that would enable men to control matter and live forever" (Cummings, 1966). The alchemist sought nothing less than "the magic of maternity" conferred upon men. This is the conclusion of scholars Sally G. Allen and Joanne Hubbs, who studied a treatise by a prominent seventeenth century alchemist. They found that it describes man's aggressive arrogation of woman's procreation power.[6] The great alchemist Paracelsus answered "yes" to the question: "Whether it was possible for art and nature that a man should be born outside a woman's body and a natural mother's." The culmination of the alchemical process is frequently depicted through the image of the birth of a male child, who, Paracelsus wrote: "By art received life, through art . . . received a body, flesh, bones and blood and through art . . . was born" (Allen and Hubbs, 1980, p. 211).

Reproductive technologists now aim to bring forth life through "art," rather than nature and enable a man to be not only the father, but also the mother of his child.

Transsexual surgery may someday help transform men into mothers. This surgery is, in the majority of cases, now performed on men in order to construct artificial females.[7] Men cut off the penises and testicles of other men, surgically construct a "vagina" and inject hormones into their patients. Fletcher comments on this surgery and then continues: "Furthermore, transplant or replacement medicine foresees the day, after the automatic rejection of alien tissues is overcome, when a uterus can be implanted in a human male's body—his abdomen has spaces—and gestation started by artificial fertilization and egg transfer." By decreasing the activity of testes, physicians could also "stimulate milk from the man's rudimentary breasts—men too have mammary glands. If surgery could not construct a cervical canal the delivery could be effected by a cesarean section and the male or transsexualized mother could nurse his own baby. . . .

"As it is at present," he continued, "women have four reproductive functions: to menstruate, ovulate, gestate and lactate—while men only impregnate. But . . . surgery may soon be trading these functions back and forth; they have already begun doing it with both surgery and hormones."

In this way, reproductive technologists, like the alchemists, would be conferring "the magic of maternity" on men.

In recent years, newspaper stories announcing that men can bear babies have appeared under these headlines: "Babies For Men," "Now Father Can Be Mother," "Scientists Reveal Proof That—MEN GIVE BIRTH." Professor Carl Wood, head of the test-tube baby team at Monash University in Australia, and senior researchers Professor Geoffrey Thorburn and Dr. Richard Harding claimed that it was theoretically possible for a male to have a baby. Dr. Harding told the tabloid *Globe:* "We've successfully transplanted mouse embryos into male mice. Although right now it might be impractical, and certainly uncomfortable, it is theoretically possible for a man to have a baby." Dr. Landrum Shettles, an American colleague who has experimented with IVF and sex predetermination, agreed: "Medical literature is loaded with cases of women who have had abdominal pregnancies. If a woman can carry a baby to full term outside the uterus [but within her abdomen], so can a man."

At a conference on test-tube babies in London in 1983, Jerome Lejeune, professor of genetics at Paris University, said an egg donated by a woman might be fertilized with a man's sperm, and implanted in his abdomen. It would be delivered nine months later by cesarean section (Veitch, 1983, May 24; Gillie, 1983, May 29).

While much experimentation remains to be done before men can indeed bear babies (if they ever really can), the fact that some researchers in reproductive technology are already predicting the advent of male mothers is noteworthy.

So too is the fact that, following public speculation on male motherhood, several men contacted Monash University and Queen Victoria Medical Centre in Melbourne volunteering for any such experiments. Dr. H. Bower, a psychiatrist working with transsexuals at the Melbourne clinic, said there are plenty more such men, that almost every man they surgically "trans-sex" at the clinic says he wants to bear a child (Roberts, 1981, July 31). "They would make excellent parents," he said. "I am quite convinced of that. I have seen several hundred of them and they are very motherly, warm creatures."

Fletcher points out that in the biblical creation story, there is no mother at all. In Genesis, God the Father was the first mother. God formed Adam artificially, from the dust. Then Adam became the second mother, birthing Eve while the male God acted as obstetrician. Only on the third round did we get a female mother with Eve birthing Cain and Abel. Fletcher writes: "Women have continued to be the mothers ever since, until now when reproduction once more takes the form of artifice as it did in the Garden of Eden—including motherless children and male mothers." We have come full circle, he writes. The new biology is restoring the modes of birth in effect before the Fall (Fletcher, 1974).

The Father God's birthing of Adam and later of Jesus, his "only-begotten" son (a phrase which does not mean "this *one*, or *only* son" but rather "alone-begotten" by the Father without a mate), are expressions of what bioethicist Dr. Janice Raymond terms a basic patriarchal myth: Single parenthood by the father. The reproductive technologies are an acting out of that myth. Fathers can be, or appear to be, the sole parent through: surrogate motherhood; destruction of the female genetic component of the egg and injection into the egg of two sperm;[8] cloning; and gestation in an artificial womb. One embryologist wonders how women will react "to being deprived of their role in reproduction not just as provider of the egg and a nine-month incubator, but also of anything to do with the process at all, from start to finish? A single male, alone on another planet, could theoretically reproduce a whole population from a piece of his own skin, given efficient incubators and a cloning technique!" (Francoeur, 1970, p. 158)[9]

If or when technology makes it possible for men to create life and give birth in their laboratories, women need not maintain their procreative capacity. Indeed, commentator Edward Grossman has written that women who use artificial wombs might choose to be sterilized.

In an article entitled "The Obsolescent Mother: A Scenario," Grossman explains approvingly how technology may destroy the awesomeness of woman's childbearing process, a spectacle "with its final event as if something were coming to inexorable term," which "still has about it a sense of prehistory, savage and elemental." This spectacle strikes both the savage and the civilized mind as awesome, he writes. Childbirth, together with the other "striking biological events" in a woman's body, may lead some to conclude that anatomy is destiny. But men are changing that. Their medicine and technology are transforming woman into a male-like being. Her cyclical, periodic nature is obliterated with hormones (such as those found in the Pill) to give her the linear biology of a man.

Still, she continues to give birth. "So long as we reproduce ourselves, we also reproduce the spectacle of a woman withdrawing into herself, becoming huge, and in blood and tumult bringing forth the succeeding generation. This is the stuff myths are made of.... Technology, which has gone part of the way toward destroying it [the myth], may yet destroy the rest" (Grossman, 1971).

To describe what we are now witnessing, "revolution" is too small a word.

If we are to understand the "metarevolution" we are now witnessing in the development of reproductive technologies, we must go back in time to an earlier phase of this revolution. During the thousands of years before paternity was discovered, and for some time thereafter, humankind revered a female deity who possessed the human mother's power to bring forth life. Perhaps even in the Upper Paleolithic period of 25,000 years ago, certainly in the Neolithic and Chalcolithic periods of the Near and Middle East, later in Classical Greece and

Rome and in Neolithic Europe, people worshiped the Great Mother as the source of all life. She was the image of origin, of genesis. She birthed all living beings as well as the sea, the earth, the heavens. People revered Her much as people now revere God the Father.

As far as we know, worship of the Earth Mother was the only religion to have ever become universal (Keeler, 1960). People saw the Goddess in many forms and called upon Her by many names, a few of which were: Anat, Nut, Ashtoreth, Ishtar, Au Set, Isis, Asherah and Hathor. The Goddess was "She of the Ten Thousand Names."

Matrilineal descent, wherein all inheritance of name, property and status was passed from mother to daughter, was a custom in the Goddess-worshiping societies, reflecting the view of the mother as the sole or most important parent.

Then the world changed. Many have hypothesized that it was the discovery of paternity that brought about that change. Once man understood that he was physically linked to the child, his altered reproductive consciousness was reflected in his religious and social institutions. Male gods overthrew the Goddess, breaking the custom of tracing descent through women. Patrilineal descent replaced matrilineal. Children were no longer the woman's, but the man's, for man appropriated them. He began stamping his children with his own name and passing his power and property down through his sons, thus achieving continuity over time, and annulling his separation from reproduction.

As legends, myths, cults and dramas reveal, this greatest of revolutions—the triumph of Father Right over Mother Right—was a violent one. Perhaps as early as 4000 to 3000 B.C., Indo-European tribes from the Caucasus and southern Russia began to invade the more southerly cultures of the Near and Middle East. From the time of their earliest records, the Indo-European tribes revered male deities and practiced patrilineal descent. As they invaded and conquered Goddess-worshiping cultures all the way from India to Greece, they imposed their own religion and social customs of paternal supremacy. Their religious legends reflect this conflict in tales of their gods marrying the Goddess and asserting their supremacy over Her, or even murdering Her, as in the accounts of Danu in the Rg Veda of India and Tiamat in the *Enuma Elish* of Babylon.[10]

The Bible represents a later stage in patriarchal development than the Babylonian text.[11] The traditions of the late Bronze and early Iron Age warriors who violently entered the sites of ancient Goddess worship have come down to us chiefly in the Old and

New Testaments and in the myths of Greece.[12]

The new father gods had no wombs but nonetheless they, like the Mother Goddess they overthrew, gave birth. Patriarchal minds devised the unlikely legends of Zeus delivering Athena from his head and Dionysus from his thigh; and Uranus producing Aphrodite from the sperm he spilled into the ocean when he was castrated by his son Cronus. Yahweh (Jehovah) is said to have made Adam out of dust and then made Eve from Adam's rib. Other male gods gave birth through their mouths, their penises, their sides, and by crude cesarean section (Walker, 1983, p. 106).

After centuries of viewing the woman as creator, then, man began to see himself as such and woman as merely a passive vessel for his seed. An old Japanese proverb exemplified this view: "A woman's womb is a borrowed vessel to beget a child" (Stannard, 1977. p. 295). (This is the view that becomes exaggerated in such new reproductive practices as surrogate motherhood, with men unapologetically referring to women as "rented wombs," "incubators," "receptacles," "vehicles.")

In antiquity, little was known of the actual process of human reproduction. Neither human sperm nor egg had been identified, nor fertilization imagined. So the ancients theorized about procreation. Hippocrates of Cos (c. 460–c. 375 B.C.), the most esteemed of early Greek physicians, believed that the female as well as the male produced seed and contributed to the procreation of the child, though male seed was "stronger." One of his speculations was that the male seed contains within it a miniature human being. This is the doctrine of preformation, which the Roman Seneca later explained in this way: "In the seed are enclosed all the parts of the body of the man that shall be formed. The infant that is borne in his mother's wombe has the rootes of the beard and hair that he shall wear one day." When, two millennia later, the microscope was invented and men examined sperm under it for the first time, some convinced themselves that they could see in the sperm head an homunculus, a tiny man (Eisenberg, 1976, p. 320).[13]

Most early scientists and philosophers, including Aristotle, liked to think of men as generating life in the female. Aristotle (384–322 B.C.), who believed that "we should look upon the female state as being as it were a deformity, though one which occurs in the ordinary course of nature," espoused the view that dominated scientific thought for centuries before the actual sight of sperm fertilizing an egg made his view untenable. Man was the life-giver, he proclaimed. With his semen, he transformed the woman's menstrual blood into a human being. He had noted that in the months before a woman birthed, she stopped menstruating and he concluded that she must be saving up the blood inside her. Like rennet, the active male semen organized the woman's passive menstrual blood, curdling it so that it grew into a body. Aristotle classed woman's menstrual fluid not as a life-giving semen, but as "prime matter." In procreation, he taught, the male, through his semen, infused the soul into the dead matter provided by the defective female. The male semen—much later identified as sperm—took on a sacred character. It was the vital spark of life. Aristotle launched an era of sperm idolatry that is ongoing.

Thomas Aquinas translated Aristotle's theory into Catholic doctrine. He explained: "Among perfect animals the active power of generation belongs to the male sex, and the passive power to the female" (quoted in Raymond, 1979, p. 57).

The *Laws of Manu*, composed in India between 100 and 300 A.D., also imputed an active role to men in procreation and a passive role to women. The rulers in India proclaimed that the Sungod created man by planting His seed in the Earthmother who merely provided fertile soil for its growth.

In the beginning, woman was the sole parent of the child. Now man was. As Apollo expressed it in *The Eumenides:*

> The mother is not the true parent of the child
> Which is called hers. She is a nurse who tends the growth
> Of young seed planted by its true parent, the male.
> So, if Fate spares the child, she keeps it, as one might
> Keep for some friend a growing plant. And of this truth,
> That father without mother may beget, we have
> Present, as proof, the daughter of Olympian Zeus [Athena]
> One never nursed in the dark cradle of the womb.
>
> (Aeschylus, pp. 169–170)

Centuries later, the brutal pornographer the Marquis de Sade, contended, just as Apollo had, that the father is the sole source of human life: "Uniquely formed of our sires' blood, we owe absolutely nothing to our mothers" (quoted in Dworkin, 1981, p. 97).

The strong desire to believe that men, not women, deserve exclusive credit for generation, that "we owe absolutely nothing to our mothers," inhibited any effort to find the female "testes" (ovary) and the female sex cell (egg), and, once found, to recognize their significance.

As long ago as 800 B.C., Hindu medical writings described the oviducts. Yet men chose to believe for centuries that the oviducts originated in the ovaries and entered the bladder so that the seed of the female was excreted and thus played no part in forming the child (Rioux, 1980).

Galen (131–201 A.D.), the great biologist of antiquity, who was the principle authority in the medical schools of medieval and renaissance Europe, discussed the ovaries, which he called the female "testes," and declared that these testes contain seed just as men's do. Though he further wrote that the male was more perfect than the female, that his testicles were stronger than hers and his seed was the formative principle of the offspring, the fact that he credited women with testes at all was offensive to medieval and renaissance physicians and philosophers. The Spanish anatomist Valverde, for example, made that clear in 1572 when he wrote: "I would have preferred to omit this chapter [on female testes], that women might not become all the more arrogant by knowing that they also, like men, have testicles, and that they not only suffer the pain of having to nourish the child within their bodies ... but also that they too put something of their own into it" (O'Faolain and Martines, 1973).

Despite their knowledge of the existence of ova (eggs) in other animals, scientists denied for centuries that ova preexisted in women. (Most seventeenth century physiologists believed that, after coitus, the sperm created an egg in the female by an action of its "effluvium.") The ovum, Stannard points out, is the largest cell in the human body. It is just barely visible to the unaided eye. But because male scientists believed it was created only after coitus by the sperm, and were therefore looking for it at the wrong time, it was not discovered for centuries.

It was the English physician William Harvey (1578–1657) who, after dissecting animals and examining deer embryos in the laboratory in the mid-1600s, rejected Aristotle's notion that menstrual blood played any part in the formation of the fetus. In 1672, dealing another blow to Aristotelian biology, Regnier de Graaf discovered that the ovary produced eggs that traveled down the oviducts to the womb. He found the ovarian follicles, the casings covering the eggs, which he mistook for the eggs themselves. Even after this discovery, many scientists refused to believe that these structures had anything to do with procreation. De Graaf himself thought they merely served a nutritive function. Finally, in 1827, Karl Ernst von Baer, an Estonian embryologist, discovered the mammalian egg. But he believed the egg was inert until the semen activated it and that its role in procreation was—once again—only nutritive.

Not until 1861 did scientists comprehend that the egg was more than a source of nourishment for the embryo, that it was actually the female sex cell. Scientists did not grasp the equal participation of egg and sperm nuclei in fertilization until the later 1870s, between 1875 and 1879.

Helping their sex deal with its separation from reproduction, Aristotle and Manu had glorified the male contribution and minimized the female's. Despite the discovery of the human egg in the nineteenth century, sperm idolatry continues. Science writer David Rorvik's contemporary description of fertilization illustrates: "At this point, the placid egg is ready to meet her mate: the sperm cell which ... is anything but placid." Rorvik writes of the sperm's odessey through the perilous female procreative tract: "Taking their size into account, again, the seven-inch journey through the birth canal and womb to the waiting egg is equivalent to a five-hundred-mile upstream swim for a salmon! Yet they often make this hazardous journey in under an hour, more than earning their title as the 'most powerful and rapid living creatures on earth.'" Rorvik describes the sperm's "heroic efforts" to penetrate the egg and "create a new human life" (Rorvik, 1967, pp. 91–92). (Meanwhile, the placid egg lies there, waiting for her prince to come.)

Eldridge Cleaver, minister of his own church in Oakland, California, shares Rorvik's reverence for sperm. Cleaver's Christlam (Christian and Islamic) church has a service auxiliary called The Guardians of Sperm, which teaches men how to conserve their sacred bodily fluids. "The dwelling place of God is in the male sperm," Cleaver said. "It is the vital life element" (Hinckle, 1980).

Just as the glorification of sperm persisted beyond discovery of the egg, so did the view of woman as a vessel for the life man generated. It was still evident in a book published by a Catholic theologian in 1967. He referred to "the man who generated the life," later writing of the life "imprisoned" in the woman's womb in the form of a seed that grew from her substance. Noting that the human brain is not fully formed at birth, he wrote: "Even biologically, the son of man still needs a protective sheath—that is, a mother—in order to attain his human form" (Guitton, p. 25, p. 29). While this theologian reduced a mother to a "protective sheath," a Catholic newspaper reporting on an antiabortion program gave her more substance. Its headline read: "Womb Is a Bank Vault; Tomorrow Stored There" (*Clarion Herald,* 1973, Oct. 4).

The view of woman as a vessel for the fetus is as evident in patriarchal obstetrics as in patriarchal religion. Obstetricians speak of "in utero transfer" of fetuses in a sentence construct that reduces the woman to a walking uterus (Chez et al., 1978). Increasingly, it is the contents of the container that matter, not the container herself. Accordingly, obstetricians are coming to view themselves as "physician to the fetus" (see Corea, 1985).

"The chief of ob/gyn won't let us answer the phone, 'Labor and Delivery' anymore," obstetric nurse Betty Wood of Vanderbilt Hospital in Nashville, told me in 1979. "We have to say, 'Fetal Intensive Care Unit.' "[14]

Notes:

1. They include: Bruno Bettelheim, Karen Horney, Wolfgang Lederer, Edith Jacobson, Ruth Mack Brunswick, Joseph Campbell, Margaret Mead (1939, pp. 33–34), G. J. Barker-Benfield and Abigail Connell.

2. He does something further. He seeks principles of continuity, what O'Brien terms "some order of procession which transcends individual life spans in some self-regenerating way." Those principles have included hereditary monarchy; primogeniture; a political community that exists before we are born and remains after we die; and the notion of eternity (O'Brien, 1981).

3. Stannard, 1977, p. 299. For more information on the father's historical right to child custody and on the specious claim by the current "fathers' rights" movement that men are unfairly disadvantaged in custody litigation, see *Women's Rights Law Reporter* 7(3), Spring 1982: Nancy D. Polikoff, "Why are mothers losing: A brief analysis of criteria used in child custody determinations," pp. 235–243; and Annamay T. Sheppard, "Unspoken premises in custody litigation," pp. 220–224.

4. The changeover from a matriarchal to a patriarchal family occurred over a period of 3,000 years and took place in different places at different times, as Barbara G. Walker, author of *The Woman's Encyclopedia of Myths and Secrets,* explained in an interview. In Egypt, both matriarchal and patriarchal families co-existed at the same time, she pointed out. Walker's guess is that the changeover occurred in the first millennium B.C. in most of the civilized world. The concept of adultery arrived with the patriarchal family.

5. We may not yet have the best handle on exactly what it is about woman's procreative power that men envy. Philosopher Mary Daly warns against womb envy theories, which "trick women into fixating upon womb, female genitalia, and breasts as our ultimately most valuable endowments." Fixating on women's procreative organs, either to disparage or glorify them, is an expression of fetishism, she adds. She argues that what men really envy is "female creative energy in *all* of its dimensions" (Daly, 1978, p. 60). Elizabeth Fisher also cautions that women are enslaved by being worshiped as mothers or breeders. "When woman is worshiped

for her 'natural powers,' woe betide her humanity" (Fisher, 1979, p. 241, p. 252).

6. During the seventeenth century, alchemists were attempting to harness natural energy for themselves. Alchemist Michael Maier wrote an alchemical treatise that used the story of Atalanta (a free Feminine spirit trapped by a cunning young man) as an allegory of technology triumphing over Mother Nature. Scholars Allen and Hubbs (1980) studied Maier's treatise.

With a series of chilling emblems (pictures suggesting ideas), Maier illustrates the stages through which the alchemical opus must proceed. The first two emblems show the assumption of maternity by the male: the birth of a child from the male and the reduction of the woman's function to that of a nurse. In the fifth emblem, a king holds a toad at a woman's breast. This king, Allen and Hubbs comment, draws into the toad, as intermediary, the maternal milk—the natural power of creation and healing—and takes that power for the male. The motto under the emblem reads:

> Place a toad at the breasts of a woman that she may nurse it
> And the woman dies, and the toad grows big from the milk.

In the later emblems, the cycle of masculine empowerment and feminine disempowerment in procreation accelerates. One emblem shows Zeus birthing Athena from his head. The final emblem, emphasizing the dispensability of the female, depicts a woman and dragon-snake (umbilicus) intertwined in a grave. Maier's commentary reads:

> Have a deep grave dug for the poisonous Dragon
> With which the woman should be tightly intertwined:
> While it rejoices in the marriage-bed, she dies.
> Have the Dragon buried with her
> Thereupon its body is abandoned to death and is imbued with blood.
> Now this is the true way of your work.

7. Raymond explains the role of the female-to-male constructed transsexual in *The Transsexual Empire* (1979).

8. The famous French biologist Jean Rostand once suggested that we can "simply do away with" the heredity from the mother's side "by extracting from the egg or destroying in it the maternal chromosome [hereditary material]: it then develops with the father's chromosomes alone." In this way, creatures with a more or less "purely paternal heredity" would be born (Rostand, 1959, p. 12).

9. Raymond also sees transsexualism as the acting out of the myth of single parenthood by the father. Here, the therapeutic fathers—psychiatrists, plastic surgeons, urologists, gynecologists, endocrinologists—make women out of men in a complicated ritual of rebirth. Mothers are blamed for the existence of transsexuals; they failed to give enough of the right hormone in utero or reared the child incorrectly. The therapeutic fathers are redeeming the biological mother's defective handiwork. The transsexual himself is a "she-male" and a "he-mother," who rejects his mothered birth and gives birth to "herself" (with the aid, of course, of the medical "father-mothers") (Raymond, 1979, p. xvi, pp. 74–75).

10. In the Babylonian text, the new god Marduk slays the ancient Mother, Tiamat: "Then Taimat advanced; Marduk as well: they approached each other for

the battle. The Lord spread his net to enmesh her and when she opened her mouth to its full, let fly into it an evil wind that poured into her belly, so that her courage was taken from her and her jaws remained open wide. He shot an arrow that tore into her, cut through her inward parts and pierced her heart. She was undone. He stood upon her carcass ... mounting upon her hinder quarters, with his merciless mace he smashed her skull. He cut the arteries of her blood and caused the north wind to bear it off to parts unknown."

Marduk then split her body, using the lower half to fashion the earth; the upper half, the heavenly roof. Marduk treated Tiamat "as raw material, making humans himself, not by generation but by killing, out of the blood of a slain enemy" (Fisher, 1979, p. 303).

The murder of the Mother continues in our time on a technologically sophisticated level. Now men bomb the ovaries of the mothers with hormones. They suck out the eggs of females. They use the eggs as raw material for the life they manufacture. They culture eggs from "slaughterhouse ovaries." They dream of penetrating eggs with dead sperm. Sometimes they kill the bovine "donors" of eggs.

11. In the Bible, the female principle is reduced to its elemental state while the male deity creates out of Himself just as the Mother alone had created in the past, Joseph Campbell points out (1964, p. 86). The Tiamat epic stands between the Mother's sole creation and the Father's sole creation along a line Campbell schematizes as follows:

1. The world born of a Goddess without a consort
2. The world born of a Goddess fecundated by a consort
3. The world fashioned from the body of a Goddess by a male warrior god
4. The world created by the unaided power of a male god alone

12. The Greek playwright Aeschylus deals with the triumph of Father Right over Mother Right in the Oresteian trilogy (Vallacott, trans., 1980). In the plays, Clytemnestra murders her husband King Agamemnon after he had outraged her motherhood by sacrificing their daughter in order to coax a fair wind from the gods and sail off to war. The son of Clytemnestra and Agamemnon, Orestes, kills his mother to avenge his father's murder. The Furies, or Eumenides, birth-goddesses and guardians of the Mother Right, punish Orestes for his matricide. But at one point he escapes them through the aid of one of the new male gods, a son of Zeus who, by his act, made "mockery of motherhood." It was not their fault that Orestes escaped punishment, the Furies assert. Indicating the violent nature of the triumph of Father Right over Mother Right, they add that the fault

lies
With younger gods who rise
In place of those that ruled before;
From stool to crown their throne
Is stained with gore.

13. The Pilaga of South America believe a man's sperm delivers a tiny, complete human being into the woman's womb. The woman merely grows it until it is ready to come out (Bettelheim, 1968, p. 131).

14. Corea, 1980. Because of the patriarchal view of a woman's body as a passive vessel, as matter upon which the male acts, many men have now, as they

did centuries ago, a distorted view of the human reproductive process. They can not imagine the female body *doing* anything. But it does. For example, the woman's cervical mucus plays an active role in fertilization. Dr. Susan Bell, who has led courses on fertility consciousness for women, writes: "The 'role' of mucus in human reproduction is to nourish and guide sperm (which would otherwise die within about one half hour or swim in circles, probably never reaching an egg.) Unlike what most of us have heard or read, sperm do not speed directly toward eggs, which await them passively" (Bell, 1981).

The secretions in the female reproductive tract also capacitate sperm. That is, they initiate physiologic changes in the sperm so the sperm is capable of penetrating the egg. Two researchers refer to capacitation as "the functional dependence of sperm upon the female reproductive tract prior to fertilization" (Soupart and Morgenstern, 1973).

As the sperm is guided to the site of fertilization, woman's reproductive tract appears to cull or select sperm. Embryologist Dr. Richard Blandau points out that, without question, "the female reproductive tract plays an active role in sperm selection, transport, and the number capacitated, an environmental phenomenon that cannot yet be duplicated in vitro," i.e., in the laboratory (Blandau, 1980). Also, the fluid in the woman's oviduct may play an important role in the separation of fertilized eggs that are developing into embryos.

Because gynecologists see the woman's body as a passive vessel, when they want to find out when or if a woman ovulates, it does not occur to them to ask the woman. But many women know. They can feel it when the egg bursts from the follicle (mittleschmerz). For centuries women like those of the Cherokee nations detected ovulation by observing changes in their cervical mucus. Women can learn that now. Susan, one of the first lesbians to bear a child conceived through artificial insemination, did. She recalls: "I studied prediction of ovulation methodically before I started [the inseminations]. I have charts I treasure which have details on my cervical mucus and the feel of my cervix and what kinds of dreams I was having, what my basal body temperature was, what my sex life was like and anything else I could think of. I had it all written there and I used to study it. So I really got tuned in. I got real good at pinpointing ovulation."

When physicians in IVF programs want to pinpoint ovulation, they do not explore the possibility that the woman who is ovulating can give them any information. Instead, they measure hormones in her urine and scan her ovaries with ultrasound machines such as the Kretz Combison 100 sector scanner to make a "diagnosis" of ovulation.

16

Reproductive Control: *The War Against the Womb*

In a study of primitive mythology, Joseph Campbell, writing of the universality of the Great Mother image in prehistory, observes that "there can be no doubt that in the very earliest ages of human history the magical force and wonder of the female was no less a marvel than the universe itself; and this gave to woman a prodigious power, which it has been one of the chief concerns of the masculine part of the population to break, control and employ to its own ends" (quoted in Rich, 1977, p. 103).

Today, it is largely the obstetrician/gynecologist who breaks, controls and employs to his own ends the magical force of the female. In controlling the female generative organs and processes, doctors are fulfilling a male need to control woman's procreative power, a need they seem to feel no less strongly than did seventeenth century alchemists or tribesmen who practiced couvade, transvestism, subincision and other initiation rites.

Margaret Mead once said that obstetrics in America reveals male jealousy of woman's ability to make a new life. She wrote: "We find the myth of the island of women all over the world; the myth that expresses men's fear that women could give birth without them. In the myth, a man finally lands and teaches the woman how to give birth properly. In the obstetrician, this male desire to take control of childbearing is expressed" (personal communication, 1976, Feb. 18).

Dr. Joan Mulligan, a nurse-midwife and associate professor of nursing and women's studies at the University of Wisconsin in Madison, and Dr. Nancy Stoller Shaw, a sociologist, made related comments after observing practices on obstetrical wards in the 1970s:

"Physician impatience with requests to wait or delay painful examinations was often expressed in crude, brutal remarks relating to the sexual activities that had resulted in the pregnancy," Mulligan wrote. "There truly seems to be something in the behavior of a pregnant woman about to birth a child which elicits brutalizing and dehumanizing physician response; it is not too extreme to suggest that uterine envy is as viable a concept as penis envy" (Mulligan, 1976, p. 232). Dr. Shaw, author of *Forced Labor*, wrote: "Most doctors appear not to want to watch and help women, but to demonstrate their power over them and the birth process. They are eager to prove that their technical power is greater than that of nature" (Shaw, 1974, p. 134).

I have also seen this male desire to control childbirth expressed in the obstetrical journals that I have been reading for more than a decade. I think of an article Dr. John Beazley wrote in the *American Journal of Obstetrics and Gynecology* in 1975 advocating "active management of labor." This means the doctor's artificial initiation, control and termination of labor with drugs, machines and surgery. In discussing "man's continued struggle for control of parturition" (the birth process), he refers to the technological developments that have led to "a greater mastery over uterine action." Planned delivery, controlled by the physician, is already approaching a practical reality, he wrote, adding: "In conclusion, the active management of labor necessitates that obstetricians take over, not just a single aspect of responsibility but the whole process of parturition. Our control of the situation must be complete" (Beazley, 1975).

Obstetrics and, later, gynecology, were specialties developed in the United States in the nineteenth century. Historian G. J. Barker-Benfield has written a book that, in part, explores the origins of these specialties. In it, he argues that what allowed men to drive women out of midwifery and formulate and practice the ob/gyn specialties at a time when extreme female modesty might have been expected to bar such a radical departure from custom was, among other factors, "their desire to conquer and control the innermost power of nature" (Barker-Benfield, 1976).

The male attack on midwives began in the second decade of the nineteenth century, but its most decisive phase came between 1900 and 1930. Midwives attended about half of all births in the United States in 1900, but only about one sixth by 1935 (Devitt, 1979). In their campaign to eliminate their competitors, physicians presented midwives as dim-witted, pestilence-carrying old hags and— in an appeal to the anti-immigrant fervor of the early twentieth century—as "unAmerican," a "foreign" element washed ashore with each wave of dirty immigrants. Asserting that the employment of midwives threatened the lives of mothers and babies, they successfully pressured states to outlaw their rivals.

It was not because it had been scientifically demonstrated that physician attendance at birth assured a better, safer outcome for mother and baby that doctors replaced midwives in America.

"They just claim that was the case, but it was not," Barker-Benfield, assistant professor of history at the State University of New York at Albany, told me. "In fact, I'm trying now to explain the proliferation of gynecological disorders very often following birth at the hands of men. Contrary to being safer, obstetricians may well have been more damaging than midwives."

The most striking example of damage done by them, he pointed out, was the epidemics of childbed fever physicians caused delivering babies with unwashed hands after attending diseased patients. The fever killed thousands of women and maimed thousands more. Furthermore, the aggressive, interventionist obstetrics of the men, with frequent use of forceps to speed up a labor process they often found tedious, lacerated cervices and tore holes in the birth canal. Powerful astringents like carbolic acid, which, at some concentrations, can burn tissues, were poured into the birth canal immediately following birth to kill a newly discovered entity: the germ (Corea, 1979).

The new specialty of "gynecology," Barker-Benfield believes, was created in the nineteenth century largely to repair the damage done to women's bodies by obstetricians. "Iatrogenesis [doctor-caused illness] was, in my view, probably a major factor in the establishment of gynecology," Barker-Benfield said. "In other words, the necessity of repairing the damage done by obstetricians provided a lot of work for gynecologists. My general impression is that doctors were very well aware that they were doing a great deal of damage even as they claimed, at the same time, that they were the only experts who should be looked to in childbirth."[1]

In the twentieth century, physicians pushed for "obstetrical reforms," which largely eliminated midwives and moved birth from home to hospital. While in 1900, fewer than 5 percent of American women delivered in hospitals, by 1940, about half did and by 1960, almost all.[2]

"The outcome of obstetrical reform," Barker-Benfield wrote, "placed women's reproductive power completely in the hands of men" (1976, p. 67).

In the hospitals, physicians turned childbirth into a technological feat performed by men on a passive, often unconscious, woman. They began performing routine episiotomies (deep cuts into the vaginal wall to widen the perineal area), "prophylactic" (that is, preventive) forceps deliveries, and inductions of labor for their convenience in 1920. Since then, physicians have added innumerable interventions in childbirth, among them: sedatives to slow labor; drugs to speed it; ultrasound; electronic fetal monitors; and liberal use of cesarean section. Interventions in normal childbirth began accelerating in the early 1980s and are now so extreme that any woman who, avoiding a cesarean, manages to actually go into labor and push a baby out of her body, can count it a victory. The damages and risks these interventions have frequently inflicted on women and their babies have been exhaustively documented.[3]

The active role taken by the doctor and the passive role imposed on the woman made it appear that it was *men*, not women, who delivered babies; that women could not deliver babies without men; that it was terribly irresponsible, even a form of child abuse, to attempt to do so. The propaganda on these points has been so thorough in recent decades that most women believe it and would be afraid to have a baby outside the male-controlled hospital.[4]

Once men moved childbirth from home to hospital, they were able to deal with another aspect of woman's procreative power: her ability to nourish a baby from her own body.

In the 1930s, physicians began replacing the woman's breast milk (which an early Gerber advertisement for baby formula called "a variable excretion") with formula, a product increasingly available from drug and milk companies. The sedating and anesthetizing of women during labor and delivery undermined a woman's efforts to nurse because the practice could impair suckling in the sedated newborn. Without the women's knowledge, physicians also sometimes gave them such hazardous medications as diethylstilbestrol (DES) and Depo-Provera to dry up their milk (Brack, 1975).

By regimenting when and under what circumstances mothers were allowed to see their babies in the hospital, physicians also made it difficult for women to breast-feed. To discourage nursing on demand, they separated mother and child. They established rules requiring feedings at intervals of no less than four hours. But many infants cry to be fed more often than that, especially in the first days of life, and the woman's breasts need the frequent suckling of the infant to stimulate milk production. In the nurseries, babies were often fed supplemental bottles without the mother's knowledge. Consequently, the babies were not hungry when brought to the mother. Without sufficient suckling, the mother's milk dried up.[5]

Once birth was moved onto male turf, physicians undermined a woman's confidence in the ability of her body to bear and nurture a child. Woman was becoming embarrassed by what earlier peoples had seen as a source of power: menstruation, pregnancy, breast-feeding.

The decline in breast-feeding began in the 1930s. By 1946, the proportion of women breast-feeding, with or without supplemental bottles, had dropped to 65 percent. By 1956, it was down to 37 percent; by 1966, 27 percent (Meyer, 1968); by 1971, 14 percent (Martinez and Nalezienski, 1979).[6] The low came around 1970, but breast-feeding has been on the increase ever since then, particularly among middle-class, educated mothers. (Evidence rolled in in the 1970s concerning the immunological factors in breast milk that protect the child.) Nationwide in 1975, 38 percent of mothers leaving hospitals after childbirth were breast-feeding (American Academy of Pediatrics, 1978).

It was not only obstetrics that expressed a male desire to control birth, but gynecological surgery as well. When gynecologists could repair woman's reproductive organs, they could not only restore her reproductive powers; "they could appear to create them" (Barker-Benfield, 1976, p. 109). The gynecologist's power came before that of the hero and the statesman because, according to an analysis by J. Marion Sims, "the father of modern gynecology," the gynecologist perpetuated society's future. In repairing woman's procreative organs and in regulating childbearing, he controlled the foundation of legal male identities through the perpetuation of names and descent of property.

Gynecologists could repair women's reproductive organs but they could also destroy those organs in women whom they wanted to control or whom they judged unfit to reproduce.

It was only in the nineteenth century, with the development of anesthesia and antiseptic techniques, that surgery became a practical method of treating ailments and gynecology could develop. Gynecologists began by repairing tissue torn in childbirth and by removing ovarian cysts, diseased ovaries, fibroid uteri and eggs trapped in oviducts. But the "indications" for pelvic operations soon increased until these men were removing both ovaries and/or the oviducts for cure of masturbation, certain "neurosis" and ovariomania, a chronic ailment of the woman's reproductive organs combined with "mental disorders."

The American Medical Association formed a section on the new specialty of obstetrics and the diseases of women and children in 1873, the same year Dr. Robert Battey of Rome, Georgia, published information on a new operation he had devised: female castration. This involved removing a woman's healthy ovaries for such indications as troublesomeness, menstrual cramps, attempted suicide, cussedness and erotic tendencies (Barker-Benfield, 1976).[7]

Surgical attacks on women's procreative organs continue today. Gynecologists are advocating and performing prophylactic hysterectomies, oophorectomies and mastectomies, arguing that by removing healthy wombs, ovaries and breasts—the seats of woman's procreative power—they are preventing the development of cancer in these organs.

In 1977, hysterectomy became the nation's most commonly performed operation and remains so as I write. In 1969, Dr. R. C. Wright, publishing in *Obstetrics and Gynecology,* advocated removal of the uterus routinely after the last planned pregnancy on the grounds that the uterus is potentially cancer-bearing. Wright claimed: "The uterus has but one function: reproduction. After the last planned pregnancy, the uterus becomes a useless, bleeding, symptom-producing, potentially cancer-bearing organ and therefore should be removed" (Wright, 1969). Such a practice cannot be logically defended as a health measure, suggesting it is exactly what one commentator has described as a "war against the womb."[8]

When doctors perform a hysterectomy, they often remove normal ovaries along with the womb to prevent cancer despite the fact that ovarian cancer is rare. It represents only 1 percent of all cancers. According to American Cancer Society figures, 17,000 women developed new cases of ovarian cancer in 1977. That same year, 60,000 men developed prostate cancer, but we hear no calls for routine "prophylactic" prostatectomies for men (Morgan, 1980, pp. 34 and 56).

In the September 1, 1977, issue of the prestigious *New England Journal of Medicine,* Dr. Robert M. Goldwyn advocated an aggressive approach to preventing breast cancer: removal of the breasts. This method, subcutaneous mastectomy with later breast reconstruction, is increasing in popularity in the United States, Goldwyn wrote. It is used by some physicians as a prophylactic measure for women considered at "high risk" of developing breast cancer. Dr. Goldwyn acknowledged that the criteria for selecting women whose breasts would be cut off are imperfect and controversial. Nonetheless, using this imperfect criteria, some doctors are indeed selecting women. Women with a family history of breast cancer or any disturbance of the breasts (and that includes large breasts) could be advised to have her breasts cut off or reduced in size. (For a more detailed critique of this practice, see Corea, 1985.)

What a U.S. Department of Health, Education and Welfare report revealed should not surprise us: Surgery on women's reproductive organs soared in the 1970s. Women had twice as many surgical procedures as men in the 15 to 44 age group. Cesarean sections were up 156 percent over the previous decade. Ovary removals were up 48 percent among older women and 23 percent among younger. Hysterectomies rose 22 percent among younger women. Dilations and curettages (D&Cs) rose 23 percent. Tubal ligations tripled (OGN, 1980, March 1).

Observations that psychiatrist Bruno Bettelheim made on emotionally disturbed boys are relevant here. The boys, he noted, exhibited a desire to be able to bear children and a feeling of having been cheated because they could not. He writes of two particular boys, aged seven and eight, who repeatedly and independently of each other stated that they felt it was a "cheat" that they did not have vaginas. Disappointed in their desire to have a vagina, and envious of women, "both boys frequently expressed a wish to tear or cut out the vaginas of girls and women." Other disturbed boys, while they did not say they wanted female sex organs, had many fantasies about cutting off and tearing out breasts and vaginas. "Certain extremely disturbed boys have for months spoken of (more accurately, screamed about) little other than this consuming desire" (Bettelheim, 1968, p. 30). Knowing how extensively male gynecologists are indeed destroying women's healthy procreative organs, I found Bettelheim's observations chilling.

In this section, I have argued that men surgically remove women's procreative organs in part to deal with their envy of female procreative power. Men developed initiation rites for boys, established customs of couvade and replaced midwifery with obstetrics out of the same motivation.

In prehistory, as we have seen, woman was revered as the life-bearer. But in recorded history, men claimed the major credit, relegating woman to the role of vessel or field for their seed. In all recorded history, there have only been a brief one hundred years when, with the discovery of the human egg, men were unable to deny woman's contribution to the child. Men grasped that the egg was the female sex cell only in 1861 and that the egg and sperm participated equally in fertilization only in the late 1870s. As soon as man understood that he was *not,* in fact, the sole real parent of the child, he began recreating the myth of single parenthood by the male, not, this time, through religious or scientific theory, but through technology.

In the nineteenth century, as some men created obstetrics and gynecology, others began developing what we have come to think of as the "new" reproductive technologies. But the "new" and "old" technologies, all of which center on controlling woman's procreative power, developed concurrently. The first attempt at in vitro fertilization occurred in 1878, just as physicians were nearing the end of their successful crusade to outlaw abortion in the United States[9] and only five years after the AMA formed a section on obstetrics and the diseases of women and children. When the first artificial insemination of a woman with donor sperm took place in 1884, castration of women for such disorders as "nymphomania" and "ovarian insanity" was at its peak in America.[10] The year embryos were first transferred among animals, 1890, the American Gynecological Society held its first discussion of birth control (Speert, 1980, p. 62). In 1912, while physicians were in the midst of their campaign against midwives, mammalian embryos were first cultured—that is, grown in a special medium in the laboratory.[11]

Men employ the "old" reproductive technologies in their obstetrics and gynecology specialty and, in this way, hold a monopoly on childbirth, contraceptive, abortion and sterilization services. So they are able to exercise a primitive control over reproduction. But soon the "new" reproductive technologies will enable them to actually take over the life-giving powers of women. "Thank you for my baby," Lesley Brown said to her obstetrician Patrick Steptoe who, with Robert Edwards, was "lab-parent" to the world's first test-tube baby.[12]

In papers reporting research on these technologies, men frequently state that they are taking control over woman's ovulation and imply that by doing so they are creating a more efficient method of reproduction. For example, a member of one test-tube baby team stated that "biological knowledge is rapidly advancing as a result of research related to in vitro fertilization and embryo transfer, and it is probable that the entire community will benefit in terms of *more efficient reproduction* [my emphasis] and family planning" (Walters, 1976). IVF pioneer Professor Carl Wood observed: "it is quite possible that the artificial system [IVF and embryo transfer] will improve natural reproduction" (Metherell, 1982).

Within the reproductive brothel I described in Chapter 14, women would be completely controlled, dominated and reduced to Matter. This would represent the culmination of a centuries-long process. When patriarchal tribes overthrew the Goddess, who included within Herself women, animals and nature, as well as men, they claimed that men were separate from and above nature, that their Father God had given men dominion over women and animals. They no longer perceived animals as being with souls or treated them as sacred. Women, as we have seen, also lost their sacred character and became vessels for the life men created.

Men have been conquering nature, women and animals ever since.

In our time, scientists write "of leading man as one biological species against the hosts of nature," of reconstructing nature for man "on an ever grander scale" (Muller, 1935), of conquering, controlling, invading, penetrating nature and stealing its secrets from it. (After describing reproductive technologies, biologist Jean Rostand wrote: "The upshot of all this is that, from now on, we possess the means of acting upon life ... due to our having penetrated into the secrets of nature. To our having laid hands on some of its mainspring. To our beginning to know at what point to strike—which are the sensitive spots. To our having stolen from life some of its recipes" [Rostand, 1959].)

Scientists write of mastering the outer world, the earth's surface, of flooding deserts, subjugating jungles, diverting ocean currents, of "plumbing the earth's interior," of mastering the upper world "through penetration of the upper air," and by projecting themselves into space. "We will control, not just biological functions on earth," one pioneer in the new reproductive technologies told me in an interview, "but we will expand in space and time to control the universe. Putting a man on the moon is nothing. We are going to colonize the universe." Other reproductive engineers, as we saw earlier, envision sending frozen human embryos or cells for clones into space to colonize planets.

The inner world, too—the cells, chromosomes, genes—must yield to man's conquest. "The fact that we ourselves involve within us a veritable cosmos is ... a cause for concern," wrote the Nobel laureate geneticist H. J. Muller, "It means that in addition to the outer world we have an inner world to understand and to administer." This inner, as well as outer, nature must be "subject to our intelligent control." How control it? First, by exploring it. "Modern genetics is already beginning to invade the ultra-microscopic land inside the eggs and sperm cells ... and to bring back from this survey what we actually call 'maps'" (Muller, 1935, p. 68, p. 22).

Muller, referring to the genetic improvement of man through the use of advanced reproductive technologies, states that these technologies will undoubtedly be used: "It is unthinkable that man will ever voluntarily relinquish his potential dominion, now that he has gone thus far. . . . Not only is our genetic improvement patently possible, but it is far surer and more feasible than any ultimate conquest of the atom, of interplanetary space, or of external nature in general. . . . And even if our conquests of external nature fail, still we shall have conquered ourselves" (Muller, 1935, p. 123).

To conquer "ourselves," men must first apply animal breeding techniques to human beings, primarily women. They must control women's biological processes more efficiently. So, in Chapter 7, we heard them speak of "man-made ovulation," of "ovulation to order," of men assuming the role of the woman's hypothalamus.

Rostand, who favored the use of the new reproductive technologies and other means to create supermen (i.e., human beings superior to those women create), wrote of human evolution controlled and directed by men: "The better to separate ourselves from the animal, shall we consent to use upon ourselves techniques that have hitherto been confined to animals?" (Rostand, 1959, p. 99).

When reproductive engineers manipulate the bodies of female animals today, they are clear, blunt and unapologetic about why they are doing it. They want to turn the females into machines for producing "superior" animals or into incubators for the embryos of more "valuable" females. They want, as one entrepreneur told me, to "manufacture embryos at a reduced cost." They aim to create beef cows yielding "quality carcasses of high cutability," and dairy cows producing more milk on the same amount of feed. H. H. Stonaker, in the 1962 textbook *Introduction to Livestock Production,* explained to students:

> Powerful means for developing more efficient farm animals lie in the hands of the breeder. Just as the designer and engineer may blueprint and develop more efficient tools and machines, the breeder may outline programs for developing improved animal tools—better equipped to produce food and fiber of higher quality and at less cost. Genetic "engineering" is a field of development barely tapped in the improvement of most farm animals.

When reproductive engineers manipulate the bodies of human

females—those beings, who, like animals, are a part of nature men must control—their language changes. Today they say they are manipulating women's bodies out of compassion; to bring new hope to the infertile; to prevent birth defects; to increase women's options, expand their freedom. Obscuring the impact of reproductive engineering on women as a class, they emphasize the "rights" of individual women to use these technologies.

The decision to change the language used when discussing the application of animal breeding techniques to women may in some cases be quite conscious. Reviewing the medical and legal literature on AID, Dr. Bernard Rubin noted that such phrases as "therapeutic donor insemination" and "semi-adoption" had been coined "to get away from the comparisons with animal husbandry" (Rubin, 1965).

Although *today,* the language men employ in speaking of the use of reproductive technology on women differs from that employed in speaking of its use on animals, it may not always be so. Women may find that the connection men have made for centuries between women and animals still lives on in patriarchal minds just as it lives on in men's laws and practices. Women and animals remain parts of nature to be controlled and subjugated (see Griffin, 1978).

Already today, one justification for using reproductive technologies in women is the same as that for using it in animals: to produce "superior" offspring. Creating a "superman" has been the dream of philosophers from Nietzsche's Zarathustra to Renan's *Dialogues philosophiques,* points out the French biologist Jean Rostand. In Zarathustra, Nietzsche writes: "Man is something that has to be surmounted. . . . What is a monkey to a man? An object of ridicule or of painful shame. And that is what man must be to superman: an object of ridicule and of painful shame." In his 1871 book, *Dialogues,* Renan wrote that a far-reaching application of germinal selection might lead to the creation of "a superior race," whose right to govern would reside in its science and "in the very superiority of its blood, its brain, its nervous system." According to Renan's conception, Rostand comments, "Superman would have domination over man as we today have over the animals" (Rostand, 1959, p. 95).

Scientific means are, and increasingly will be, available to make the dream of the (male) philosophers come true, Rostand wrote in 1959. He outlines the biological methods by which man could be modified. These include many of the technologies discussed in this book. His outline, he concludes, "shows plainly that the idea of a creature superior to man emerges quite naturally from the facts." Such creatures would be what he calls "denatured men," men removed from, and holding themselves above, nature. The traditional notions of parenthood, maternity and sex are, he observes, "in the process of being denatured." These "denatured men," let us note, are brought forth by wombless men, not by women, and are superior to the pitiful specimens mere "natured" woman can produce. She births "natural man, seedling man," as Rostand calls him, and it may be that the best men of this sort, compared to the potential supermen, are "no more than the wild pears of the woodlands, with their small, sour, uneatable fruit, to the huge William pears that melt in one's mouth" (Rostand, 1959, p. 57). Men, then, can manufacture a life better than that which women can birth.

Now men are far beyond the stage at which they expressed their envy of woman's procreative power through couvade, transvestism, subincision. They are beyond merely giving spiritual birth in their baptismal-font wombs, beyond giving physical birth with their electronic fetal monitors, their forceps, their knives.

Now they have laboratories.

Notes

1. In the early twentieth century, doctors were equally aware of the harm they were doing. Dr. J. Whitridge Williams, professor of obstetrics at the prestigious Johns Hopkins, investigated the teaching of obstetrics in American medical schools in 1912. His study had an enormous impact on obstetrical teaching in this country. Dr. Williams concluded in his report that doctors—inadequately trained in obstetrics in all but one American medical school—were inferior to midwives. The average medical student, he found, delivered only one baby during his training.

His study showed, Dr. Williams wrote, that most medical schools "are each year turning loose on the community, hundreds of young men whom they have failed to prepare properly for the practice of obstetrics, and whose lack of training is responsible for unnecessary deaths of many women and infants, not to speak of a much larger number, more or less permanently injured by improper treatment." Many of his respondents directed attention "to the unnecessary death of large numbers of children, as the result of unnecessary or improper operating." He concludes that "most of the ills of women result from poor obstetrics" (Williams, 1912).

It was widely recognized by doctors that the obstetrical training of American medical students was "a farce and a disgrace to a great nation," as Dr. Charles Ziegler, professor of obstetrics at the University of Pittsburgh, put it. Nonetheless, Dr. Ziegler wrote in a 1913 issue of the *Journal of the American Medical Association:* "The argument that large numbers of physicians do as poor obstetrics as the midwives is entirely beside the question. We are quite ready to admit this, but to claim that for this reason we must retain the midwife, if we retain the physician, is absurd. . . . We can get along very nicely without the midwife, whereas all are agreed that the physician is indispensable. It thus seems that the sensible thing to do is to train the physician until he is capable of doing good obstetrics, and then make it financially possible for him to do it, by eliminating the midwife" (Ziegler, 1913).

Dr. Williams, recognizing the superiority of the midwife's skills, recommended in his report that she be abolished. Dr. Ziegler joined him in this. Both wanted to use the women then attended by midwives to teach medical students obstetrics so the students could deliver more than one baby before beginning their practices.

So the midwife was eliminated. Doctors lobbied legislatures and legislatures outlawed midwives, who were never organized enough to resist the campaign against them. Maternity hospitals were set up where poor women could get "free," "charity" care. These women—consistently referred to by both Williams and Ziegler as "clinical material," "obstetric material," or, simply "the material"—were used to teach young men obstetrics. This is how the move from home to hospital birth began.

2. Devitt, 1979. Increased physician attendance at birth did not result in improved outcome for mothers and babies. As the percentage of births attended by midwives decreased from 50 to 15 percent, perinatal infant mortality increased. During this first decade of the twentieth century, midwives in New York were significantly superior to doctors in preventing stillbirths and childbed fever. For example, Newark's maternal mortality rate of 1.7 per 1000 from 1914 to 1916 among mothers delivered by midwives compared most favorably to the 6.5 per 1000 rate in Boston, where midwives were banned (Kobrin, 1966).

3. A small sampling: Suzanne Arms, *Immaculate Deception* (Boston: Houghton Mifflin, 1975); Harrison, 1982; Brewer and Brewer, 1977; Corea, 1985; Nancy Cohen and Lois Estner, *Silent Knife* (South Hadley, Mass.: J. F. Bergin Publishers, Inc., 1983); Lee and David Stewart, *21st Century Obstetrics Now!* (Chapel Hill, N.C.: NAPSAC Publication, vols. I, II, and III, 1978); *Obstetrical Practices in the United States, 1978,* hearing before the Subcommittee on Health and Scientific Research of the Committee on Human Resources, U.S. Senate, U.S. Government Printing Office. Washington, D.C., April 17, 1978.

4. There are exceptions. Since the 1970s, there has been a revival of midwifery and home birth, a revival the ob/gyn profession is fighting with every tool at its disposal (see Corea, 1979).

5. Physicians also prescribed antiseptic "care" of the woman's breasts—washing breasts with hexachlorophene or soap and water three or four times a day—a treatment that could lead to dried, cracked and bleeding nipples. Nursing became painful.

The emotional tension, exhaustion, frustration and fear of failure young mothers could experience on obstetrics wards could inhibit the let-down reflex. This reflex is a physical sensation that occurs when the sphincter muscles are relaxed to let the milk flow. It is like an orgasm in that it is triggered when the woman is both relaxed and stimulated. Women in one survey on breast-feeding reported joking put-downs from doctors not calculated to encourage the self-confidence that would have helped put the woman at the ease necessary for nursing: "What are you trying to prove?" "My God, Alberta, at thirty?" And, tellingly: "Well, aren't we the little earth mother?" (Brack, 1975).

In 1932, the American Medical Association Committee on Foods published advertising guidelines for infant foods that insisted that physicians should supervise the feeding of *all* infants, even when women were breast-feeding. It stated that "every infant, breast-fed and doubly so the artificially fed, should be under the supervision of the physician who is experienced and skilled in the care and feeding of infants" (Apple, 1980).

6. Estimates of the percentage of women breast-feeding differ for the same years in various surveys. Some surveys count only those women who are breast-feeding without supplemental bottles, while others include the women who also use some bottle feedings. Some give the percentage of women breast-feeding in the hospital. Others give figures for some months after the women have left hospital, when the rate may have changed.

Other figures: By some estimates, only 18 percent of American babies were breast-fed in the 1960s (Brack, 1978). A 1975 study in an urban Chicago hospital with a low-income black population found that only 4 percent of pregnant women planned unsupplemented breast-feeding (Aquino, 1979).

According to Gwen Gotsch, research librarian of the La Leche League, it is difficult to cite an overall breast-feeding rate for the country because there are such enormous variations in different areas. In some hospitals, 85 to 90 percent of women will breast-feed while in others, like Cook County Hospital in Chicago, almost none will. In each area, the rate depends on the attitudes of physicians to breast-feeding, how active the La Leche League is, and how many childbirth organizations are active.

7. An operation performed less frequently than ovariectomy was clitoridectomy—removal of the clitoris with scissors or a knife. Dr. Isaac Baker Brown, senior surgeon to the London Surgical Home, devised the operation. From his case histories, which he published, it is clear that when presented with almost any symptom in a woman (including clammy skin, sterility, indigestion, a tendency toward miscarriage, and headache), he cured the patient by destroying her sex organ.

Let me tell you about a few of Dr. Brown's patients. In 1863, he visited a 20-year-old patient who had an irritable temper, experienced sleepless nights, and had been "disobedient to her mother's wishes." She suffered from a "restless desire for society," the doctor reported and, in her quieter moments, "spent much time in serious reading." Clearly an alarming case. After an examination, Dr. Brown determined that the woman's symptoms had been caused by masturbation. He removed her clitoris with a pair of scissors and then reported that "all her delusions disappeared."

Dr. Brown records many other miraculous cures in his book: A woman could not walk. He cut out her clitoris and she walked. A woman could not see. He cut out her clitoris and she saw. A 25-year-old woman was "melancholy." He cut out her clitoris and she cheered up. His operation even improved the moral sense of a 19-year-old. He recorded on her chart: "Has a daily clearer notion of right and wrong."

Rebellious or unhappy women seemed particularly vulnerable to the surgeon's scissors. For example, Brown records the case of a 57-year-old woman who had "fits" during which she scratched and tore at her husband. "In the paroxysm," Brown wrote, "the desire was always to destroy the husband." Brown cut out her clitoris. She "sleeps well, and for many hours, but will not admit to being better," he reported. She remained "sulky," and complained that the doctor had unsexed her. But her husband considered her greatly improved. Weeks later, he stopped by to thank Dr. Brown for restoring his wife to health. "For whereas his nights were passed in constant fear, rendering his life most wretched," the doctor wrote, "his home was now one of comfort and happiness both night and day" (Brown, 1866).

8. Dr. Phillip Cole of Harvard School of Public Health has demonstrated that if prophylactic hysterectomies were performed on one million women, the average gain in life expectancy would be about two months, "or about the time it takes to go through the operation and convalescence" (Brown and Druckman, 1976). The fact that most militates against the "prophylactic hysterectomy" is this: The mortality rate of uterine cancer is less than the mortality rate of hysterectomy.

Nonetheless, the majority of doctors present at a 1971 meeting of the American College of Obstetrics and Gynecology registered approval of prophylactic hysterectomy for relief of anxiety, sterilization or prevention of cancer (MWN, 1972). Six years later, Dr. James Sammons, the AMA's senior staff physician, testifying before a House commerce committee hearing, said that hysterectomy may be acceptable as a treatment for anxiety. He advocated this major surgical procedure as the treatment of choice for "fear of pregnancy" (Sammons, 1977). If the present hysterectomy rate continues, half the women in this country will have lost their wombs by age 65, victims of what one author has termed "the war against the womb" (Morgan, 1982).

According to the latest (1979) figures from the National Center for Health Statistics, 800,000 hysterectomies are performed a year in the United States. The actual number is much higher because that figure leaves out the hysterectomies done on Indian reservations and the very large number done in military hospitals.

When physicians remove the ovaries as well as the uterus, the woman undergoes instant menopause. The sudden change in her hormonal equilibrium has profound effects on her entire body, on her emotions and on her relationships with family and friends. Many women find these changes, which many physicians do not warn them of, devastating (see the forthcoming book on hysterectomy by Nora Coffey).

9. The crusade to outlaw abortion took place between 1857 and 1880 (see Mohr, 1978).

10. The peak of the "ovariectomy" craze was from 1880 to 1900, according to Barker-Benfield; also see Scully, 1980, p. 48.

11. Brachet, in 1912 and 1913, made the first recorded attempt to culture mammalian embryos. He tried to maintain 5-day rabbit embryos on plasma clots.

12. In an essay on IVF, Rev. Albert S. Moraczewski refers to "R. G. Edwards, one of the two principal 'lab-parents' of Louise Brown."

Afterword: Crystallization

The new reproductive technologies have developed at breathtaking speed and with essentially no controls. In the six short years since the first test-tube baby was born, pharmacrats have frozen human embryos, used donor eggs with IVF, and flushed embryos from women and implanted them into other women. They are on the verge of sexing and twinning human embryos, as they have acknowledged at their professional meetings.

Various ethics committees and commissions, composed predominantly of male professionals who often share the values of the pharmacrats, have hardly slowed the speed. Indeed, the role such commissions play in legitimating the new technologies needs to be studied. Most often the commissions are helpful to the pharmacrats, who can point to them and assert that they are acting responsibly in following commission guidelines.

But the technologies need not continue to expand at such a breakneck pace. Opposition is gathering and it is coming from women. In the spring of 1984, Australian Dr. Robyn Rowland, chairwoman of the committee co-ordinating social/psychological research into donor programs at Queen Victoria Medical Centre, resigned her position, terming research into various reproductive technologies "morally reprehensible." That research was being advanced by stealth, she charged. The IVF team, she said, put out carefully constructed press releases that, catching the public by surprise, informed it of breakthroughs in each new step while providing no opportunity for discussion of whether the research was needed or wanted (SMH, 1984, May 25). Rowland's resignation, which sent shock waves throughout Australia, stimulated a national

318

debate on the reproductive technologies.

Women from fourteen countries spoke out as well at the Second International Interdisciplinary Congress on Women in Groningen, the Netherlands, in April 1984. Alarmed at the implications of these technologies for women's future as presented on a panel entitled "Death of the Female," they formed the Feminist International Network on the New Reproductive Technologies. Through the Network, these 542 women (Rowland and myself among them) are monitoring developments in such areas as IVF, sex predetermination and human/animal hybrids. We are also involved in organizing women's conferences where we can plan our response to the technologies. British women have already held two such conferences, one in Leeds and another in London, both in 1984. A Women's Emergency Conference on the New Reproductive Technologies is to be held in Sweden in 1985 with women from as many countries as possible participating.

Something else gives me hope that, to some degree, the technologies can be controlled. It is an approach suggested by Patricia Hynes, an environmental engineer from Massachusetts. In a series of conversations with me, Hynes said that a possible model for the control of reproductive technology exists in the federal hazardous waste program where she works. The model—which is a model of regulation, not prohibition—involves no infringement of the right to free scientific inquiry.

This is the approach: A regulatory body comparable to the Environmental Protection Agency could be instituted to control the medibusiness that is marketing the new reproductive technologies.

Hazardous substances and wastes have come under government control, Hynes explained, because of this insight: Unregulated applied science has developed many chemical compounds that, even when used well, have proved to be harmful to human health and the environment.

Since the end of World War II, there had been a pioneering industrial spirit in the United States, a country that has prided itself on a tradition of free enterprise. Therefore, in the late 1950s and early 1960s, the notion that the government had the right to regulate the chemical industry to the degree that it does now would have been nearly inconceivable, Hynes said. However, environmental statutes with the authority to control industry's use of chemical compounds were passed in the 1970s.

What happened to create such a dramatic turnaround in public opinion? Values were crystallized, Hynes explained. These values—

human health and the environment—were so important that society would control industry for the sake of preserving them. We had come to see the environment as valuable in and of itself.

Before we could crystallize the environment as a value, we had to undergo a consciousness raising. It was Rachel Carson's *Silent Spring*, published in 1962, that heightened consciousness on the danger of pesticide use in the United States.

In Carson's time, the Department of Agriculture, which favored use of pesticides, regulated them. It was clear to Carson that as long as that was the case, there would be no sincere regulation of pesticides. She advocated the establishment of an independent agency for the regulation of any harmful substance. That idea eventually bore fruit in the creation of the Environmental Protection Agency, which is not affiliated to any particular industry.[1]

If we can compare the perceived good for the few (i.e., the infertile) in the biomedical technologies with the larger harm to the many, and demonstrate that there is a greater harm than good, then we can argue that there has to be a regulatory framework to prevent that harm.[2]

"It would be edifying and shocking for there to be, side by side with the medical profession and in theoretical conflict with it, a regulatory body which had enough power to control it," Hynes said. "It is not yet conceivable because it hasn't existed. I think the same situation must have been true twenty years ago with respect to the chemical industry."

The enormous power that industry had then, she added, is comparable to the power the medical profession has now. Similarly, medicine has become allied with applied science in the same way that agriculture did when it became a market for the chemical industry, an alliance that propelled agriculture into agribusiness. Biotechnology is imitating the same model as agriculture in becoming a product-oriented business.

An editorial in *Fertility and Sterility*, gives weight to Hynes's observation. In that editorial, Dr. Alan H. DeCherney, a member of the Yale University School of Medicine's in vitro fertilization team, wrote: "The engagement of industry and academic medicine has been announced, with marriage planned soon. What better area could there be to test out commercialized medical crafts than the area of IVF. This field is potentially highly profitable, limited in scope, and based on high technology."

One possible path for the commercial distribution of IVF was an IVF industry, he wrote, observing that kidney dialysis had already become an industry. "Professionally planned IVF centers, managed and marketed, seem a likely extension of this concept." This "controversial and yet creative" concept threatened "to catapult the obstetric-gynecologic community into . . . [the] medical industrial complex" (DeCherney, 1983).[3]

Before statutes controlling the medical-industrial complex can be conceived, the value such a statute would be designed to protect would have to be crystallized.

"That means, then, that we would have to elevate the well-being of women to the status of the environment?" I asked Hynes.

She nodded.

But given the fact that the patriarchy had managed to roll along, century after century, without seeing women's well-being as anything of any value whatsoever, wasn't that a formidable task?

Hynes felt hope tempered with realism. What she found so significant about the statutes she enforces, she said, is that something as intangible and, only twenty years ago, as undervalued as the environment, gained so much value in such a short time that statutes giving the government control over industry were created. This made her optimistic about accomplishing the same in terms of safeguarding women.

But our task, she told me, was more difficult than the environmentalists' had been. The environmental movement is perceived as a people's movement dealing with a people's issue. In contrast, what we are advocating—the crystallization of the health and well-being of women as a value—is being advocated primarily by women. This was much more threatening and would be more arduous.

Despite this fact and the existence of other problems common to any regulatory agency,[4] I share Hynes's "realistic optimism." While the clean-up of toxic waste is far too slow, still, the fact that earth-poisoning is now an issue of public concern means an extraordinary change of consciousness has occurred.

The challenge for those of us concerned about biotechnologies is to bring about another change of consciousness by clearly articulating the values we want to uphold and by demonstrating how the technologies impair the well-being of women.

And of animals too. We need to crystallize the notion that animals have a value in and of themselves, that, for example, cattle are *not* "intrinsically worth only the meat or milk they produce," but have a value beyond their usefulness to us. Various feminist writers and the animal liberation movement are beginning to crystallize this.[5]

We can all contribute to the crystallization. How? By breaking silence.

The runaway development of the new reproductive technologies has taken place in a culture where women have been silenced (see Dworkin, 1982, pp. 255–258). It is true that we are allowed to speak, even taken along by pharmacrats to talk on television programs, if we say the right things such as: "I will go through *anything,* including IVF, to bear a child and be grateful for it." Or, "I have always felt an empathy for infertile women, I love to be pregnant, and by serving as a rented womb, I am giving the gift of life." But there is much less readiness to allow us a public platform when we look to our own experiences—for example, surgical ones—and say such things as Julie Melrose did in articulating the threat to woman's well-being posed by such "minor" manipulations as those involved in IVF: "The human body has an integrity of its own and it can not be violated, even in a way that the doctor may see as minor, without there being physical and emotional consequences for the person on whom the surgery is being performed."

Women have been silenced partly by the accusation that, in questioning the reproductive technologies, we are being insensitive to the needs of infertile women. Dr. Robyn Rowland has seen through this silencing technique and spoken up: "Over a period of two years, I have developed an overwhelming sympathy and empathy for the plight of the infertile. But I cannot divorce this from the feeling that they are being used by the medical profession in order to gain funding for research which is not necessarily intended to help the infertile person" (Rowland, 1984).

Despite the unwillingness of a male supremacist society to hear us, we must speak. We can speak out against any injustice suffered by women and, in doing so, contribute to the crystallization of woman's well-being as a value. We can speak out in our conversations with others—on the telephone, at a party, in line at the post office or the grocery store, in the office, the factory.

It will not be easy for us to speak at first. The issues surrounding the new reproductive technologies are confusing. Sometimes our heads spin. The benevolent rationales for the technologies and images of kindly, smiling pharmacrats swirl around in our brains along with our sense that when we are called "living incubators" and "oocytes donors," all is not well. We are *supposed* to be confused. The confusion keeps us speechless and powerless. It is as a Native American friend once told me: Confusion is a tool of oppression.

While we are struggling out of our confusion and into speech, we must stubbornly stay with our sense of uneasiness and think it through. We can not allow ourselves to be bullied into acquiescence with a "tolerant" view of the technologies simply because we are not yet able to fully articulate why the benevolent rationales for these technologies clash with our sense of our own dignity and worth. We can stand stubbornly and say: "Something is wrong here," and explain that "something" to the best of our ability. Each time we do it, we will get better at it.

When many women break silence, when many women finally speak their truth, and speak it again and again and again, the world will have to change.

Notes

1. The EPA is not free of the potential for conflicts of interest, Hynes said. Its administrator is appointed by the president. So there is that political affiliation or loyalty. Also, EPA employees, like employees of any regulatory agency, are capable of having personal ties or of making unethical sweetheart deals with an industry against which they are supposed to be applying the statutes.

"What probably separates EPA from such agencies as the Department of Agriculture and the Food and Drug Administration is that its founding philosophy and purpose were inspired by *Silent Spring*," she said. "It seems to have a more idealistic spirit than other federal agencies."

2. There may be some limited good to the bio-technologies, just as there may be certain good uses of hazardous substances. Rachel Carson recognized that there might be minor and beneficial uses of pesticides when used carefully. But Carson also said a lot of the good technology based on biology for "pest control," like sterilization of male insects, had not been seriously tried. In the same way, systematic attempts to prevent infertility have not been tried.

3. Emphasizing that the new reproductive technology is accompanied by a new way of thinking about medical practice, DeCherney observed that the UCLA–Harbor Group had applied for a patent for its embryo transfer process. "I wonder whether trenchant evaluation of the market for in vitro services will cause us to determine the proper commercial course" (DeCherney, 1983).

A statement by Dr. Richard Seed, the embryo transfer pioneer, also makes Hynes's observation on the transformation of biotechnology into an industry seem apt. Seed, who works with the UCLA–Harbor group, sees no reason why his company's patent application should not be approved: "I like to think of the procedure in terms of industry, where large numbers of process patents have been granted. Medical procedures are not that much different than industrial procedures" (Merz, 1984).

4. Problems: Who would work in the agency? Would some of them make sweetheart deals with the medibusiness they were supposed to regulate? Would they

be bribed with offers of lucrative jobs for serving medibusiness well while employed in the agency?

5. See, for example: Cantor, Aviva, 1983, August, "The club, the yoke and the leash: what we can learn from the way a culture treats animals, *Ms.;* Griffin, 1978; André Collard, 1983, Spring, "Rape of the wild," *Trivia: A Journal of Ideas,* 2; Mason and Singer, 1980; Singer, 1975; Godlovitch, S. and R. and J. Harris, eds., 1971, *Animals, Men and Morals,* Grove Press, New York.

Some addresses for further information on animal liberation:

—*Agenda: News Magazine of the Animal Rights Network.* P.O. Box 5234, Westport, Ct. 06881. Subscription $15/year in the U.S., $25 elsewhere.

—*FARM* (Farm Animal Reform Movement) *Report.* P.O. Box 70123, Washington, D.C. 20088.

—People for the Ethical Treatment of Animals (PETA), P.O. Box 56272, Washington, D.C. 20011.

Chronology

Most of us have become aware of the new reproductive technologies only in the last decade or so. The dramatic birth of the world's first "test-tube" baby, the establishment of sperm and embryo banks, and the opening of businesses that rent women's bodies for reproductive services drew our attention to the technologies in the late 1970s. But scientists have been working on them for more than a century. As the following brief overview demonstrates, progress has been steady.

1870s

In vitro fertilization. A Viennese embryologist made the first attempt at external fertilization. He used rabbit eggs.

1890s

Embryo transfer. Walter Heape performed the first embryo transfer in animals.

1900

Artificial wombs. At the turn of the twentieth century, premature babies were displayed at state fairs and in Coney Island in incubators, primitive forms of the artificial womb.

1920s

Sex predetermination. In 1923, scientists learned that there are two kinds of sex chromosomes responsible for the child's gender. This discovery made techniques to separate gynosperm (X) and androsperm (Y) seem possible.

In vitro fertilization. In order to fertilize eggs in a laboratory dish, scientists had to retrieve eggs from females. So they needed to control ovulation, the process by which an egg is released from an ovary. In 1927, they discovered that gonadotropins (hormones produced by the pituitary gland) affect the ovaries. That same year, they purified preparations of gonadotropins and superovulated mice, forcing the production of large numbers of eggs, which could be used in research.

1930s

Sex predetermination. Researchers experimented with various techniques, primarily the acid-alkali method. A German physician reported that he had observed a high correlation between alkalinity of the woman's vaginal secretions and the birth of male babies. He and others tried to help patients conceive males by the use of alkaline douches. (In the early 1940s, after repeated tests had not borne out earlier results, interest in this method faded.) Also during this decade, a Soviet biochemist separated rabbit androsperm and gynosperm on the basis of the sperm's supposed electrical charges and reported success in controlling the sex of the offspring in 80 percent of cases. (American researchers, obtaining less impressive results, abandoned the method.)

In vitro fertilization. In the 1930s, scientists began learning how to "culture" eggs, that is, propagate them in a special substance conducive to their growth. This was an important technique to master if eggs were ever to be fertilized in the laboratory because eggs extracted directly from women's ovaries are too immature to be fertilized. Researchers began with rabbits. They found that if they placed such immature eggs into a culture medium in the lab, the eggs would complete the maturation process outside the body. The first instance of human eggs maturing outside a woman's body was also reported in the 1930s.

Hormonal research. The 1930s was the decade of the sex hormones. Researchers discovered a simple way to manufacture progesterone, a hormone that would later be used in the oral contraceptive. The first estrogen, diethylstilbestrol (DES), was synthesized in 1938, the same year it was discovered that it caused cancer in mice. Gynecologists and obstetricians introduced sex hormones, including DES, into their medical practices at the end of the decade for such indications as lactation suppression and prevention of miscarriage.

Artificial insemination. Farmers began to use artificial insemination commercially with their livestock.

Transsexualism. The first transsexual operation was performed in an attempt to transform a man into a woman by cutting off male organs and constructing female ones.

1940s

In vitro fertilization. Rabbits, sheep, cows and goats were super-ovulated. During this decade, one physician, in an attempt at in vitro fertilization, cultured human eggs from the ovary in the presence of sperm. However, he could not demonstrate to his colleagues that the sperm fertilized the eggs.

Artificial insemination. A few physicians in Europe and the United States began using artificial insemination in women but it was a rare practice. In England, researchers found that glycerol protects sperm so that it can be stored in dry ice after slowly freezing it. This discovery of a sperm freezing method opened the way for the development of sperm banks.

Embryo transfer. A researcher attempted to transfer embryos from one cow to the uteri of other cows. Attempts to freeze animal embryos also began during the 1940s.

1950s

Sex predetermination. Researchers tried to physically separate androsperm and gynosperm according to their size and weight using a method of differential centrifugation. In centrifugation, materials are separated from a mixture by spinning a solution at high speeds so that the heavier materials settle out faster than the lighter ones. Differential centrifugation is a more sophisticated form. It allows the separation of several materials at once into a number of layers.

In vitro fertilization. Men discovered that before the sperm of certain animals could penetrate the egg, it had to be triggered or "capacitated" by exposure to fluid from the female reproductive tract.

During this decade, a researcher succeeded in fertilizing the eggs of a rabbit in the lab. He transferred embryos to surrogate rabbit mothers who subsequently produced healthy litters of offspring. For the first time, evidence for the in vitro fertilization of a mammalian egg was incontestable. Another researcher attempted the in vitro fertilization of human eggs but did not demonstrate that he had succeeded.

Hormonal research. Scientists at Worcester Foundation in Massachusetts tested compounds for inhibiting ovulation. Elsewhere, an active hormonal ingredient (progesterone) in the Pill was synthesized. In 1959, the U.S. Food and Drug Administration approved the oral contraceptive, a combination of hormones that prevent conception by suppressing ovulation.

Artificial insemination. Frozen human sperm was used for the first time, producing a normal child.

Transsexualism. Hormonal and surgical techniques for transsexual operations were refined and made public. George Jorgensen was transsexed into "Christine" in Denmark.

Embryo transfer. Embryo transfers were successfully carried out in animals in the United States and England.

Cloning. Scientists in Philadelphia cloned tadpoles.

1960s

Artificial wombs. A variety of researchers conducted experiments in attempts to make sundry apparatuses perform functions of the uterus and placenta.

Sex determination. Two British researchers announced that they had, for the first time, controlled the sex of a mammal's offspring (see Chapter 10, p. 197).

In vitro fertilization. At Vanderbilt University Medical Center, scientists conducted basic research on the in vitro fertilization of laboratory animals. In Australia, a researcher reported the fertilization of mouse eggs in the lab. Elsewhere, scientists fertilized golden hamster eggs in the lab and implanted them in a surrogate hamster mother. Other scientists simplified cross-fertilization between different animal species by removing the outer membrane from the egg before in vitro fertilization.

Research on the superovulation of women moved ahead in the 1960s.

Dr. Robert G. Edwards, British reproductive physiologist, formed a team of scientists to achieve the in vitro fertilization of human eggs. Later in the decade, he launched his collaboration with obstetrician/gynecologist Patrick Steptoe, which would lead to the birth of the world's first test-tube baby ten years later. In the 1960s, Edwards extracted immature egg cells from the human ovary and cultured them up to the point of ripeness for fertilization. He subsequently succeeded in fertilizing human eggs in a dish.

Artificial insemination. The Feversham Committee, appointed by the British government to look into human artificial insemination, issued a disapproving report on the controversial practice. Meanwhile, the introduction of liquid nitrogen as a medium for freezing sperm perfected the deep-frozen technique for use with human sperm.

Transsexualism. Treatment for transsexualism through surgery and hormones became more common. The Harry Benjamin Foundation, which brought together professionals from many specialties to research transsexualism, was founded. In 1967, the Johns Hopkins Gender Identity Clinic opened in Baltimore, helping to make transsexualism a legitimate medical problem. At that time, no other reputable medical center permitted the surgery.

Embryo transfer. In 1962, a researcher reported that fertilized sheep eggs were placed in the oviducts of a rabbit. The rabbit, used as an incubator for the sheep eggs, was crated to South Africa. There, the embryos were surgically transferred into two ewes whose uteri had been prepared for implantation by the injection of hormones. The ewes later delivered two lambs. Since that report, there has been speculation on the possibility of using animals as incubators for human embryos.

Late in the 1960s, men conducted numerous experiments in embryo culture and transfer in animals.

Cloning. Professor F. C. Steward cloned a carrot. Dr. J. B. Gurdon cloned frogs.

Artificial wombs. The first medical clinic (Yale–New Haven) put into operation an intensive care prenatal unit for electronically monitoring human fetuses from onset of labor through to birth. Some of the knowledge gained in this may prove useful in monitoring fetuses in artificial wombs.

Chimeras. Researchers formed what are called "chimeric" embryos by fusing together several growing embryos or by placing cells in embryos of an early developmental stage. In 1965, the first mosaic mouse, which had four parents, was born.

1970s

Sex predetermination. In 1969 and 1970, two discoveries making it possible to count androsperm and gynosperm gave major impetus to the study of sex predetermination. Researchers discovered how to stain chromosomes and locate a spot on the stained sperm indicating the presence of the Y chromosome. These discoveries made it possible to identify androsperm simply and cheaply.

Researchers worked on the antigen-antibody reaction between sperm and egg as a possible method of controlling sex. Other researchers attempted to detect fetal sex by examining the mother's saliva, cervical mucus or blood.

Dr. Ronald Ericcson introduced a new technique of sex predetermination, which involves an attempt to separate sperm on the basis of swimming ability. Sperm are placed on top of a dense liquid in a test tube. The method is based on the hypothesis that androgenic sperm would be able to swim faster through this suspension and reach the bottom earlier than gynogenic sperm. Ericsson and colleagues reported getting suspensions containing up to 80 percent Y sperm with the method in 1973. He introduced his technique that year and four years later took out a patent on a "Y sperm isolation kit" for increasing the incidence of males among offspring in cows, humans and other mammals. He opened up a clinic, Gametrics, Inc., in Sausalito, California, offering selection for boy babies. Several centers in France and Taiwan and nine centers in the United States—in Louisiana, Pennsylvania, Oregon, California, New York and Illinois—are using the method. Ericsson's results have been confirmed by some (including Dmowski, 1979) but not others (including Evans et al., 1975; Ross et al., 1975).

In vitro fertilization. Louise Brown, the world's first test-tube baby, was born as a result of the work of Edwards and Steptoe. She was delivered by cesarean section and nurtured in the first hours of her life with sterile water and dextrose.

Research teams around the world formed clinics for human in vitro fertilization.

Artificial insemination. A commercial sperm bank using frozen sperm opened in Maryland. In England, the Peel Committee, appointed by the British Medical Association, recommended that the National Health Service provide AID. Its positive report on artificial insemination contrasted sharply with the negative report of the Feversham Committee a decade earlier.

Embryo transfer. Attempts to freeze animal embryos, begun after World War II, were finally successful. The first mammalian embryos frozen and thawed were those of mice. In 1974, the first large mammal, a bull, was born from a deep-frozen embryo in Cambridge, England. The embryo was removed from one cow, frozen, thawed six days later, and transferred into a surrogate cow mother. That same year, the International Embryo Transfer Society formed to further the use of embryo transfer throughout the livestock industry. By the decade's end, embryo transfer in livestock had become a multimillion-dollar industry. In the late 1970s, the Reproduction and Fertility Clinic Inc. opened in Chicago to attempt embryo transfer in women.

Breeder women. For the first time, a "surrogate mother" bore a baby for payment for a man who had advertised for a human breeder in the *San Francisco Chronicle*. Several more such births followed in 1978 and 1979.

1980s

Sex predetermination. Some physicians in India and in China began detecting fetal sex with the use of prenatal diagnostic techniques and, at the request of the parents, aborting females.

In vitro fertilization. By 1984, more than a hundred IVF clinics were operating around the world though the success rate for the procedure was still very low. One clinic in Australia, experimenting in the freezing of human embryos, opened an embryo bank. This clinic also reported the first successful birth with a donor egg taken from one woman, fertilized in the lab, and then transferred into another woman.

Artificial insemination. A sperm bank was established to collect and distribute the semen of allegedly superior men, including Nobel laureates.

Embryo transfer. Embryo transfer technology, long used in cattle, was successfully applied to women for the first time in 1984. Dr. John E. Buster of the University of California at Los Angeles School of Medicine headed the embryo transfer team.

In an experiment conducted by Dr. Gary D. Hodgen of the National Institute of Child Health and Human Development, monkeys with their ovaries removed gave birth to normal offspring. Fertilized donor eggs had been transferred into the monkeys. The animals were treated with two hormones necessary for pregnancy. Dr. Buster announced that his embryo transfer team planned to use a similar technique soon on women.

Breeder women. By 1984, there were at least sixteen American firms selling the reproductive services of women as surrogate mothers.

Cloning. Biologist Peter C. Hoppe and microsurgeon Karl Illmensee reportedly succeeded in producing the first true clone of a mammal. To date, these experiments have not been replicated.

Researchers James McGrath and Davor Solter reported a significant advance in nuclear transplantation, the procedure used in one form of cloning.

Bibliography

Code for abbreviations

AJOG   *American Journal of Obstetricians and Gynecologists*
Appendix Appendix: HEW Support of Research Involving Human In Vitro
        Fertilization and Embryo Transfer. Ethics Advisory Board.
        Department of Health, Education and Welfare. U.S. Government
        Printing Office.
BMJ   *British Medical Journal*
BJOG   *British Journal of Obstetrics and Gynaecology*
COG   *Contemporary Ob/Gyn*
JAMA   *Journal of the American Medical Association*
NEJM   *New England Journal of Medicine*
NYT   *The New York Times*
OGN   *Ob/Gyn News*

AASPEC. 1977. The Ann Arbor Science for the People Editorial Collective. *Biology As a Social Weapon.* Burgess Publishing Co. Minneapolis.

AATB. 1980, November. *American Association of Tissue Banks Newsletter.* 4(Supplement): 37.

ABC. 1980, October 23. ABC News. Media Transcript of 20/20.

———. 1978, July 13. Brenda Shapiro, producer. Bob Clark, correspondent. Test Tube Baby: Brave New World or Nightmare Alley? *Directions.*

ABS. 1981, April 4. Australian Women's Broadcasting Cooperative, producer. Australian Broadcasting System. Madonna of the 21st Century. *Coming Out.*

ABT, ISAAC A. 1917, August 11. The Technique of Wetnurse Management in Institutions. JAMA.

ADELMAN, STUART and ROSENZWEIG, SAUL. 1978. Parental Predetermination of the Sex of Offspring: II. The Attitudes of Young Married Couples with High School and with College Education. *J. Biosoc. Sci.* 10: 235–247.

AESCHYLUS. 1980. Philip Vallacott, translator. *The Oresteian Trilogy.* Penguin Books. New York.

THE AGE. 1981, July 25. The Ethics of Aiding Nature.

ALEXANDER, NANCY J., et al. Undated. *Artificial Insemination.* Booklet prepared by staffers in Infertility Laboratory, departments of obstetrics, gynecology and urology. University of Oregon Health Sciences Center. Portland, Oregon.

ALLEN, SALLY G. and JOANNA HUBBS. 1980. Outrunning Atalanta: Feminine Destiny in Alchemical Transmutation. *Signs.* 6(21):210–229.

ALTUS, WILLIAM D. 1966, January 7. Birth Order and Its Sequelae. *Science.* 151: 44–49.

AMERICAN ACADEMY OF PEDIATRICS. 1978. Breast-Feeding. *Pediatrics* 62(4): 591–600.

AMA. 1973, June. Human Artificial Insemination: Report of the Judicial Council. Adopted by the American Medical Association House of Delegates, June 1974.

AMN. 1980, October 11. Human Sperm Is a Medicine, Pharmacists Say. *American Medical News.*

ANDERSON, CAROLE with SUE CAMPBELL and MARY ANNE COHEN. 1981. Eternal Punishment of Women: Adoption Abuse. Pamphlet available from Concerned United Birthparents. P.O. Box 573. Milford, Mass. 01757.

ANDREWS, MASON. 1979, October 18. Letter to *The Virginia–Pilot.*

———. 1979, October 31. Testimony submitted in response to Health Systems Agency public hearing.

AQUINO, AMY. 1979, May. What they don't know won't hurt them. Unpublished paper presented to the Department of Biology. Harvard/Radcliffe College.

ARDITTI, RITA, RENATE DUELLI KLEIN and SHELLEY MINDEN, eds. 1984. *Test-Tube Women: What Future for Motherhood?* Pandora Press. London. Boston. Melbourne and Henley.

ANNAS, GEORGE. 1979, August. Artificial Insemination: Beyond the Best Interest of the Donor. *Hastings Center Report.*

———. 1981, April. Contracts to Bear a Child: Compassion or Commercialism? *The Hastings Report:* 23–24.

ANONYMOUS, SARAH and MARY. 1979. *Woman Controlled Conception.* Womanshare Books.

APPLE, RIMA D. 1980. "To Be Used Only Under the Direction of a Physician": Commercial Infant Feeding and Medical Practice, 1870–1940. *Bull. Hist. Med.* 54: 402–417.

AVERY, T. L., FAHNING, M. L. and GRAHAM, E. F. 1962. Investigations Associated with the Transplantation of Bovine Ova: II. Superovulation. *J. Reprod. Fertil:* 212–217.

——— and Graham, E. F. 1962. Investigations Associated with the Transplanting of Bovine Ova: III. Recovery and Fertilization. *J. Reprod. Fertil:* 212–217.

BAKER, BARBARA. 1984. Attempt to patent embryo transfer procedure sparks strong objections. OGN 19(7).

BAKER, JILL. 1981, March 31. More join test-tube baby race. *The Australian.*

———. 1981, April 6. Human embryos frozen for test-tube program. *The Australian.*

———. 1981, April 9. Test-tube babies puzzle for legislators. *The Australian.*

———. 1981, October 28. Embryo experiments: Test-tube team calls for independent inquiry. *The Australian.*

———. 1981, October 28. Test-tube babies—Call for controls. *The Sydney Morning Herald.*

BAKSYS, SANDY. 1979, September 29. Woman seeks chance to bear her own child. *The Ledger–Star* (Norfolk, Va.).

———. 1979, November 24. Future of test tube baby clinic remains uncertain. *The Ledger–Star.*

BANTA, DAVID H. and STEPHEN B. THACKER. 1979, April. Costs and benefits of electronic fetal monitoring: a review of the literature. Department of Health, Education and Welfare Publication No. (PHS) 79-3245.

BALLANTYNE, SHEILA. 1975. *Norma Jean the Termite Queen.* Doubleday & Co. Garden City, New York.

BARKER-BENFIELD, G. J. 1976. *The Horrors of the Half-Known Life.* Harper & Row. New York.

BARLOW, SUSAN and FRANK SULLIVAN. 1982. *Reproductive Hazards of Industrial Chemicals.* Academic Press. New York.

BARNES, GEORGE, et al. 1953, Jan. 17. Management of breast-feeding. JAMA: 192–199.

BARROMES, BERNARD. 1981. Transplanting bovine embryos: test tube calves in mass production. Copyright: Agence Gamma.

BEARDEN, H. JOE and JOHN FUQUAY. 1980. *Applied Animal Breeding.* Reston Publishing Co., Inc. Reston, Va.

BEAZLEY, JOHN M. 1975, May 15. Active Management of Labor. AJOG: 161–168.

BEHRMAN, S. J. and D. R. ACKERMAN. 1969, Jan.–April. AJOG: 103.

BELL, SUSAN E. 1981, June. Feminist self-help: The case of fertility consciousness woman controlled natural birth control groups. *Radical Teacher.*

BERRY, AILEEN. 1982, May 24. Egg donor move by test tube baby team. *The Melbourne Age.*

BETTELHEIM, BRUNO. 1968. *Symbolic Wounds: Puberty Rites and the Envious Male.* Collier Books. New York.

BETTERIDGE, K. J. 1981. An historical look at embryo transfer. *J. of Reprod. Fert.* 62: 1–13.

BHATTACHARYA, B. C. 1964, Oct. 15. Pre-arranging the sex of offspring. *New Scientist.* 413: 151–152.

———. 1979, March. A convectional counter-stream sedimentation process for separating biological isotopes. *IEEE Transactions on Biomedical Engineering.* BME-26(3): 160–164.

——— and B. M. EVANS and P. SHOME. Semen separation technique monitored with greater accuracy by B-body test. *Int. J. Fertility.* 24(4): 256–259.

BIGGERS, JOHN D. 1979. In vitro fertilization, embryo culture and embryo transfer in the human. *Appendix.*

————. 1981. In vitro fertilization and embryo transfer in human beings. NEJM. 304(6): 336–342.

BLACKSTONE, WILLIAM. 1788. *Commentaries on the Laws of England in Four Books*. Reprinted from the British edition. Philadelphia.

BLAIR, BETTY J. 1982, Nov. 24. Surrogate motherhood: Controversy and a dilemma. *Detroit News.*

BLAKE, MARTIN. 1984, May 19. In vitro row—woman quits. *Geelong Advertisen* (Australia).

BLANDAU, RICHARD J. 1980. In vitro fertilization and embryo transfer. *Fertility and Infertility*. 33(1): 3–11.

BMJ. 1960, July 30. Human artificial insemination: Feversham committee's report. BMJ: 379–380.

BRACK, DATHA. 1975. Social forces, feminism and breastfeeding. *Nursing Outlook*. 23:556–561.

————. 1978, Sept. Breast-feeding: A function of women's power in social exchange. Prepared for presentation, Sociology for Women in Society meeting, San Francisco.

BREO, DENNIS L. 1980, October 21. Pair brave criticisms to produce a new life. *Chicago Tribune.*

BREWER, GAIL SFORZA with TOM BREWER. 1977. *What Every Pregnant Woman Should Know*. Random House. New York.

BRIGGS, R. and T. J. KING. 1952. Transplantation of living nuclei from blastula cells into enucleated frogs' eggs. *Proc. Natl. Acad. Sci. U.S.* 38: 455–463.

BROMHALL, J. D. 1975, Dec. 25. Nuclear transplantation in the rabbit egg. *Nature*. 258: 719–721.

BROOKS-GUNN, JEANNE and WENDY MATTHEWS. 1980. But we wanted a ... *Hard Choices*. William Bennet and Barbara Gale, eds. Copyright by KCTS/9, The Regents of the University of Washington. Seattle.

BROTMAN, HARRIS. 1983, June 8. Human embryo transplants. *New York Times Magazine.*

————. 1983, May 15. Engineering the birth of cattle. *New York Times Magazine.*

BROWN, ISAAC BAKER. 1866. *On the Curability of Certain Forms of Insanity, Epilepsy, Catalepsy and Hysteria in Females*. R. Hardwicke, publishers. London.

BROWN, LESLEY and JOHN, with SUE FREEMAN. 1979. *Our Miracle Called Louise, a Parents' Story*. Paddington Press Ltd. New York and London.

BROWN, P. and E. DRUCKMAN, editors. 1976. Elective hysterectomy: Pro and con. NEJM. 295(5): 264–268.

BROWN, SUSAN. 1977, Feb. 4. Bear our baby, couple ask. *Detroit Free Press.*

BROZAN, NADINE. 1984, Feb. 27. Surrogate mothers: problems and goals. NYT.

BUDGE, E. A. WALLIS. 1969. *The Gods of the Egyptians*. Vol. 1. Dover Publications. New York.

Bullseye. 1973, June 15. *Nature.* 243: 371.

BUNGE, R. G. and J. K. SHERMAN. 1954. Frozen human semen. *Fertility and Sterility.* 5: 193–194.

BURTON, F. G., et al. 1978. Role of controlled drug delivery in contraception. Reprinted in *Fertility and Contraception in America. Domestic Fertility Trends and Family Planning Services, Hearings before the Selection Committee on Population.* 3: 366–416.

BUSTER, JOHN E., et al. 1983, July 23. Non-surgical transfer of in vivo fertilised donated ova to five infertile women: Report of two pregnancies. *The Lancet:* 223–224.

BUSTILLO, MARIA, et al. 1984. Nonsurgical ovum transfer as a treatment in infertile women. JAMA. 251(9): 1171–1173.

CALLAGHAN, J. C., et al. 1962. Study of prepulmonary bypass in the development of an artificial placenta for prematurity and respiratory distress syndrome of the newborn. *Journal of Thoracic and Cardiovascular Surgery.* 44(5): 600–607.

———— and EARL A. MAYNES and HENRY R. HUG. 1965. Studies on lambs of the development of an artificial placenta. *Canadian Journal of Surgery.* 8: 208–213.

CALLAHAN, SHEILA. 1981, July 1. Ob. starts prenatal counseling before conception. OGN.

————. 1982, May 1. In vitro fertilization no longer considered experimental. OGN. 17(9).

CAMPBELL, JOSEPH. 1964. *The Masks of God: Occidental Mythology.* The Viking Press. New York.

CARBINES, LOUISE. 1983, March 12. Pregnant—with egg from another woman. *Melbourne Age.*

CASTILLO, ANGEL. 1981, Jan. 28. Kentucky attorney general calls surrogate motherhood illegal. NYT.

CEDERQVIST, LARS L. and FRITZ FUCH. 1970. Antenatal sex determination: A historical review. *Clin. Obstet. Gynec.* 13: 159–177.

CEQ. 1981, Jan. *Chemical Hazards to Human Reproduction.* President's Council on Environmental Quality. 1981-337-130/8008. U.S. Government Printing Office. Washington, D.C. 20402.

CHASE, Alan. 1980. *The Legacy of Malthus.* University of Illinois Press. Urbana.

CHATTERJEE, MOLLY S. 1983, May. Paternal age and Down's syndrome. COG.

CHEDD, GRAHAM, producer. 1981. *Hard Choices: Boy or Girl?* Copyright by KCTS/9 and The Regents of the University of Washington. Seattle.

CHEZ, R. A. et al. 1978, February 28. Monitor every patient in labor? *Patient Care.*

CHILDS, BARTON. 1978, Sept. 16. Testimony before the Ethics Advisory Board. Unpublished.

CLARE, JEANNE E. and CLYDE V. KISER. 1951, October. Social and psychological factors affecting fertility, XIV. Preferences for children of given sex in relation to fertility. *Milbank Memorial Fund Quarterly.* XXIX(4): 440–492.

CLARK, JOHN F. J. 1982. Embryo transfer in vivo. *Journal of the National Medical Association.* 74(8).

CLEWE, THOMAS H. and LARRY MORGENSTERN, et al. 1971. Searches for ova in the human uterus and tubes. AJOG. 109(2): 313–334.

COG. 1977, October. Beyond in vitro fertilization: A progress report.

———. 1979, April. Gonadotropins: Their role in inducing ovulation. Symposium.

———. 1979, June. Fertility and infertility: What's new?

———. 1984, Jan. Referring your patient for in vitro fertilization.

———. 1984, Feb. A British view of IVF issues.

COHEN, MARK E. 1978, Fall. The 'brave new baby' and the law: Fashioning remedies for the victims of IVF. *Am. J. Law Med.*

COLE, H. H., ed. 1962. *Introduction to Livestock Production.* Second Edition. W. H. Freeman & Co. San Francisco.

COLEN, B. D. 1979, September 28. Norfolk doctors ready to implant human embryos. *The Washington Post.*

COLLIGAN, DOUGLAS. 1977, Nov. 7. Tipping the balance of the sexes. *New York.*

CONNORS, DENISE. 1981. Sex preselection response. In H. Holmes, B. Hoskins and M. Gross, eds. *The Custom-Made Child.* Humana Press, Inc. Clifton, N.J.

COREA, GENA. 1985. *The Hidden Malpractice.* Harper & Row. New York.

———. 1979, April. Childbirth 2000. *Omni.*

———. 1980a, July. The cesarean epidemic. *Mother Jones.*

———. 1980b. The Depo-Provera weapon. In H. Holmes, B. Hoskins and M. Gross, eds. *Birth Control and Controlling Birth.* Humana Press. Clifton, New Jersey.

———. 1984. Dominance and control. *Agenda: News Magazine of the Animal Rights Network.* P.O. Box 5234, Westport, Ct. 06881.

COREN, TERRI. 1979, June 15. Model law is drafted to protect against liability for in vitro fertilization. OGN.

CRAFT, IAN and JOHN YOVICH. 1979, September 22. Implications of embryo transfer. *The Lancet.*

CROXATTO, HORACIO, et al. 1969. Fertility control in women with a progestogen released in microquantities from subcutaneous capsules. AJOG. 1(7).

———. 1972. A simple nonsurgical technique to obtain unimplanted eggs from human uteri. AJOG. 112(5): 662–668.

CUMMINGS, RICHARD. 1966. *The Alchemists: Fathers of Practical Chemistry.* David McKay Co., Inc. New York.

CUNNINGHAM, F. GARY. 1979, September. Treating infections following cesarean section. COG. 14: 77–82.

CURIE-COHEN, MARTIN, LESLEIGH LUTTRELL and SANDER SHAPIRO. 1979. Current practice of artificial insemination by donor in the United States. NEJM. 300(11): 585–590.

CUSINE, DOUGLAS J. 1979, August 25. Some legal implications of embryo transfer. *The Lancet.*

DALTON, BILL. 1977, Feb. 1. Couple seeks woman to bear their child. *Ann Arbor News.*

DALY, MARY. 1973. *Beyond God the Father.* Beacon Press. Boston.

———. 1978. *Gyn/Ecology.* Beacon Press. Boston.

DANIEL, WILLIAM J. 1982. Sexual ethics in relation to in vitro fertilization and embryo transfer: The fitting use of human reproductive power. In W. A. W. Walters and P. Singer, eds. *Test-Tube Babies.* Oxford University Press. Oxford.

DAVIS, ANGELA. 1981. *Women, Race and Class.* Random House. New York.

DAVIS, KINGSLEY. 1937. Reproductive institutions and the pressure for population. *The Sociological Review.*

DE BEAUVOIR, SIMONE. 1970. *The Second Sex.* Bantam. New York.

DE CHATEAU, P., et al. 1977. A study of factors promoting and inhibiting lactation. *Develop. Med. Child Neurol.* 19: 575–584.

DECHERNEY, ALAN H., et al. 1981. Diethylstilbestrol and the fallopian tube. *Fertility and Sterility.* Abstract Supplement. 35(2): 261.

———. 1983. Doctored babies. *Fertility and Sterility.* 40(6): 724–726.

DECROW, KAREN and ROBERT SEIDENBERG. 1982. *Women Who Marry Houses.* McGraw Hill. New York.

DEL ZIO, DORIS, as told to SUZANNE WILDING. 1979, March. I was cheated of my test-tube baby. *Good Housekeeping.*

DEMETER, ANNA. 1977. *Legal Kidnapping.* Beacon Press. Boston.

DES. 1981. DES and science. *DES Action Voice.* 3(2).

DEVELOPMENTS. 1978, May 31. Developments in cell biology and genetics: hearing before the subcommittee on health and the environment of the Committee on Interstate and Foreign Commerce, House of Representatives. Serial No. 95-105. U.S. Government Printing Office. Washington, D.C.

DEVITT, N. 1979. The statistical case for elimination of the midwife: Fact versus prejudice, 1890–1935. *Women & Health.* 4.

DHEW. 1979, June 18. Protection of human subjects: HEW support of human in vitro fertilization and embryo transfer. Report of the Ethics Advisory Board. *Federal Register.*

DIASIO, ROBERT B. and ROBERT H. GLASS. 1971. *Fertility and Sterility.* 22(5): 303–305.

DJERASSI, CARL. 1979. *The Politics of Contraception.* W. W. Norton & Co. New York. London.

DMOWSKI, W. PAUL. 1979. Use of albumin gradients for X and Y sperm separation and clinical experience with male sex preselection. *Fertility and Sterility.* 31(1): 52–57.

Donahue transcript. Interview with Dr. William Shockley. Available from Multimedia Program Productions. Syndication Services. 140 W. Ninth Street. Cincinnati, Ohio 45202.

———. Donahue transcript #02260

———. Donahue transcript #04150

———. Donahue transcript #12170

———. Donahue transcript #07290

———. Donahue transcript #06161

———. Donahue transcript #02023

———. Donahue transcript #02033

———. Donahue transcript #08223

DONOWITZ, LEIGH G. and RICHARD P. WENZEL. 1980. Endometritis following cesarean section. AJOG. 137(4): 467–469.

DRANOV, PAULA. 1980, Sept. The artificial baby game. *Cosmopolitan.*

DREIFUS, CLAUDIA. 1980, March. Intrauterine devices: A story of pain— and risk. *Redbook.*

DT. 1980, June 24. Candice is a world first. *Daily Telegraph* (Sydney).

DWORKIN, ANDREA. 1974. *Woman Hating.* E. P. Dutton. New York.

———. 1976. *Our Blood.* Harper & Row. New York.

———. 1982. For men, freedom of speech; for women, silence please. In Laura Lederer, ed., *Take Back the Night: Women on Pornography.* Bantam Books. New York.

———. 1983. *Right-Wing Women.* Perigee Books. New York.

EBON, MARTIN. 1978. *The Cloning of Man.* New American Library. New York.

EDMAN, IRWIN, ed. 1956. *The Republic.* In *The Philosophy of Plato.* The Modern Library. New York.

EDWARDS, R. G. 1966. Preliminary attempts to fertilize human oocytes matured in vitro. AJOG. 96(2): 192–200.

——— and B. D. BAVISTER and P. C. STEPTOE. 1969. Early stages of fertilization in vitro of human oocytes matured in vitro. *Nature.* 221: 632–635.

———. 1979. Correspondence with Patrick Steptoe and R. G. Edwards. *Appendix.*

——— and P. C. STEPTOE and J. M. PURDY. 1970. Fertilization and cleavage in vitro of preovular human oocytes. *Nature.* 227: 1307–1309.

——— and RUTH E. FOWLER. 1970. Human embryos in the laboratory. *Scientific American.* 223(6): 44–54.

——— and DAVID SHARPE. 1971. Social values and research in human embryology. *Nature.* 231: 87–91.

———. 1974, March. Fertilization of human eggs in vitro: Morals, ethics and the law. *Quarterly Review of Biology.* 49: 3–6.

——— and PATRICK STEPTOE. 1977, Jan. The relevance of the frozen storage of human embryos. *Ciba, Foundation and Symposium*. 52: 235–250.

——— and PATRICK STEPTOE. 1980. *A Matter of Life*. William Morrow and Co., Inc. New York.

——— and J. M. PURDY. 1980. Establishing full-term human pregnancies using cleaving embryos grown in vitro. BJOG 87(9).

EISENBERG, LEON. 1976. The outcome as cause: predestination and human cloning. *Journal of Medicine and Philosophy*. 1(4): 318–331.

ELIAS, DAVID. 1978, Nov. 2. Test-tube pioneer furious at doubt on technique. *The Australian*.

ELLIOTT, JOHN. 1979. Abortion for "wrong" fetal sex: An ethical-legal dilemma. JAMA. 242(14).

ELLIOTT, JOHN P. 1982, June. The case for antibiotic prophylaxis before some cesareans. COG. 19: 117–127.

ELSDEN, PETER. 1978, Feb. 10. Advances in embryo transfer techniques. *Holstein Friesian World*.

———. 1979, March. Cost, success and advisability of embryo transfer for your herd. *Hereford Journal*.

———. Undated. Embryo transfer and the beef cattle industry. Photocopied sheet obtained from the International Embryo Transfer Society.

EMECHETA, BUCHI. 1979. *The Joys of Motherhood*. George Braziller. New York.

ENGELS, FREDERICK. 1972. *The Origin of the Family, Private Property and the State*. Eleanor Burke Leacock, ed. International Publishers. New York.

ERICSSON, RONALD. 1977, Feb. 22. U.S. Patent 4,009,260.

ETZIONI, AMITAI. 1968, Sept. Sex control, science and society. *Science*.

EVANS, J. M., T. A. DOUGLAS and J. P. RENTON. 1975, Jan. 31. An attempt to separate fractions rich in human Y sperm. *Nature*.

EVHSA. 1979, Sept. 20. *Minutes: Project Review Committee: EVHSA* (Eastern Virginia Health Systems Agency).

———. 1979, Nov. 9. *Staff Recommendation: Certificate of Need Request No. VA-1285, Norfolk General Hospital, Norfolk, Virginia*.

———. Undated. *Consent Form #3, Entitled: Title of Study: Vital Initiation of Pregnancy*. Form filed with EVHSA along with Norfolk General Hospital's application for a Certificate of Need.

FAULKNER, WILLIAM L. and HOWARD W. ORY. 1976. Intrauterine devices and acute pelvic inflammatory diseases. JAMA. 235(17): 1851–1853.

FELDMAN, DAVID M. 1975. *Marital Relations, Birth Control, Abortion in Jewish Law*. Schocken Books. New York.

FEVERSHAM. 1960, July. Report of the Departmental Committee on human artificial insemination. Earl of Feversham, chairman. Her Majesty's Stationery Office. London.

FIGES, EVA. 1970. *Patriarchal Attitudes*. Fawcett Publications, Inc. Greenwich, Conn.

FINKEL, MARION J., presiding. 1978, June 21. *Hearings on Elective Induction of Labor: Injectable Oxytocic Drugs.* Food and Drug Administration. Rockville, Maryland.

FISHER, ELIZABETH. 1979. *Woman's Creation.* McGraw-Hill Book Company. New York.

FLEMING, ANNE TAYLOR. 1980, July 20. New frontiers in conception. *The New York Times Magazine.*

FLEMING, JENNIFER BAKER and CAROLYN WASHBURN. Undated. *For Better or For Worse: A Feminist Handbook for Marriage and Other Options.* Charles Scribners Sons. New York.

FLEMING, SUSAN. 1978, Jan. 4. Babies by proxy: A quandary. *Detroit News.*

FLETCHER, JOHN C. 1979. Sounding board: Ethics and amniocentesis for fetal sex identification. NEJM. 301(10): 550–553.

FLETCHER, JOSEPH. 1974. *The Ethics of Genetic Control: Ending Reproductive Roulette.* Anchor Press/Doubleday. Garden City, New York.

———. 1976. Ethical aspects of genetic controls. In Thomas A. Shannon, ed. *Bioethics.* Paulist Press. New York/Ramsey, N.J.

FOLSOME, CLAIR E. 1943. The status of artificial insemination. AJOG. 45(6): 915–927.

FOOTE, ROBERT H. 1979. In vitro fertilization in perspective, relative to the science and art of domestic animal reproduction. *Appendix.*

FOSS, G. L. 1982. Artificial insemination by donor: A review of 12 years' experience. *J. Biosoc. Sci.* 14: 253–262.

FNP. 1979, Feb. 15. Child from donor insemination legally illegitimate. *Family Practice News.*

FRANCOEUR, ROBERT T. 1970. *Utopian Motherhood.* Doubleday and Co., Inc. Garden City, New York.

FRAZER, JAMES GEORGE. 1972. *The New Golden Bough.* T. H. Gaster, ed. S. G. Phillips, Inc. New York.

FREEDMAN, DEBORAH S., RONALD FREEDMAN and PASCAL K. WHELPTON. Size of family and preference for children of each sex. *Am. J. of Sociology.* 66:141–146.

FREITAS, ROBERT A., JR. 1980, May/June. Fetal adoption: a technological solution to the problem of abortion ethics. *The Humanist.*

FRYE, MARILYN. 1983. *The Politics of Reality: Essays in Feminist Theory.* The Crossing Press. Trumansburg, New York.

GAIR, GEORGE F. 1981. Extract from a report by the National Health and Medical Research Council, which surveyed the status of in vitro fertilization programs in Australia in 1980. Contained in the report of George F. Gair, New Zealand Minister of Health, to Marilyn Waring, Member of Parliament. New Zealand. October 1, 1981.

GARDNER, R. L. and R. G. EDWARDS. 1968. Control of the sex ratio at full term in the rabbit by transferring sexed blastocysts. *Nature.*

GAYLIN, WILLARD. 1972, March 5. We have the awful knowledge to make exact copies of human beings. *New York Times Magazine.*

————. 1974, Feb. On the borders of persuasion: a psychoanalytic look at coercion. *Psychiatry.* 37: 1–9.

GAYNES, MINDY. 1981, July/August. Legal questions surround surrogate parenting. *State Legislatures.*

GILLIE, OLIVER. 1983, May 29. Could a man be a mother? *The Sunday Times* (London): 14.

GLASS, ROBERT H. 1977, January. Sex preselection. *Obstetrics and Gynecology.*

Globe. 1981, Jan. 25. Court orders cesarean if needed to save baby. *Boston Sunday Globe.*

GOGOI, M. P. 1971. Maternal morbidity from cesarean section in infected cases. *J. Obstet. Gynecol.* (Britain) 78: 373.

GOLBUS, MITCHELL, S., et al. 1974. Intrauterine diagnosis of genetic defects: results, problems and follow-up of one hundred cases in a prenatal genetic detection center. AJOG. 118(7): 897–905.

GOLDSTEIN, ARTHUR I., ROBERT C. LUCKESH and MYRNA KETCHUM. 1973, March 15. Prenatal sex determination by fluorescent staining of the cervical smear for the presence of a Y chromosome: An evaluation. AJOG.

GOLDWYN, ROBERT M. Subcutaneous mastectomy. NEJM. 297(9): 503–505.

GOODLIN, ROBERT C. 1963. An improved fetal incubator. *Trans. Amer. Soc. Artif. Int. Organ.* IX: 348–350.

GORDON, A. D. G. 1978, May. Bicarbonate for a boy, vinegar for a girl. *Nursing Times.*

GORDON, LINDA. 1977. *Woman's Body, Woman's Right.* Penguin Books. New York.

GOULD, KENNETH G. 1979. Fertilization in vitro of nonhuman primate ova; present status and rationale for further development of the technique. *Appendix.*

GOULD, STEPHEN JAY. 1981. *The Mismeasure of Man.* W. W. Norton & Company. New York.

GRAHAM, ROBERT KLARK. 1981. *The Future of Man.* Foundation for the Advancement of Man. Escondido, California.

GRAY, ELMER and N. MARLENE MORRISON. 1974. Influence of combinations of sexes of children on family size. *The Journal of Heredity.* 65: 169–174.

GREENHILL, J. P. 1947. Artificial insemination: its medicolegal implications: A symposium. *Amer. Prac.* I(5):227–241.

GREGOIRE, A. T. and ROBERT C. MAYER. 1965. The impregnators. *Fertility and Sterility.* 16(1): 130–134.

GREINER, TED. 1975. The promotion of bottle feeding by multinational corporations: How advertising and the health professions have contributed. Booklet.

GRIFFIN, SUSAN. 1978. *Woman and Nature.* Harper & Row. New York.

GROBSTEIN, CLIFFORD. 1979. External human fertilization. *Scientific American.*

————. 1981. *From Chance to Purpose: An Appraisal of External Human Fertilization.* Addison-Wesley Publishing Co. Reading, Mass.

GROSSET, L., V. BARRELET, and N. ODARTCHENKO. 1974. Antenatal fetal sex determination from maternal blood during early pregnancy. AJOG. 120(1): 60–63.

GROSSMAN, EDWARD. 1971. The obsolescent mother. *The Atlantic Monthly.* 227(5).

GUERREO, RODRIGO. 1974, Nov. 14. Association of the type and time of insemination within the menstrual cycle with the human sex ratio at birth. NEJM.

GUITTON, JEAN. 1967. *Feminine Fulfillment.* Paulist Press Deus Books. New York.

GUNBY, PHIL. 1979. Sex selection before child's conception. JAMA. 241(12): 1220–1226.

GUPTA, RANJAN. 1981, June 26. Jibes put test-tube baby pioneer on path to suicide. *Sydney Morning Herald.*

GURDON, J. B. 1962. The developmental capacity of nuclei taken from intestinal epithelium cells of feeding tadpoles. *J. Embryol. Exp. Morph.* 10(4): 622–640.

HAGEN, D. 1975. Maternal febrile morbidity associated with fetal monitoring and cesarean section. *Obstet. Gynecol.* 46: 260.

HALES, DIANNE. 1981, Aug. 26. Surrogate moms' motivation complex, but money figures. *Medical Tribune.*

HALLER, MARK H. 1963. *Eugenics: Hereditarian Attitudes in American Thought.* Rutgers University Press. New Brunswick, N.J.

HANMER, JALNA. 1984. A womb of one's own. In R. Arditti, R. Duelli-Klein and S. Minden, eds., *Test Tube Women.* Routledge & Kegan Paul. Boston and London.

————. 1981. Sex predetermination, artificial insemination and the maintenance of male-dominated culture. In H. Roberts, ed., *Women, Health and Reproduction.* Routledge & Kegan Paul. London.

———— and PAT ALLEN. 1980. Reproductive engineering—the final solution? In Brighton Women and Science Collective, ed., *Alice Through the Microscope: The Power of Science over Women's Lives.* Virago. London.

HARLAP, SUSAN. 1979, June 28. Gender of infants conceived on different days of the menstrual cycle. NEJM.

HARRIS, MURIEL. 1978, Nov. 2. Louise: the test-tube miracle. *Nursing Mirror.*

HARRIS, SEALE. 1950. *Woman's Surgeon.* Macmillan Co. New York.

HARRISON, MICHELLE. 1982. *A Woman in Residence.* Random House. New York.

HARTLEY, RUTH E., FRANCIS P. HARDESTY and DAVID S. GORFEIN. 1962. Children's perceptions and expressions of sex preference. *Child Development.* 33: 221–227.

HAYS, H. R. 1964. *The Dangerous Sex.* G. P. Putnam's Sons. New York.

HERON, FRAN. 1981, May 26. Carla is born—and she's a little miracle. *Daily Mirror* (Sydney).

HIBBARD, LESTER T. 1976. Changing trends in cesarean section. AJOG. 125(6).

HICKS, RON. 1980, Dec. 23/30. Australia leads world in "test tube" baby techniques. *The Bulletin* (Australia).

HILLEL, MARC and CLARISSA HENRY. 1976. *Of Pure Blood.* McGraw-Hill Book Company. New York.

HINKLE, WARREN. 1980, May 13. Why Eldridge Cleaver is a wife-beater. *San Francisco Chronicle.*

HIRSCHHORN, KURT. 1968, May 17. On re-doing man. *Commonweal.* 260.

HOBBINS, JOHN C., et al. 1979. How safe is ultrasound in obstetrics? COG. 14. Special issue.

HODGEN, GARY D. 1983. Surrogate embryo transfer combined with estrogen-progesterone therapy in monkeys. JAMA. 250(16): 2167–2171.

HOOBLER, B. RAYMOND. 1917, April 11. Problems connected with the collection and production of human milk. JAMA.

HOWARD, TED and JEREMY RIFKIN. 1977. *Who Should Play God?* Dell Publishing Co. New York.

HUBBARD, RUTH. 1981. The case against in vitro fertilization. In H. Holmes, B. Hoskins and M. Gross, eds., *The Custom-Made Child?* Humana Press. Clifton, N.J.

——— and MARY SUE HENIFIN and BARBARA FRIED, eds. 1979. *Women Look at Biology Looking at Women.* Schenkman Publishing Co. Cambridge, Mass.

HULL, GLORIA T., et al., 1981. *All the Women Are White, All the Blacks are Men, But Some of Us Are Brave.* The Feminist Press. Old Westbury, New York.

HULKA, J. F. Report of the Ad Hoc Committee on Artificial Insemination. American Fertility Society. Committee formed in 1980 and chaired by Hulka.

HUTCHINS, ROBERT MAYNARD, ed. 1952. *Summa Theologica.* Great Books of the Western World. 19. Thomas Aquinas: I. Vol. I. Encyclopedia Britannica Co., Inc. Chicago.

ILLMENSEE, KARL and PETER C. HOPPE. 1981. Nuclear transplantation in Mus Musculus: Developmental potential of nuclei from preimplantation embryos. *Cell.* 23: 9–11.

INCE, SUSAN. 1984. Inside the surrogate industry. In R. Arditti, R. Duelli-Klein and S. Minden, eds., *Test-Tube Women.* Routledge & Kegan Paul. Boston and London.

INTERNATIONAL EMBRYO TRANSFER SOCIETY (IETS). 1981 Directory of Members. (LaPorte, Colorado).

———. IETS PROCEEDINGS, 1982, Jan. 17. Proceedings of the owners and managers workshop: 8th annual meeting of the International Embryo Transfer Society. Denver, Colorado.

JAMA. 1939, May 6. Artificial insemination and illegitimacy. JAMA. 112(18): 1832–1833.

———. 1972, June 5. Genetic engineering: Reprise. JAMA. 220(10): 1356–1357.

———. 1979, March 23. Artificial insemination by donor: Survey reveals surprising facts. JAMA. 241(12): 1219.

———. 1979, March 23. Sex selection before child's conception. JAMA. 241(12).

———. 1982, April 23/30. Question of risk still hovers over routine prenatal use of ultrasound. JAMA. 247(16): 2195–2197.

JANSEN, ROBERT P. S. 1982. Spontaneous abortion incidence in the treatment of infertility: Addendum on in vitro fertilization. AJOG. 144(6): 738–739.

JASZCZAK, S. E. and E. S. E. HAFEZ. Undated. Factors affecting in situ recovery of embryos in human and nonhuman primates. *Archives of Andrology.* 5(1): 90.

JME. 1978. Case conference, "Lesbian couples: Should help extend to AID? *Journal of Medical Ethics.* 4: 91–95.

JOHNSTON, IAN. 1981. Selection of patients and the place of spontaneous or stimulated cycles. In A. W. Walters and Carl Wood, eds., *VII Asian and Oceanic Congress of Obstetrics and Gynaecology, Melbourne, 1981, Scientific Proceedings.* Printed by Ramsay Ware Stockland Pty. Ltd. Melbourne.

JONES, Ann. 1980. *Women Who Kill.* Holt, Rinehart and Winston. New York.

JONES, HOWARD W., JR. 1982. The ethics of in vitro fertilization—1982. *Fertility and Sterility.* (37)2: 146–149.

———. 1983. Variations on a theme. JAMA. 250(16): 2182–2183.

——— et al. 1983. What is a pregnancy? A question for programs of in vitro fertilization. *Fertility & Sterility.* 40(6): 728–733.

JONES, O. HUNTER. 1976. Cesarean section in present-day obstetrics. AJOG. 126(5): 521–530.

JONES, R. C. 1971, Feb. 19. Uses of artificial insemination. *Nature.* 229.

JONES, ROGER J. 1973, June. Sex predetermination and the sex ratio at birth. *Social Biology.* 20(2): 203–211.

JONES, SYL. 1980, Aug. Playboy interview: William Shockley. *Playboy.*

JRM. 1973. In vitro fertilization of human ova and blastocyst transfer: An invitational symposium. *J. of Reproductive Medicine.* 11(5): 192–204.

KAMIN, L. 1974. *The Science and Politics of IQ.* Halsted Press, New York. Quoted in Lewontin, R. C., Biological Determinism as a social weapon. In Ann Arbor Science for the People, ed. *Biology As a Social Weapon.* Burgess, Minneapolis.

KANDELL, JONATHAN. 1974, March 17. Argentina, hoping to double her population in this century, is taking action to restrict birth control. NYT.

———. 1978, June 6. French ex-premier seeking to foster population growth. NYT.

KAP SOON JU, et al. 1976. Prenatal sex determination by observation of the x-chromatin and the y-chromatin of exfoliated amniotic fluid cells. *Obstetrics and Gynecology.* 47(3): 287–290.

KAPLAN, BRUCE. 1981, July 5. Frozen baby soon: Brave new world coming closer. *Daily Telegraph* (Sydney).

KARP, LAURENCE E. 1978, Oct. Novel mechanisms of reproduction: Preimplantational ectogenesis. *Postgraduate Medicine.*

——— and ROGER P. DONAHUE. 1976. Preimplantation ectogenesis. *The Western Journal of Medicine.* 124(4).

KASAI, M., K. NIWA and A. IRITANI. 1981. Effects of various cryoprotective agents in the survival of frozen mouse embryos. *J. of Reproduction and Fertility.* 63:175–180.

KASS, LEON. 1971. Babies by means of in vitro fertilization: Unethical experiments on the unborn? NEJM. 285: 1174–1179.

———. 1972. Making babies. The new biology and the "old" morality. *Public Interest.* 26: 19–56.

———. 1979, Winter. "Making babies" revisited. *The Public Interest.* 54.

———. 1979. Ethical issues in human in vitro fertilization, embryo culture and research, and embryo transfer. *Appendix.*

KASSELL, PAULA. 1982, March/April. Male pride equals too many children. *New Directions for Women.*

KATZ, BARBARA F. 1979, May 4. Legal implications of in vitro fertilization and its regulation. *Appendix.*

KEANE, NOEL P., with DENNIS L. BREO. 1981. *The Surrogate Mother.* Everest House. New York.

KEELER, CLYDE E. 1960. *Secrets of the Cuna Earthmother.* Exposition Press. New York.

KENNEDY, JOSEPH F. and ROGER P. DONAHUE. 1969, June 13. Human oocytes: maturation in chemically defined media. *Science.* 164: 1292–1293.

KERN, PATRICIA A. and KATHLEEN M. RIDOLFI. 1982. The Fourteenth Amendment's protection of a woman's right to be a single parent through artificial insemination by donor. *Women's Rights Law bReporter.* 7(3): 251–284.

KEYE, WILLIAM R. 1982, March. Strategy for avoiding iatrogenic infertility. COG. 19: 185–195.

KIEFFER, GEORGE H. 1979. *Bioethics: A Textbook of Issues.* Addison-Wesley Publishing Co. Reading, Mass.

KITZINGER, SHELIA. 1978. *Women As Mothers.* Vintage Books. New York.

KLEIMAN, DENA. 1979, Dec. 16. Anguished search to cure infertility. *New York Times Magazine.*

KLEMESRUD, JUDY. 1983, Jan. 17. Fertilization clinic to open in New York. NYT.

KOBRIN, FRANCES E. 1966, July/August. The American midwife controversy: A crisis of professionalization. *Bulletin of the History of Medicine.* 40: 350–363.

KOLATA, GINA. 1983. In vitro fertilization goes commercial. *Science.* 221: 1160–1161.

KRANZ, KERMIT E., THEODORE C. PANOS and JAMES EVANS. 1962. Physiology of maternal–fetal relationship through extracorporeal circulation of the human placenta. AJOG 86(9): 1214–1228.

KRIER, BETH ANN. 1981, Nov. 10. The moral and legal problems of surrogate parenting. *Los Angeles Times.*

KRITCHEVSKY, BARBARA. 1981. The unmarried woman's right to artificial insemination: A call for an expanded definition of family. *Harvard Women's Law Journal.* 4(1).

KRUCOFF, CAROL. 1980, Nov. 9. Surrogate parenting is controversial birth technique. *Hartford Courant* (Connecticut).

LANGER, G., et al. 1969. Artificial insemination: A study of 156 successful cases. *Int. J. of Fertility.* 14(3): 232–240.

LAPPE, MARC. 1974, Feb. Choosing the sex of our children. *Hastings Center Report.*

LAUDERDALE, JAMES W., and JAMES H. SOKOLOWSKI, eds. 1979, Aug. 6–8. A historical overview of estrus control in the bovine. *Proceedings of the Lutalyse Symposium.* The Upjohn Co.

LAUERMAN, CONNIE. 1977, Dec. 4. Surrogate-mother law: Will it be conceived? *Chicago Tribune.*

LAUERSEN, NIELS and EILEEN STUKANE. 1982, Nov. New ways of making babies: How science can help! *Cosmopolitan.* 193: 262.

LAWN, L., and R. A. McCANCE. 1961. Ventures with an artificial placenta. I. Principles and preliminary results. 155: 500–509. In *Proceedings of the Royal Society: Series B: Biological Sciences.* London. April 10, 1962.

LEACH, GERALD. 1970. *The Biocrats.* McGraw-Hill Book Company. New York.

LEDERBERG, JOSHUA. 1966, Oct. Experimental genetics and human evolution. *Bulletin of the Atomic Scientists.* Pp. 4–11.

LEDERER, WOLFGANG. 1968. *The Fear of Women.* Harcourt Brace Jovanovich, Inc. New York.

LEE, BRIAN. 1980, Dec. 18/25. And now—test tube twins on the way. *New Scientist.*

LEETON, JOHN. 1981, June. The transfer of human embryos. *Modern Medicine of Australia.* Pp. 32–35.

LEHEW, WILLETTE L. 1979, Oct. 31. Testimony presented at public hearing held by the Eastern Virginia Health Systems Agency, Norfolk, Va.

LEIBO, S. P. and PETER MAZUR. 1978. Methods for the preservation of mammalian embryos by freezing. In Joseph C. Daniel, Jr., ed., *Methods in Mammalian Reproduction.* Academic Press, Inc. New York.

LEIMAN, SID Z. 1979. Human in vitro fertilization: A Jewish perspective. *Appendix.*

LERNER, GERDA. 1973. *Black Women in White America.* Vintage Books. New York.

LEVIE, L. H. 1972. Donor insemination in Holland. *World Medical Journal.* 19(5).

LEVIN, ARTHUR. 1978, Nov. Artificial fertilization: The newest therapy. *Parents.*

LICHTMAN, WENDY. 1982. *The Boy Who Wanted a Baby.* The Feminist Press. Old Westbury, New York.

LIEDHOLM, P., P. SUNDSTRÖM and H. WRAMSKY. Undated. A model for experimental studies on human egg transfer. *Archives of Andrology.* 5(1): 92.

Life. 1965, Sept. 10. A test-tube colony.

LISTER, JOHN. 1978, Sept. 28. Extrauterine conception—More uniformity?— Operation dump. NEJM: 705–707.

LOCHBILER, PETER R. 1978, May 4. Proxy moms bear babies for two childless couples. *Detroit News.*

LOCKAMY, SUSAN. 1979, Dec. 5. Health board to ask genetics lab approval. *Virginian–Pilot.*

LOPATA, A., et al. 1978. In vitro fertilization of preovulatory human eggs. *J. Reprod. Fert.* 52: 339–342.

———. 1980. Pregnancy following intrauterine implantation of an embryo obtained by in vitro fertilization of a preovulatory egg. *Fertility and Sterility.* 33(2).

———. 1982. Embryonic development and blastocyst implantation following in vitro fertilization and embryo transfer. *Fertility and Sterility.* 38(6): 682.

LUCE, CLARE BOOTHE. 1978, Aug. 6. Fewer moms would slow pop clock. *Seattle Times.*

LYGRE, DAVID G. 1979. *Life Manipulation: From Test-Tube Babies to Aging.* Walker and Co. New York.

LYNCH, PAUL. 1983, April 27. Peril seen in donor system of in-vitro birth. *The Australian.*

LYONS, RICHARD D. 1983, July 22. 2 women become pregnant with transferred embryos. NYT.

MACKINNON, CATHARINE A. 1979. *Sexual Harassment of Working Women.* Yale University Press. New Haven and London.

MALHOTRA, INDER. 1982, July 19. Alarm at girl foetus scandal. *The Guardian.*

MANUEL, MAY, I. J. PARK and HOWARD W. JONES, JR. 1974, July 15. Prenatal sex determination by fluorescent staining of cells for the presence of y chromatin. AJOG.

MARGO, JILL. 1981, July 31. Men can bear children ... at least that's the theory. *Sydney Morning Herald.*

MARIESKIND, HELEN I. 1979, June. An evaluation of cesarean section in the United States. Report submitted to the U.S. Department of Health, Education and Welfare.

MARKLE, GERALD E. and CHARLES B. NAM. 1971. Sex predetermination: Its impact on fertility. *Social Biology.* 18(1): 73–83.

MARTINEZ, GILBERT A. and JOHN P. NALEZIENSKI. 1979. The recent trend in breast-feeding. *Pediatrics.* 64(5): 686–715.

MARX, JEAN L. 1983, June 17. Bar Harbor investigation reveals no fraud. *Science.* 220: 1254.

MASON, JIM and PETER SINGER. 1980. *Animal Factories.* Crown Publishers, Inc. New York.

MASTROIANNI, LUIGI. 1979, May 4. In vitro fertilization and embryo transfer. *Appendix.*

—— and CARLOS NORIEGA. 1970. Observations on human ova and the fertilization process. AJOG. 107(5): 682–690.

MAULE, JAMES EDWARD. 1982, Sept. Federal tax consequences of surrogate motherhood. *Taxes—The Tax Magazine.* Pp. 656–668.

McCARTHY, DON. 1980, May. Parenting and technology. *Boston Pilot.*

McCORDUCK, PAMELA. 1981, June. Babies from the lab. *Redbook.*

McGRATH, JAMES and DAVOR SOLTER. 1983, June 17. Nuclear transplantation in the mouse embryo by microsurgery and cell fusion. *Science.* 220: 1300–1302.

McLAUGHLIN, LORETTA. 1982. *The Pill, John Rock, and the Church.* Little, Brown & Company. Boston. Toronto.

McLEAN, STUART. 1980, June 24. Tiny test tube baby beating all odds. *Daily Telegraph* (Sydney).

——. 1981, March 30. Third test tube baby's 'a little Ripper.' *Daily Telegraph.*

McMASTER, R., et al. 1978. Penetration of human eggs by human spermatozoa in vitro. *Biology of Reproduction.* 19: 212–216.

McMULLEN, JAY, reporter. 1979, Oct. 30. Transcript of CBS Reports: The Babymakers.

McNULTY, FAITH. 1981. *The Burning Bed.* Bantam Books. New York.

MEAD, MARGARET. 1939. *From the South Seas.* William Morrow & Co., Inc. New York.

MEHLER, BARRY. 1983, May/June. The new eugenics: Academic racism in the U.S. today. *Science for the People.*

MELROSE, JULIE. Preface to, *The Harp That's Singing: Interviews with Feminist Writers.* Forthcoming.

MENKIN, MIRIAM F. and JOHN ROCK. 1948. IVF and cleavage of human ovarian eggs. AJOG. 55(3): 440–452.

MENNING, BARBARA ECK. 1977. *Infertility.* Prentice-Hall, Inc. Englewood Cliffs, New Jersey.

——. 1980, Oct. The emotional needs of infertile couples. *Fertility and Sterility.* 34(4): 313–319.

————. 1981. In defense of in vitro fertilization. In H. Holmes, B. Hoskins and M. Gross, eds., *The Custom-Made Child?* The Humana Press. Clifton, New Jersey.

————. 1981, Oct. Donor insemination: the psychosocial issues. COG. 18: 155–172.

MERZ, BEVERLY. 1984. Stock breeding technique applied to human infertility. JAMA. 250(10): 1257.

METHERELL, MARK. 1982, Sept. 1. Test-tube ethics: Doctor calls for study. *The Age* (Melbourne).

————. 1983, March 3. Female babies dominate world of the test tube. *The Age.*

METTLER, L. and K. SEMM. 1980. Follicular puncture for human ovum recovery via pelviscopy. *Archives of Andrology.* 5(1): 87–89.

MEYER, HERMAN F. 1968. Breast-feeding in the United States: Report of a 1966 national survey with comparable 1946 and 1956 data. *Clinical Pediatrics.* 7(12): 708–715.

MILLER, ROBERT H. 1983. Surrogate parenting: An infant industry presents society with legal, ethical questions. OGN. 18(3).

MILLET, KATE. 1970. *Sexual Politics.* Doubleday. Garden City, N.Y.

MILLIGAN, DEBI. 1981, June. Sexually transmitted diseases: Neglected concerns in infertility. *Resolve.* P. 5.

MILLINER, KAREN. 1984, May 17. In-vitro babies better adjusted: team leader. *Canberra Times* (Australia).

MINDEN, SHELLEY. 1981, Nov. Sex selection. *Second Opinion.*

MOHR, JAMES C. 1978. *Abortion in America.* Oxford University Press. New York.

MONAGHAM, PATRICIA. 1981. *The Book of Goddesses and Heroines.* E. P. Dutton, New York.

MORAGA, CHERRIE and GLORIA ANZALDINA. 1981. *This Bridge Called My Back.* Persephone Press. Watertown, Mass.

MORAN, JOHN F. 1915, Jan. 9. The endowment of motherhood. JAMA.

MORGAN, ROBIN. 1970. *Sisterhood Is Powerful.* Vintage Books. New York.

————. 1982. *The Anatomy of Freedom.* Anchor Press/Doubleday. New York.

MORGAN, SUSANNE. 1982. *Coping with a Hysterectomy.* The Dial Press. New York.

————. 1978. *Hysterectomy.* A pamphlet that is a collaborative effort of the Feminist History Research Project and the Boston Women's Health Book Collective, Inc.

MULLAN, PATRICIA A. 1980, May 1. Surrogate parenting association sparks interest at AFS meeting. OGN.

————. 1980. Experts consider Nobel Prize winners' sperm bank a sham. OGN. 15(10).

MULLER, H. J. 1935. *Out of the Night: A Biologist's View of the Future.* The Vanguard Press, Inc. New York.

———. 1959. The guidance of human evolution. *Perspectives in Biology and Medicine.* III(1).

———. 1961. Human evolution by voluntary choice of germ plasm. *Science.* 134(348).

MULLIGAN, JOAN E. 1976. Professional transition: Nurse to nurse-widwife. *Nursing Outlook.* 24(4): 228–233.

MURCHE, JOHN. 1978, July 27. Test-tube baby brings hope to childless women. *Daily Telegraph.*

MURRAY, FINNIE A. 1978. Embryo transfer in large domestic mammals. In Joseph C. Daniel, Jr., ed. *Methods in Mammalian Reproduction.* Academic Press. New York.

MWN. 1979, Feb. 19. Dr. Steptoe's full report—at last. *Medical World News.*

NATHANSON, BERNARD, with RICHARD N. OSTLING. 1979. *Aborting America.* Pinnacle Books. New York.

Nature. 1973, June 15. *Bullseye.* 243: 371.

NBC. 1980, Nov. 8. "Surrogate mother: Elizabeth Kane." *NBC Magazine.*

NESBITT, R. E. L., JR., et al. 1970. In vitro perfusion studies of the human placenta; a newly-designed apparatus for extracorporeal perfusion achieving dual closed circulation. *Gynec. Invet.* 1: 185–203.

NETWIG, RUTH E. 1980. Technical aspects of sex preselection. In H. Holmes, B. Hoskins and M. Gross, eds., *The Custom-Made Child?* Humana Press. Clifton, N.J.

NEUMANN, ERICH. 1974. *The Great Mother.* Princeton University Press. Princeton, N.J.

Newsweek. 1982, July 16. The sperm-bank scandal.

NIH. 1984. The use of diagnostic ultrasound imaging in pregnancy. Draft. National Institutes of Health Consensus Development Conference Tentative Consensus Statement.

———. NIH Publication No. 79-1973. 1979, April. *Antenatal Diagnosis.* U.S. Department of Health, Education and Welfare.

NJI. 1978. Welcome, Miss Test-Tube! *The Nursing Journal of India.* LXIX(8).

NORMAN, COLIN. 1984, March 2. No fraud found in Swiss study. *Science.* 223: 913.

NOYES, R. W., et al. 1965, Feb. Pronuclear ovum from a patient using an interuterine contraceptive device. *Science.* Pp. 744–745.

NT. 1981, March 15. Aborigines given birth control drug banned in the U.S. *National Times* (Australia).

NYT. 1980, May 17. Surrogate mothers: a controversial solution to infertility.

———. 1980, Nov. 23. Gestation, Inc.

———. 1981, March 8. Woman gives birth to boy in disputed surrogate case.

———. 1981, March 25. Surrogate mother-to-be fights to keep unborn child.

———. 1981, April 2. Love for sale.

———. 1981, June 5. Baby's father agrees to withdraw his suit over surrogate birth.

———. 1981, Oct. 28. A surrogate mother proposal.

———. 1982, Jan. 29. Embryo "donation" criticized.

———. 1984, June 18. Embryos' future in question.

———. 1984, June 23. Australia dispute arises on embryos.

O'BRIEN, MARY. 1981. *The Politics of Reproduction.* Routledge & Kegan Paul, Ltd. London and Boston.

O'FAOLAIN, JULIA and LAURO MARTINES, eds. 1973. *Not in God's Image.* Harper & Row. New York.

OGN. 1980, Jan. 1. Laws on donor insemination held weak. 15(1).

———. 1980, April 15. Unmarried woman to become surrogate mother.

———. 1980, June 1. PID epidemic today, infertility tomorrow.

———. 1980, June 1. Predictions of fetal sex: A cautionary tale.

———. 1980, June 1. "Vasectomy insurance" misleading because future fertility of sperm not guaranteed.

———. 1980, Dec. 1. Suit impels fertility clinic to alter stand on marital status.

———. 1980, May 15. Fertilized human eggs can be recovered but not yet transferred.

———. 1981, Feb. 15. Ob. Gyns disagree over benefit/risk value of using ultrasound routinely in pregnancy.

———. 1981, May 15. Surrogate mother's right to renege is challenged.

———. 1981, Aug. 15. Most potential surrogate mothers deny they would feel loss.

———. 1981, Nov. 15. Sonography termed accurate to establish optimal time for harvesting an oocyte.

———. 1983, Feb. 15. Bonding held greater in fathers of infants delivered by cesarean.

———. 1983, April 1. Deformed infant rejection may spur Mich. surrogate parent law.

———. 1983, June 1. Maintenance of brain-dead gravida held viable course.

———. 1983, July 1. Australia studying ethics of using donor oocytes.

———. 1983, Aug. In-vitro fertilization nearly as efficient as normal reproduction. 18(15).

———. 1983, Aug. 15. Obs face ethical questions raised by in-vitro, in-vivo fertilization.

———. 1983, Dec. 1. Ovum donor transfer may see wide use in treating infertility.

OPPENHEIMER, W. 1959. Prevention of pregnancy by the Grafenberg ring method: A re-evaluation after 28 years' experience. AJOG. 87: 446–454.

PACKARD, VANCE. 1977. *The People Shapers.* Bantam Books. New York.

PARENTS. 1978, Nov. Test tube babies: For or against?

PARKER, PHILIP J. Undated. Surrogate motherhood—an opinion essay.

———. 1982. Surrogate motherhood: The interaction of litigation, legislation, and psychiatry. *International Journal of Law and Psychiatry.* 5(2/4).

———. 1982, Nov. 20. The psychology of surrogate motherhood: An updated report of a longitudinal pilot study. Presented at the Inter-Disciplinary Surrogate Mother Symposium at Wayne State University.

———. 1983. Motivation of surrogate mothers: Initial findings. *American Journal of Psychiatry.* 140(1).

PARKER, ROY. 1979, Oct. 31. Testimony presented at Eastern Virginia Health Systems Agency public hearing.

———. 1979, Nov. 22. To aid childless couples. *Virginian–Pilot.*

PB. 1978, Jan. Boys or girls? Parents' preferences and sex control. *Population Bulletin.*

PEARCE, DIANA and HARRIETTE MCADOO. 1981, Sept. Women and children: Alone and in poverty. Pamphlet prepared for the National Advisory Council on Economic Opportunity. Available for $2 from Diana Pearce, The Center for National Policy Review. Catholic University Law School. Washington, D.C. 20064.

PEEL REPORT. 1973, April 7. Appendix V: Report of panel on human artificial insemination. *British Medical Journal Supplement.*

PEMBREY, MARCUS. 1979, Oct. 13. Letter. *Lancet.*

People. 1983, Aug. 8. A UCLA doctor, first to transplant human embryos, offers hope to infertile women. 20(6).

PEPPERELL, ROGER J. 1983. A rational approach to ovulation induction. *Fertility & Sterility.* 40(11): 1–14.

PERSSON, P. H., et al. Undated. Ultrasonic determination of the optimal time for harvesting human eggs. *Archives of Andrology.* 5(1): 93–94.

PFAFFLIN, FRIEDEMANN. 1983, Nov. 22–26. The connection between eugenics, sterilisation and mass murder in Germany 1933–1945. Paper read at the annual meeting of the International Academy of Sex Research. Arden House, New York. Translation by Derek Brunt.

——— and JAN GROSS. 1982. Involuntary sterilization in Germany from 1933 to 1945 and some consequences for today. *Int. J. of Law and Psychiatry.* 5: 419–423.

PICKERING, GEORGE. 1966, July. Reflections on research and the future of medicine. *Science.*

PINCUS, GREGORY and BARBARA SAUNDERS. Undated. The comparative behavior of mammalian eggs in vivo and in vitro. VI. The matural of human ovarian ova. *The Anatomical Record.* 75(4) and supplement: 537–545.

POHLMAN, EDWARD. 1967. Some effects of being able to control sex of offspring. *Eugenics Quarterly.* 14(4): 274–281.

POMEROY, SARAH B. 1975. *Goddesses, Whores, Wives and Slaves.* Schocken Books. New York.

POSTGATE, JOHN. 1973, April 5. Bat's chance in hell. *New Scientist.*

POWLEDGE, TABITHA N. 1978, Oct. A report from the Del Zio trial. *Hastings Center Report.*

————. 1981. Unnatural selection: on choosing children's sex. In H. Holmes, B. Hoskins and M. Gross, eds., *The Custom-Made Child?* The Humana Press, Inc. Clifton, N.J.

PROCEEDINGS. 1919. *The proceedings of the International Conference of Women Physicians.* The Woman's Press. New York. Available at the Rudolf Matas Medical Library, Elizabeth Bass Collection, Tulane Medical School, New Orleans.

RAMANAMMA, A. and USHA BAMBAWALI. 1980. The mania for sons: an analysis of social values in South Asia. *Social Science and Medicine.* 14B: 107–110.

RAMSEY, PAUL. 1970. *Fabricated Man: The Ethics of Genetic Control.* Yale University Press. New Haven, Conn.

————. 1972. Shall we "reproduce"? JAMA. 220.

RANDEL, JUDITH. 1981. Breeding the perfect cow. *Science.* 2(9).

RASSABY, ALAN A. 1982. Surrogate motherhood: The position and problems of substitutes. In W. Walters and P. Singer, eds., *Test-Tube Babies.* Oxford University Press. Melbourne.

RAYMOND, JANICE. 1979. Fetishism, feminism and genetic technology. Paper given at American Association for the Advancement of Science meeting in Houston, Texas.

————. 1979. *The Transsexual Empire.* Beacon Press. Boston.

————. 1981. Sex preselection: A response. In H. B. Holmes, B. Hoskins and M. Gross, eds., *The Custom-Made Child?* The Humana Press. Clifton, N.J.

RCOG. 1983, March. Report of the RCOG Ethics Committee on in vitro fertilization embryo replacement or transfer. Royal College of Obstetricians and Gynaecologists. Available from: RCOG, 27 Sussex Place, Regent's Park, London NW1 4RG.

REED, SHELDON C. 1968. Eugenics tomorrow. In K. R. Dronamraju, ed., *Haldane and Modern Biology.* The Johns Hopkins Press. Baltimore, Md.

RENT, CLYDA S. and GEORGE S. RENT. 1977. More on offspring-sex preference: A comment on Nancy E. Williamsons' "Sex preferences, sex control, and the status of women." *Signs.* 3(2).

REVELLE, ROGER. 1974, Nov. 14. On rhythm and sex ratio. NEJM.

RHEINGOLD, JOSEPH C. 1964. *The Fear of Being a Woman: A Theory of Maternal Destructiveness.* Grune & Stratton, Inc. New York.

RHINE, SAMUEL A., et al. 1975. Prenatal sex detection with endocervical smears: Successful results utilizing Y-body fluorescence. AJOG. 122(2): 155–160.

RICE, THURMAN B. 1929. *Racial Hygiene.* Macmillan. New York.

RICH, ADRIENNE. 1977. *Of Woman Born.* Bantam. New York.

————. 1980. Compulsory heterosexuality and lesbian existence. In Catharine R. Stimpson and Ethel Spector Person, eds., *Women: Sex and Sexuality.* University of Chicago Press. Chicago.

RICHART, RALPH M., ed. 1980, Oct. Uterine anomalies of DES progeny. COG.

———. 1981, Jan. Ovarian abscesses in IUD wearers. COG.

RIFKIN, JEREMY. *Algeny.* The Viking Press. New York.

RIOUX, JACQUES-E. 1980. 100 Years/1001 methods of female sterilization. Paper presented at the Centennial Conference on Voluntary Sterilization for Women, June 12–13, 1980 in Monterey, California.

RINEHART, WARD. 1975, May. Sex preselection: not yet practical. *Population Reports.* 1(2).

ROBERTS, ALUN M. 1978. The origins of fluctuations in the human secondary sex ratio. *J. Biosoc. Sci.* 10: 169–182.

ROBERTS, KATHERINE. 1977, July. The intrauterine device as a health risk. *Women and Health.*

ROBERTS, PETER. 1981, July 25. One small miracle of creation. *The Age* (Australia).

———. 1981, July 30. Men may be able to bear children. *The Age.*

———. 1981, July 31. Some men keen to volunteer as mothers. *The Age.*

ROBERTSON, WILLIAM C. 1961. Breast-feeding practices: Some implications of regional variations. *American Journal of Public Health.* 51(7): 1035–1042.

ROCK, JOHN and ARTHUR T. HERTIG. 1948. The human conceptus during the first two weeks of gestation. AJOG. 55(1): 6–17.

ROCK, JOHN and MIRIAM F. MENKIN. 1944. In vitro fertilization and cleavage of human ovarian eggs. *Science.* 100(2588): 105–107.

———. 1948. In vitro fertilization and cleavage of human ovarian eggs. AJOG. 55(3): 440–452.

ROHLEDER, HERMANN. 1934. *Test Tube Babies.* Panurge Press. New York.

RORVIK, DAVID. 1971, May 18. The test tube baby is coming. *Look.*

———. 1981, May. Penthouse interview: Dr. Shettles. *Penthouse.* 12.

——— with LANDRUM B. SHETTLES. 1971. *Your Baby's Sex: Now You Can Choose.* Bantam. New York.

ROSE, HILARY and JALNA HANMER. 1976. Women's reproduction and the technological fix. In D. Barker and S. Allen, eds., *Sexual Divisions and Society: Process and Change.*

ROSENZWEIG, SAUL and STUART ADELMAN. 1976. Parental predetermination of the sex of offspring: The attitudes of young married couples with university education. *J. Biosoc. Sci.* 8: 335–346.

ROSNER, FRED. 1979. The biblical and Talmudic secret for choosing one's baby's sex. *Israel J. Med. Sci.* 15(9): 784–787.

ROSS, A. and J. A. ROBINSON and H. J. EVANS. 1975, Jan. 31. Failure to confirm separation of X-and-Y-bearing human sperm using BSA gradients. *Nature.* 253: 354–355.

ROSTAND, JEAN. 1959. *Can Man Be Modified?* Basic Books. New York.

RTC. 1981. Depo report. *Right To Choose.* (Australia) 22.

RUBIN, BERNARD. 1965, Aug. Psychological aspects of human artificial insemination. *Arch. Gen. Psychiat.* 13.

SACKETT, GENE P. 1979. A nonhuman primate research model of developmental risk following in vitro fertilization and embryo transfer. *Appendix.*

SAMMONS, JAMES H. 1977, May 9. Testimony. House Hearings on Costs and Quality of Surgery. I.

SANDLER, BERNARD. 1972. Donor insemination in England. *World Medical Journal.* 19(5).

SANTAMARIA, B. A. 1982, Oct. 5. Producing embryos for the Strangelove society? *The Australian.*

SARMA, VIMALA. 1982, Dec. 30. Ethical problems of "test-tube" children under scrutiny. *The Canberra Times* (Australia).

SCHAUBLE, JOHN. 1984, May 17. Babies: They're better from glass. *Sydney Morning Herald* (Australia).

SCHEIDT, PETER C., et al. 1978. One-year follow-up of infants exposed to ultrasound in utero. AJOG. 131(7): 743–781.

SCHLEIFER, HARRIET. 1982, July. Reviews. *Agenda.*

SCHLESSELMAN, JAMES. 1979. How does one assess the risks of abnormalities from human in vitro fertilization? AJOG. 135(1): 135–148.

SCHMECK, HAROLD M., JR. 1981, Aug. 10. Frozen mice embryos banked. NYT.

——. 1983, June 14. "Prenatal adoption" is the objective of new technique. NYT.

——. 1983, Oct. 28. Births to monkeys without ovaries may offer hope to infertile women. NYT.

SCHOTTEN, ANNEMARIE and CHRISTA GIESE. 1980. The "female echo": Prenatal determination of the female fetus by ultrasound. AJOG. 138.

SCHRODER, JIM and LEONARD A. HERZENBERG. 1980. Fetal cells in the maternal circulation: Prenatal diagnosis by cell sorting under a fluorescence-activated cell sorter (FACS). In Aubrey Milunsky, ed., *Genetic Disorders and the Fetus.* Plenum Publishing Co. New York.

SCHROEDER, LEHA OBIER. 1974, May. New life: Person or property? *Am. J. Psychiatry.* 131(5): 541–544.

SCHULMAN, JOANNE. 1980. The marital rape exemption in the criminal law. *Clearinghouse Review.* 14(6): 538–540.

SCOTT, RUSSELL. 1981. *The Body As Property.* The Viking Press. New York.

SCULLY, DIANA. 1980. *Men Who Control Women's Health.* Houghton Mifflin Co. Boston.

SEAMAN, BARBARA. 1980. *The Doctor's Case Against the Pill.* Doubleday & Co., Inc. Garden City, New York.

—— and GIDEON SEAMAN. 1977. *Women and the Crisis in Sex Hormones.* Rawson Associates Publishers, Inc. New York.

SEDGWICK, J. P. and E. C. FLEISCHNER. 1921, Feb. Breast-feeding in the reduction of infant mortality. *Am. J. of Public Health.* 11: 153–157.

SEED, R. G. and RANA WEISS. 1980. Embryo adoption—technical, ethical and legal aspects. *Archives of Andrology.* 5(1).

SEED, RANDOLPH W. and RICHARD G. SEED. 1978, Oct. 13. Statement before the Ethics Advisory Board of the Department of Health, Education and Welfare.

SEED, RICHARD G. and DONALD S. BAKER and RANDOLPH W. SEED. 1977, June. Aspects of bovine embryo transplant directly applicable to humans—a report on over 300 procedures. *Fertility & Sterility.* 23.

SEIDEL, GEORGE E., JR. 1975, April/May. Embryo Transfer. *Charolais Bull-O-Gram.*

———. 1975, Aug./Sept. Embryo transfer III, embryo recovery. *Charolais Bull-O-Gram.*

———. 1975. Embryo transfer V: future developments. *Charolais Bull-O-Gram.*

———. 1980, Nov. Embryo transfer, a growing concept. *Guernsey Breeder's Journal.*

———. 1981a. Superovulation and embryo transfer in cattle. *Science.* 211(4479): 351–358.

———. 1981b. Critical review of embryo transfer procedures with cattle. In Luigi Mastroianni, Jr., and John D. Biggers, eds., *Fertilization and Embryonic Development In Vitro.* Plenum Publishing Co. New York.

———. Undated. Applications of embryo preservation and transfer. In Harold Hawk, ed., *Animal Reproduction.* BARC, Symposium Number 3. Copyright Allanheld, Osmun, Montclair.

——— with L. L. LARSON and R. H. FOOTE. 1971. Effects of age and gonadotropin treatment on superovulation in the calf. *Journal of Animal Science.* 33(3): 617–622.

——— with S. M. SEIDEL. 1978. Bovine embryo transfer: Costs and success rates. *The Advanced Animal Breeder.* XXVI(8).

SGVT. 1977, Feb. 4. "Donor" sought to carry, deliver baby. *San Gabriel Valley Tribune.*

SHAPIRO, SANDER S. 1981, Jan. Some unresolved questions about artificial insemination. COG. 17.

SHASTRY, PADMA R., UMASHASHI C. HEGDE and SHANTA S. RAO. 1977, Sept. 1. Use of ficoll-sodium metrizoate density gradient to separate human X-and-Y-bearing spermatozoa. *Nature.* 269: 58–60.

SHAW, MARGERY W. 1980, Oct. In vitro fertilization: For infertile married couples only? *Hastings Center Report.* P. 4.

SHAW, NANCY STOLLER. 1974. *Forced Labor: Maternity Care in the United States.* Pergamon Press Inc. New York.

SHEPHERD, STEPHEN A. 1981, Jan. 6. Heavy response reported to surrogate mother ad. *Patriot Ledger* (Quincy, Massachusetts).

SHERMAN, J. K. 1964. Research on frozen human semen: Past, present and future. *Fertility & Sterility.* 15(5): 485–499.

———. 1973. Synopsis of the use of frozen human semen since 1964: State of the art of human semen banking. *Fertility & Sterility.* 24(5): 397–412.

SHETTLES, LANDRUM. 1953. Observations on human follicular and tubal ova. AJOG. 66(2): 235–247.

———. 1955. A morula stage of human ovum developed in vitro. *Fertility & Sterility.* 6(4): 287–289.

———. 1958. Corona radiata cells and zona pellucida of living human ova. *Fertility & Sterility.* 9(2): 167–170.

SHORT, ROGER V. 1979a. Human in vitro fertilization and embryo transfer. *Appendix.*

———. 1979b. Summary of the presentation by Dr. P. C. Steptoe and Dr. R. G. Edwards at the Royal College of Obstetricians. *Appendix.*

———. 1979c. Sex determination and differentiation. *British Medical Bulletin.* 35(2): 121–127.

SHULMAN, JOSEPH. 1978, Sept. Testimony before the Ethics Advisory Board of the U.S. Department of Health, Education and Welfare.

SHULTZ, GLADYS DENNY. 1958, Dec. Cruelty in maternity wards. *Ladies' Home Journal.*

———. 1959, May. Journal mothers report on cruelty in maternity wards. *Ladies' Home Journal.*

SIMPSON, JOE LEIGH. 1979. More than we ever wanted to know about sex. NEJM. 300: 1483–1484.

SINGER, PETER. 1975. *Animal Liberation.* Avon Books. New York.

SMH. 1982, May 5. Can a woman give another her test-tube baby? *Sydney Morning Herald.*

———. 1984, May 25. Test tube doctors clash at meeting. *Sydney Morning Herald.*

SMITH, BARBARA. 1983. *Home Girls: A Black Feminist Anthology.* Kitchen Table: Women of Color Press, Inc. New York.

SMT. 1980, Jan. Frozen embryos for in vitro babies. *Sexual Medicine Today.*

SNIDER, ARTHUR J. 1980, Sept. 6. New technique may help women who are infertile. *The Boston Globe.*

SNOWDEN, ROBERT and DUNCAN MITCHELL. 1980, March 13. Anonymous AID for the childless couple. *New Scientist.*

SOBEL, DAVA. 1981, June 29. Surrogate mothers: Why women volunteer. NYT.

SOUPART, PIERRE. 1978, Sept. 15. Cytogenetics of human preimplantation embryos. Presentation of a research proposal for consideration by the National Ethics Advisory Board at the National Institutes of Health. Bethesda, Maryland.

——— and LARRY L. MORGENSTERN. 1973. Human sperm capacitation and in vitro fertilization. *Fertility & Sterility.* 24(6): 462–478.

——— and PATRICIA ANN STRONG. 1974. Ultrastructural observations on human oocytes fertilized in vitro. *Fertility & Sterility.* 25(1): 11–44.

SPEERT, HAROLD. 1980. *Obstetrics and Gynecology in America: A History.* Copyright by the American College of Obstetricians and Gynecologists. Printed at Waverly Press, Inc. Baltimore.

SPENDER, DALE. 1982. *Women of Ideas and What Men Have Done to Them.* Routledge & Kegan Paul. London.

SPN. 1983. Embryo transplant fails in Calif. *Surrogate Parenting News.* 1(2): 20.

———. 1983. Embryo transfer for women without ovaries. *Surrogate Parenting News.* 1(4): 40–42.

———. 1983. Oklahoma A. G. bans fees for surrogates. *Surrogate Parenting News.* 1(6).

SPRETNAK, CHARLENE. 1978. *Lost Goddesses of Early Greece.* Beacon Press. Boston.

ST. 1980, Dec. 14. Volunteer surrogates pour in. *Sunday Telegraph* (Sydney, Australia).

STANNARD, UNA. 1977. *Mrs. Man.* Germainbooks. San Francisco.

STANTON, JOSEPH R. 1979, Oct. 31. Testimony presented at Eastern Virginia Health Systems Agency hearing.

Star-Ledger. (Newark, N.J.). 1983, March 31. Brain dead woman gives birth.

STEINBACHER, ROBERTA. 1981. Futuristic implications of sex preselection. In H. B. Holmes, B. Hoskins and M. Gross, eds., *The Custom-Made Child.* Humana Press, Inc. Clifton, N.J.

STEPTOE, PATRICK and R. G. EDWARDS. 1970, April 4. Laparoscopic recovery of preovulatory human oocytes after priming of ovaries with gonadotrophins. *The Lancet.* 683–689.

———. 1976, April 24. Reimplantation of a human embryo with subsequent tubal pregnancy. *The Lancet.* 880–882.

STERN, SANDER, teleplay writer. 1981, Aug. 12. The seeding of Sarah Burns. CBS movie.

STEWARD, F. C. 1970. From cultured cells to whole plants: The induction and control of their growth and differentiation. *Proceedings of the Royal Society [Biology].* 175: 1–30.

STONE, MERLIN. 1978. *When God Was a Woman.* A Harvest/HBJ Book. Harcourt Brace Jovanovich, Inc. New York.

———. 1979. *Ancient Mirrors of Womanhood.* Vols. I and II. New Sibylline Books. New York.

STRICKLER, RONALD C., et al. 1975. Artificial insemination with fresh donor semen. NEJM. 295(17): 848–853.

SULLIVAN, WALTER. 1981, Dec. 29. A test tube baby born in U.S., joining successes around the world. NYT.

SUNDSTROM, P., P. LIEDHOLM and O. NILSSON. 1980. Ultrastructure of in vitro fertilized human eggs. *Archives of Andrology.* 5(1): 94–95.

SUSSKIND, DAVID. 1981, Dec. 6. Rented Wombs. *The David Susskind Show.*

SUTHERST, JOHN R. and BARBARA D. CASE. 1975. Caesarean section and its place in the active approach to delivery. *Clinics in Obstetrics and Gynaecology.* 2(1): 241–261.

TAYMOR, M. L., et al. 1980. Use of rapid RIA for LH in the harvesting of maturing human oocytes. *Archives of Andrology.* 5(1): 86–87.

TEITUNG HOSPITAL of Anshan Iron and Steel Company. 1975. Fetal sex prediction by sex chromatin of chorionic villi cells during early pregnancy. *Chinese Medical Journal.* 1: 117–125.

THORNE, ROGER W. 1982, Feb. 1. Choosing child's sex a possibility in the 80's with new techniques. OGN.

THORSTEN, GERALDINE. 1980. *God Herself.* Avon Books. New York.

TIMSON, JOHN. 1979, Dec. 13. Lazzaro Spallanzani's seminal discovery. *New Scientist.*

UDDENBERG, N., P.-E. ALMGREN and A. NISSON. 1971, July. Preferences for sex of the child among pregnant women. *J. Biosoc. Sci.* 3: 267–280.

UP. 1978, June 6. Judge rules vice girl can keep pair's tube baby. *United Press.* London.

Upjohn, 1979. Beef cattle reproduction with A.I. and Lutalyse: The dawn of an era new in cattle breeding management. Booklet copyrighted by The Upjohn Company. (In the booklet, Upjohn thanks the National Association of Animal Breeders for permission to reprint most of the Association's "Better Beef with A.I." booklet.)

U.S. 1981, June. The Equal Rights Amendment: guaranteeing equal rights for women under the constitution. U.S. Commission on Civil Rights Clearinghouse Publication 68. U.S. Government Printing Office. Washington, D.C. 20402.

VAN STRUM, CAROL. 1983. *Bitter Fog: Herbicides and Human Rights.* Sierra Club Books. San Francisco.

VEITCH, ANDREW. 1983, April 23. Doctors clash over test-tube ethics. *The Guardian* (England).

———. 1983, April 27. Gynaecologists' report sets limits for work with test tube babies. *The Guardian.*

———. 1983, May 13. Doctors given go-ahead to store embryos "on ice." *The Guardian.*

———. 1983, May 24. How men might be able to give birth. *The Guardian.*

———. 1983, June 25. Doctors ready to divide embryos. *The Guardian.*

———. 1983, June 25. Test tube baby doctors urge clinic controls. *The Guardian.*

———. 1983, June 25. Father of the century. *The Guardian.*

WALKER, ALICE. 1983. *In Search of Our Mothers' Gardens.* Harcourt Brace Jovanovich. San Diego.

WALKER, BARBARA G. 1983. *The Woman's Encyclopedia of Myths and Secrets.* Harper & Row. San Francisco.

WALLACE, JULIA. 1979, Jan. 10. EVMS must warn of research danger. *Ledger–Star* (Norfolk, Va.)

WALLACH, EDWARD E. 1982. In vitro fertilization and embryo transfer in 1982—random thoughts. *Fertility & Sterility.* 38(6).

WALLIS, CLAUDIA, with reporting by MARY CRONIN, PATRICIA DELANEY and RUTH MEHRTENS GALVIN. 1984, Sept. 10. The new origins of life. *Time.*

WALTERS, LEROY. 1979, May 4. Ethical issues in human in vitro fertilization, embryo culture and research, and embryo transfer. *Appendix.*

————. 1983. Ethical aspects of surrogate embryo transfer. JAMA. 250(16): 2183–2184.

WALTERS, WILLIAM A. W. 1976, June. Ethical and legal problems of in vitro fertilization and embryo transplants. Typescript.

———— and PETER SINGER, eds. 1982. *Test-Tube Babies.* Oxford University Press. Melbourne.

WATSON, JAMES D. 1971, May. Moving toward the clonal man. *The Atlantic.*

WEBB, JOHN and JILL BAKER. 1981, June 20. Funds pleas by test-tube baby teams. *The Australian.*

WEBSTER, BAYARD. 1981, Aug. 14. Bronx Zoo birth could aid rare species. NYT.

WEINER, STEPHEN M. and JAN M. LEVINE. 1979. Legal control on use of human tissue in experimentation. *Appendix.*

WELDNER, BRITTE-MARIE. 1981. Accuracy of fetal sex determination by ultrasound. *Acto. Obstet. Gynecol. Scand.* 60: 333–334.

WESTIN, BJÖRN, RUNE NYBERG and GÖRAN ENHÖRNING. 1958. A technique for perfusion of the previable human fetus. *Acta Paediatrica.* 47: 339–349.

WESTMORE, ANN. 1981, June 15. But just whose baby is it? *The West Australian.*

WESTOFF, CHARLES F. 1978. Some speculations on the future of marriage and fertility. *Family Planning Perspectives.* 10(2): 79–83.

———— and RONALD R. RINDFUSS. 1974, May. Sex preselection in the United States: Some implications. *Science.*

WHELAN, ELIZABETH. 1977. *Boy or Girl?* Pocket Books. New York.

WHITLOCK, FIONA. 1984, May 25. Test-tube "miracle workers" attacked. *The Australian.*

————. 1984, May 17. Test-tube babies are smarter and stronger. *The Australian.*

WHITNEY, LEON F. 1934. *The Case for Sterilization.* Frederick A. Stokes Co. New York.

WHITTINGHAM, D. C. 1971, Sept. 10. Survival of mouse embryos after freezing and thawing. *Nature.* 233: 1250–1260.

————. 1979. In vitro fertilization, embryo transfer and storage. *British Medical Bulletin.* 35(2): 105–111.

———— and W. K. WHITTEN. 1974. Long-term storage and aerial transport of frozen mouse embryos. *J. Reprod. Fert.* 36: 433–435.

WILLADSEN, S. M. 1979, Jan. 25. A method for culture of micromanipulated sheep embryos and its use to produce monozygotic twins. *Nature.* 227: 298–300.

———— and C. B. FEHILLY and R. NEWCOMB. 1981. The production of monozygotic twins of preselected parentage by micromanipulation of nonsurgically collected cow embryos. *Theriogenology.* 15(1): 23–27.

WILLIAMS, J. WHITRIDGE. 1912. Medical education and the midwife problem in the United States. JAMA. 58: 1–7.

WILLIAMSON, NANCY E. 1976. *Sons or Daughters: A Cross-Cultural Survey of Parental Preferences.* Vol. 31. Sage Library of Social Research. Sage Publications. Beverly Hills and London.

—— and T. H. LEAN and D. VENGADASALAM. 1978. Evaluation of an unsuccessful sex preselection clinic in Singapore. *J. Biosoc. Sci.* 10: 375–388.

WOLSTENHOLME, GORDON, ed. 1963. *Man and His Future.* A Ciba Foundation Volume. J. & A. Churchill Ltd. London.

WOOD, ANN DOUGLAS. 1973. "The fashionable diseases": Women's complaints and their treatment in nineteenth century America. *Journal of Interdisciplinary History.* IV(1): 25–52.

WOOD, CARL and ANN WESTMORE. 1983. *Test-Tube Conception.* Hill of Content Publishing Co. Pty. Ltd. Melbourne.

WOODSIDE, MOYA. 1950. *Sterilization in North Carolina.* University of North Carolina Press. Chapel Hill.

WOOLF, VIRGINIA. 1966. *Three Guineas.* Harcourt Brace Jovanovich. New York and London.

WREN, CHRISTOPHER S. 1982, Aug. 1. Old nemesis haunts China on birth plan. NYT.

WRIGHT, BRETT. 1983, June 4. Test-tube doctor threatens to resign. *Sydney Morning Herald.*

WRIGHT, R. C. 1969. Hysterectomy: Past, present and future. *Obstetrics and Gynecology.* 33: 560–563.

WS. 1976, Nov. 19. Rented mother has a baby girl. *Washington Star.*

YOUNG, LETTIE. 1982, Nov. 16. Memo to members of the [Michigan State] Assembly Judiciary Committee Concerning Hearing on Surrogate Parenting Contracts.

ZAPOL, WARREN M., THEODOR KOLOBOW, JOSEPH E. PIERCE, GERALD G. VUREX and ROBERT L. BOWMAN. 1969, Oct. 31. Artificial placenta: two days of total extrauterine support of the isolated premature lamb fetus. *Science.* 166: 617–618.

ZIEGLER, CHARLES E. 1913. The elimination of the midwife. JAMA. 60: 32–38.

ZION, BEN-RAFAEL, et al. 1983. Abortion rate in pregnancies following ovulation induced by human menopausal gonadotropin/human chorionic gonadotropin. *Fertility & Sterility.* 39(2).

INDEX